Jillian D.

Nursing Diagnoses in Psychiatric Nursing:
— • —

Care Plans and Psychotropic Medications

EIGHTH EDITION

Mary C. Townsend, DSN, PMHCNS-BC
Clinical Specialist/Nurse Consultant
Adult Psychiatric Mental Health Nursing

Former Assistant Professor and
Coordinator, Mental Health Nursing
Kramer School of Nursing
Oklahoma City University
Oklahoma City, OK

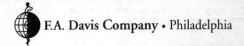

F.A. Davis Company • Philadelphia

F. A. Davis Company
1915 Arch Street
Philadelphia, PA 19103
www.fadavis.com

Printed in the United States of America

Last digit indicates print number: 10 9 8 7 6 5 4 3 2

Publisher, Nursing: Robert G. Martone
Director of Content Development: Darlene D. Pedersen
Sr. Project Editor: Padraic J. Maroney
Design and Illustration Manager: Carolyn O'Brien

As new scientific information becomes available through basic and clinical research, recommended treatments and drug therapies undergo changes. The author(s) and publisher have done everything possible to make this book accurate, up to date, and in accord with accepted standards at the time of publication. The author(s), editors, and publisher are not responsible for errors or omissions or for consequences from application of the book, and make no warranty, expressed or implied, in regard to the contents of the book. Any practice described in this book should be applied by the reader in accordance with professional standards of care used in regard to the unique circumstances that may apply in each situation. The reader is advised always to check product information (package inserts) for changes and new information regarding dose and contraindications before administering any drug. Caution is especially urged when using new or infrequently ordered drugs.

Library of Congress Cataloging-in-Publication Data

Townsend, Mary C., 1941-
  Nursing diagnoses in psychiatric nursing : care plans and psychotropic medications / Mary C. Townsend. – 8th ed.
    p. ; cm.
  Includes bibliographical references and index.
  ISBN 978-0-8036-2506-8 (alk. paper)
  1. Psychiatric nursing–Diagnosis–Handbooks, manuals, etc.
  2. Mental illness–Diagnosis–Handbooks, manuals, etc.
  3. Nursing diagnosis–Handbooks, manuals, etc. I. Title.
  [DNLM: 1. Mental Disorders–nursing–Handbooks.
  2. Nursing Diagnosis–Handbooks. 3. Patient Care
Planning–Handbooks. 4. Psychotropic Drugs–therapeutic
use–Handbooks. WY 49]
  RC440.T69 2011
  616.89'0231–dc22

                                            2010034291

This Book Is Dedicated:

To my husband, Jim, who encourages and supports me throughout all my writing projects, and whose love continues to nurture and sustain me, even after 49 years.

To my daughters, Kerry and Tina, my grandchildren, Meghan and Matthew, and my sons-in-law, Ryan and Jonathan. You are the joys of my life.

To my faithful and beloved companions, Chiro, Angel, and Max, who make me laugh and bring pure pleasure into my life each and every day.

And finally, to the memory of my father and mother, Francis and Camalla Welsh, who reared my sister Francie and me without knowledge of psychology or developmental theories but with the kind of unconditional love I have come to believe is so vital to the achievement and maintenance of emotional wellness.

MCT

Consultants

Maude H. Alston, RN, PhD
Assistant Professor of Nursing
University of North Carolina at Greensboro
Greensboro, North Carolina

Betty J. Carmack, RN, EdD
Assistant Professor
University of San Francisco
School of Nursing
San Francisco, California

Doris K. DeVincenzo, PhD
Professor
Lienhard School of Nursing
Pace University
Pleasantville, New York

Mary Jo Gorney-Fadiman, RN, PhD
Assistant Professor
San Jose State University
School of Nursing
San Jose, California

Mary E. Martucci, RN, PhD
Associate Professor and Chairman
Saint Mary's College
Notre Dame, Indiana

Sheridan V. McCabe, BA, BSN, MSN, PhD
Assistant Professor of Nursing
University of Virginia
School of Nursing
Charlottesville, Virginia

Elizabeth Anne Rankin, PhD
Psychotherapist and Consultant
University of Maryland
School of Nursing
Baltimore, Maryland

Judith M. Saunders, DNS, FAAN
Postdoctoral Research Fellow
University of Washington
School of Nursing
Seattle, Washington

Gail Stuart, RN, CS, PhD
Associate Professor
Medical University of South Carolina
College of Nursing
Charleston, South Carolina

Reviewers

Susan Atwood
Faculty
Antelope Valley College
Lancaster, California

Jaynee R. Boucher, MS, RN
St. Joseph's College of Nursing
Syracuse, New York

Sherry Campbell
Allegany College of Maryland
Cumberland, Maryland

Lorraine Chiappetta
Professor
Washtenaw Community College
Ann Arbor, Michigan

Ileen Craven
Instructor
Roxborough Memorial Hospital
Philadelphia, Pennsylvania

Marcy Echternacht
College of St. Mary
Omaha, Nebraska

Susan Feinstein
Instructor Psychiatric Nursing
Cochran School of Nursing
Yonkers, New York

Mavonne Gansen
Northeast Iowa Community College
Peosta, Iowa

Diane Gardner
Assistant Professor
University of West Florida
Pensacola, Florida

Jo Anne C. Jackson, EdD, RN
Middle Georgia College
Cochran, Georgia

Elizbeth Kawecki
South University
Royal Palm Beach, Florida

Florence Keane, DNSc, MSN, BSN
Assistant Professor
Florida International University
Miami, Florida

Gayle Massie, MSN, RN
Professor
Shawne, State University
Portsmouth, Ohio

Mary McClay
Walla Walla University
Portland, Oregon

Judith Nolen
Clinical Assistant Professor
University of Arizona
Tucson, Arizona

Pamela Parlocha
California State University–East Bay
Hayward, California

Joyce Rittenhouse
Burlington County College
Pemberton, New Jersey

Phyllis Rowe, DNP, RN, ANP
Riverside Community College
Riverside, California

Georgia Seward
Baptist Health Schools Little Rock
Little Rock, Arkansas

Anna Shanks
Shoreline Community College
Seattle, Washington

Rhonda Snow
Stillman College
Tuscaloosa, Alabama

Karen Tarnow, RN, PhD
Clinical Associate Professor
University of Kansas Medical Center
Kansas City, Kansas

Shirley Weiglein
South University
Tampa, Florida

Tammie Willis
Penn Valley Community College
Kansas City, Missouri

Acknowledgments

My special thanks and appreciation:

To Bob Martone, who patiently provides assistance and guidance for all my writing projects.

To the editorial and production staffs of the F.A. Davis Company, who are always willing to provide assistance when requested and whose consistent excellence in publishing makes me proud to be associated with them.

To the gracious individuals who read and critiqued the original manuscript, providing valuable input into the final product.

And finally, a special acknowledgment to the nurses who staff the psychiatric units of the clinical agencies where nursing students go to learn about psychiatric nursing. To those of you who willingly share your knowledge and expertise with, and act as role models for, these nursing students. If this book provides you with even a small amount of nursing assistance, please acknowledge it as my way of saying, "thanks."

MCT

Contents

UNIT THREE

SPECIAL TOPICS IN PSYCHIATRIC/ MENTAL HEALTH NURSING

UNIT FOUR

PSYCHOTROPIC MEDICATIONS

Index of DSM-IV-TR Psychiatric Diagnoses

Classification: Axes I and II Categories and Codes

Introduction

● **HOW TO USE THIS BOOK**

NANDA International (NANDA-I) describes its purpose as follows:

> NANDA International exists to develop, refine and promote terminology that accurately reflects nurses' clinical judgments. This unique, evidence-based perspective includes social, psychological and spiritual dimensions of care (NANDA-I, 2009).

Standardization of nursing actions and common terminology is important in the provision of consistent care over time, among nurses, across shifts, and even between different health care agencies. This text incorporates the nomenclature of Taxonomy II that has been adopted by NANDA-I.

There are those individuals who believe that NANDA's list is incomplete. My intent is not to judge the completeness of this list but rather to suggest the need for clinical testing of what is available. NANDA encourages nurses to submit new diagnoses for consideration, after testing and research of that diagnosis has been conducted in the clinical setting.

There are three essential components in a nursing diagnosis, which comprise the *PES format*. The "P" identifies the problem (or human issue of concern), the "E" represents the etiology (or cause) of the problem, and the "S" describes a cluster of signs and symptoms, or what has come to be known as "defining characteristics." These three parts are combined into one statement by the use of "connecting words." The diagnosis would then be written in this manner: Problem (or issue of concern) "related to" etiology "evidenced by" signs and symptoms (defining characteristics).

The problem can be identified as the human response to actual or potential health problems as assessed by the nurse. The etiology may be represented by past experiences of the individual, genetic influences, current environmental factors, or pathophysiological changes. The defining characteristics describe what the client says and what the nurse observes that indicate the existence of a particular problem.

Nursing diagnoses, then, become the basis for the care plan. This book may be used as a guide in the construction of care plans for various psychiatric clients. The concepts are presented in such a manner that they may be applied to various types of health care settings: inpatient hospitalization, outpatient clinic, home health, partial hospitalization, and private practice, to name a few. Major divisions in the book are identified by psychiatric diagnostic categories, according to the order in which they appear in the *Diagnostic and Statistical Manual of Mental Disorders, Fourth Edition, Text Revision (DSM-IV-TR, APA, 2000)*. The use of this format is not to imply that nursing diagnoses are based on, or flow from, medical diagnoses; it is meant only to enhance the usability of the book. In addition, I am not suggesting that those nursing diagnoses presented with each psychiatric category are all-inclusive.

It is valid, however, to state that certain nursing diagnoses are indeed common to individuals with specific psychiatric disorders. The diagnoses presented in this book are intended to be used as guidelines for construction of care plans that must be individualized for each client, based on the nursing assessment. The interventions can also be used in areas in which interdisciplinary treatment plans take the place of the nursing care plan.

Each chapter in Unit II begins with an overview of information related to the medical diagnostic category, which may be useful to the nurse as background assessment data. This section includes:

1. **The Disorder:** A definition and common types or categories that have been identified.
2. **Predisposing Factors:** Information regarding theories of etiology, which the nurse may use in formulating the "related to" portion of the nursing diagnosis, as it applies to the client.
3. **Symptomatology:** Subjective and objective data identifying behaviors common to the disorder. These behaviors, as they apply to the individual client, may be pertinent to the "evidenced by" portion of the nursing diagnosis.

Information presented with each nursing diagnosis includes the following:

1. **Definition:** The approved NANDA definition is included for each of the accepted NANDA nursing diagnoses. Any additions or alterations made by the author to the NANDA definition are identified by brackets [ ].
2. **Possible Etiologies ("related to"):** This section suggests possible causes for the problem identified. Those not approved by NANDA are identified by brackets [ ]. **Related/Risk Factors** are given for diagnoses for which the client is at risk. *Note*: **Defining characteristics are replaced by "related/risk factors" for the "Risk for" diagnoses.**

3. **Defining Characteristics ("evidenced by"):** This section includes signs and symptoms that may be evident to indicate that the problem exists. Again, as with definitions and etiologies, those not approved by NANDA are identified by brackets [ ].
4. **Goals/Objectives:** These statements are made in client behavioral objective terminology. They are measurable, short- and long-term goals, to be used in evaluating the effectiveness of the nursing interventions in alleviating the identified problem. There may be more than one short-term goal, and they may be considered "stepping stones" to fulfillment of the long-term goal. For purposes of this book, "long-term," in most instances, is designated as "by discharge from treatment," whether the client is in an inpatient or outpatient setting.
5. **Interventions with *Selected Rationales:*** Only those interventions that are appropriate to a particular nursing diagnosis within the context of the psychiatric setting are presented. Rationales for selected interventions are included to provide clarification beyond fundamental nursing knowledge, and to assist in the selection of appropriate interventions for individual clients. Important interventions related to communication may be identified with the icon.
6. **Outcome Criteria:** These are behavioral changes that can be used as criteria to determine the extent to which the nursing diagnosis has been resolved.

To use this book in the preparation of psychiatric nursing care plans, find the section in the text applicable to the client's psychiatric diagnosis. Review background data pertinent to the diagnosis, if needed. Complete a biopsychosocial history and assessment on the client. Select and prioritize nursing diagnoses appropriate to the client. Using the list of NANDA-approved nursing diagnoses, be sure to include those that are client-specific, and not just those that have been identified as "common" to a particular medical diagnosis. Select nursing interventions and outcome criteria appropriate to the client for each nursing diagnosis identified. Include all of this information on the care plan, along with a date for evaluating the status of each problem. On the evaluation date, document success of the nursing interventions in achieving the goals of care, using the desired client outcomes as criteria. Modify the plan as required.

Unit III deals with client populations with special psychiatric nursing needs. These include victims of abuse or neglect, clients with premenstrual dysphoric disorder or HIV disease, clients who are homeless, and clients who are experiencing bereavement. Topics related to forensic nursing, psychiatric home nursing care, and complementary therapies are also included.

Unit IV, Psychotropic Medications, has been updated to include new medications that have been approved by the U.S. Food and Drug Administration (FDA) since the last edition. This information should facilitate use of the book for nurses administering psychotropic medications and also for nurse practitioners with prescriptive authority. The major categories of psychotropic medications are identified by chemical class. Information is presented related to indications, actions, contraindications and precautions, interactions, route and dosage, and adverse reactions and side effects. Examples of medications in each chemical class are presented by generic and trade name, along with information about half-life, controlled and pregnancy categories, and available forms of the medication. Therapeutic plasma level ranges are provided, where appropriate. Nursing diagnoses related to each category, along with nursing interventions, and client and family education are included in each chapter.

Another helpful feature of this text is the table in Appendix N, which lists some client behaviors commonly observed in the psychiatric setting and the most appropriate nursing diagnosis for each. It is hoped that this information will broaden the understanding of the need to use a variety of nursing diagnoses in preparing the client treatment plan.

This book helps to familiarize the nurse with the current NANDA-approved nursing diagnoses and provides suggestions for their use within the psychiatric setting. The book is designed to be used as a quick reference in the preparation of care plans, with the expectation that additional information will be required for each nursing diagnosis as the nurse individualizes care for psychiatric clients.

MCT

● **NANDA-I NURSING DIAGNOSES TAXONOMY II (2009–2011)**

Domain 1: Health Promotion

Ineffective **health** maintenance
Ineffective **self health** management
Impaired **home** maintenance
Readiness for enhanced **immunization** status
Self neglect
Readiness for enhanced **nutrition**
Ineffective family **therapeutic** regimen management
Readiness for enhanced **self health** management

Domain 2: Nutrition

Ineffective infant **feeding** pattern
Impaired **swallowing**
Imbalanced **nutrition**: Less than body requirements

Imbalanced **nutrition**: More than body requirements
Risk for imbalanced **nutrition**: More than body requirements
Risk for unstable blood **glucose** level
Neonatal **jaundice**
Risk for impaired **liver** function
Risk for **electrolyte** imbalance
Deficient **fluid** volume
Risk for deficient **fluid** volume
Excess **fluid** volume
Risk for imbalanced **fluid** volume
Readiness for enhanced **fluid** balance

Domain 3: Elimination and Exchange

Impaired **urinary** elimination
Urinary retention
Functional urinary **incontinence**
Stress urinary **incontinence**
Urge urinary **incontinence**
Reflex urinary **incontinence**
Risk for urge urinary **incontinence**
Readiness for enhanced **urinary** elimination
Overflow urinary **incontinence**
Bowel incontinence
Diarrhea
Constipation
Risk for **constipation**
Perceived **constipation**
Dysfunctional gastrointestinal **motility**
Risk for dysfunctional gastrointestinal **motility**
Impaired **gas** exchange

Domain 4: Activity/Rest

Insomnia
Disturbed **sleep** pattern
Sleep deprivation
Readiness for enhanced **sleep**
Risk for **disuse** syndrome
Impaired physical **mobility**
Impaired bed **mobility**
Impaired wheelchair **mobility**
Impaired **transfer** ability
Impaired **walking**
Deficient **diversional** activity
Delayed **surgical** recovery
Sedentary **lifestyle**
Disturbed **energy** field
Fatigue

Decreased **cardiac** output
Ineffective **breathing** pattern
Activity intolerance
Risk for **activity** intolerance
Risk for **bleeding**
Impaired spontaneous **ventilation**
Dysfunctional **ventilatory** weaning response
Ineffective peripheral tissue **perfusion**
Risk for decreased cardiac tissue **perfusion**
Risk for ineffective cerebral tissue **perfusion**
Risk for ineffective gastrointestinal **perfusion**
Risk for ineffective renal **perfusion**
Risk for **shock**
Readiness for enhanced **self-care**
Dressing **self-care** deficit
Bathing **self-care** deficit
Feeding **self-care** deficit
Toileting **self-care** deficit

Domain 5: Perception/Cognition

Unilateral **neglect**
Impaired **environmental** interpretation syndrome
Wandering
Disturbed **sensory** perception (specify: visual, auditory, kinesthetic, gustatory, tactile, olfactory)
Deficient **knowledge** (specify)
Readiness for enhanced **knowledge** (specify)
Acute **confusion**
Chronic **confusion**
Impaired **memory**
Risk for acute **confusion**
Readiness for enhanced **decision-making**
Ineffective **activity** planning
Impaired verbal **communication**
Readiness for enhanced **communication**

Domain 6: Self-Perception

Disturbed personal **identity**
Powerlessness
Risk for **powerlessness**
Readiness for enhanced **power**
Hopelessness
Readiness for enhanced **hope**
Risk for **loneliness**
Readiness for enhanced **self-concept**
Chronic low **self-esteem**
Situational low **self-esteem**

Risk for situational low **self-esteem**
Risk for compromised human **dignity**
Disturbed **body** image

Domain 7: Role Relationships

Caregiver role strain
Risk for **caregiver** role strain
Impaired **parenting**
Risk for impaired **parenting**
Readiness for enhanced **parenting**
Interrupted **family** processes
Readiness for enhanced **family** processes
Dysfunctional **family** processes
Risk for impaired **attachment**
Effective **breastfeeding**
Ineffective **breastfeeding**
Interrupted **breastfeeding**
Ineffective **role** performance
Parental role **conflict**
Impaired **social** interaction
Readiness for enhanced **relationship**

Domain 8: Sexuality

Sexual dysfunction
Ineffective **sexuality** pattern
Readiness for enhanced **childbearing** process
Risk for disturbed **maternal/fetal** dyad

Domain 9: Coping/Stress Tolerance

Relocation stress syndrome
Risk for **relocation** stress syndrome
Rape-trauma syndrome
Post-trauma syndrome
Risk for **post-trauma** syndrome
Fear
Anxiety
Death **anxiety**
Chronic **sorrow**
Ineffective **denial**
Grieving
Complicated **grieving**
Risk for complicated **grieving**
Impaired individual **resilience**
Readiness for enhanced **resilience**
Risk for compromised **resilience**
Risk-prone health **behavior**

Ineffective **coping**
Stress overload
Disabled family **coping**
Compromised family **coping**
Defensive **coping**
Ineffective community **coping**
Readiness for enhanced **coping**
Readiness for enhanced family **coping**
Readiness for enhanced community **coping**
Autonomic dysreflexia
Risk for **autonomic** dysreflexia
Disorganized **infant** behavior
Risk for disorganized **infant** behavior
Readiness for enhanced organized **infant** behavior
Decreased **intracranial** adaptive capacity

Domain 10: Life Principles

Readiness for enhanced **spiritual** well-being
Readiness for enhanced **hope**
Spiritual distress
Risk for **spiritual** distress
Decisional **conflict**
Noncompliance
Risk for impaired **religiosity**
Impaired **religiosity**
Readiness for enhanced **religiosity**
Moral **distress**

Domain 11: Safety/Protection

Risk for **infection**
Impaired **oral** mucous membrane
Risk for **injury**
Risk for perioperative positioning **injury**
Risk for **falls**
Risk for **trauma**
Risk for vascular **trauma**
Impaired **skin** integrity
Risk for impaired **skin** integrity
Impaired **tissue** integrity
Impaired **dentition**
Risk for **suffocation**
Risk for **aspiration**
Ineffective **airway** clearance
Risk for **peripheral** neurovascular dysfunction
Ineffective **protection**
Risk for sudden infant **death** syndrome
Risk for **self-mutilation**

Self-mutilation

Risk for other-directed **violence**

Risk for self-directed **violence**

Risk for **suicide**

Risk for **poisoning**

Latex **allergy** response

Risk for latex **allergy** response

Risk for imbalanced **body** temperature

Ineffective **thermoregulation**

Hypothermia

Hyperthermia

Readiness for enhanced **immunization** status

Risk for **contamination**

Contamination

Domain 12: Comfort

Acute **pain**

Chronic **pain**

Nausea

Impaired **comfort**

Readiness for enhanced **comfort**

Social isolation

Domain 13: Growth/Development

Delayed **growth** and development

Risk for disproportionate **growth**

Adult **failure** to thrive

Risk for delayed **development**

Source: *NANDA International nursing diagnoses: Definitions and classification 2009-2011.* (2009). Hoboken, NJ: Wiley-Blackwell. With permission.

 INTERNET REFERENCES

- http://www.apna.org
- http://www.nanda.org
- http://www.nursecominc.com

THE FOUNDATION FOR PLANNING PSYCHIATRIC NURSING CARE

CHAPTER 1

Nursing Process: One Step to Professionalism

Nursing has struggled for many years to achieve recognition as a profession. Out of this struggle has emerged an awareness of the need to do the following:

1. Define the boundaries of nursing (What is nursing?).
2. Identify a scientific method for delivering nursing care.

In its statement on social policy, the American Nurses Association (ANA) presented the following definition:

> Nursing is the protection, promotion, and optimization of health and abilities, prevention of illness and injury, alleviation of suffering through the diagnosis and treatment of human response, and advocacy in the care of individuals, families, communities, and populations (ANA, 2010, p. 10).

The nursing process has been identified as nursing's scientific methodology for the delivery of nursing care. The curricula of most nursing schools include nursing process as a component of their conceptual frameworks. The National Council of State Boards of Nursing (NCSBN) has integrated the nursing process throughout the test plan for the National Council Licensure Examination for Registered Nurses (NCSBN, 2010). Questions that relate to nursing behaviors in a variety of client situations are presented according to the steps of the nursing process:

1. **Assessment:** Establishing a database on a client
2. **Diagnosis:** Identifying the client's health care needs and selecting goals of care
3. **Outcome identification:** Establishing criteria for measuring achievement of desired outcomes
4. **Planning:** Designing a strategy to achieve the goals established for client care
5. **Implementation:** Initiating and completing actions necessary to accomplish the goals
6. **Evaluation:** Determining the extent to which the goals of care have been achieved

By following these six steps, the nurse has a systematic framework for decision-making and problem-solving in the delivery of nursing care. The nursing process is dynamic, not static. It is an ongoing process that continues for as long as the nurse and client have interactions directed toward change in the client's physical or behavioral responses. Figure 1-1 presents a schematic of the ongoing nursing process.

Diagnosis is an integral part of the nursing process. In this step, the nurse identifies the human responses to actual or potential health problems. In some states, diagnosing is identified within the Nurse Practice Acts as a legal responsibility of

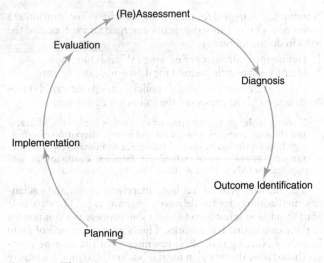

Figure 1-1: The ongoing nursing process.

the professional nurse. Nursing diagnosis provides the basis for prescribing the specific interventions for which the nurse is accountable.

As an inherent part of the nursing process, nursing diagnosis is included in the ANA Standards of Practice. These standards provide one broad basis for evaluating practice and reflect recognition of the rights of the person receiving nursing care (ANA, 2010).

● CONCEPT MAPPING

Concept mapping is a diagrammatic teaching and learning strategy that allows students and faculty to visualize interrelationships between medical diagnoses, nursing diagnoses, assessment data, and treatments. The concept map care plan is an innovative approach to planning and organizing nursing care. Basically, it is a diagram of client problems and interventions. Compared to the commonly used column-format care plans, concept map care plans are more succinct. They are practical, realistic, and time-saving, and they serve to enhance critical-thinking skills and clinical reasoning ability.

The nursing process is foundational to developing and using the concept map care plan, just as it is with all types of nursing care plans. Client data are collected and analyzed, nursing diagnoses are formulated, outcome criteria are identified, nursing actions are planned and implemented, and the success of the interventions in meeting the outcome criteria is evaluated.

The concept map care plan may be presented in its entirety on one page, or the assessment data and nursing diagnoses may appear in diagram format on one page, with outcomes, interventions, and evaluation written on a second page. Additionally, the diagram may appear in circular format, with nursing diagnoses and interventions branching off the "client" in the center of the diagram. Or, it may begin with the "client" at the top of the diagram, with branches emanating in a linear fashion downward.

As stated previously, the concept map care plan is based on the components of the nursing process. Accordingly, the diagram is assembled in the nursing process stepwise fashion, beginning with the client and his or her reason for needing care, nursing diagnoses with subjective and objective clinical evidence for each, nursing interventions, and outcome criteria for evaluation.

Various colors may be used in the diagram to designate various components of the care plan. Lines are drawn to connect the various components to indicate any relationships that exist. For example, there may be a relationship between two nursing diagnoses (e.g., there may be a relationship between the nursing diagnoses of pain or anxiety and disturbed sleep pattern). A line between these nursing diagnoses should be drawn to show the relationship.

Concept map care plans allow for a great deal of creativity on the part of the user, and they permit viewing the "whole picture" without generating a great deal of paperwork. Because they reflect the steps of the nursing process, concept map care plans also are valuable guides for the documentation of client care. Doenges, Moorhouse, and Murr (2008) state,

> As students, you are asked to develop plans of care that often contain more detail than what you see in the hospital plans of care. This is to help you learn how to apply the nursing process and create individualized client care plans. However, even though much time and energy may be spent focusing on filling the columns of traditional clinical care plan forms, some students never develop a holistic view of their clients and fail to visualize how each client need interacts with other identified needs. A new technique or learning tool [concept mapping] has been developed to assist you in visualizing the linkages, enhance your critical thinking skills, and to facilitate the creative process of planning client care (p. 35).

An example of one format for a concept map care plan is presented in Figure 1-2.

The purpose of this book is to assist students and staff nurses as they endeavor to provide high-quality nursing care to their psychiatric clients. The following is an example of a nursing history and assessment tool that may be used to gather information about the client during the assessment phase of the nursing process.

● NURSING HISTORY AND ASSESSMENT TOOL
I. General Information

Client name: _____	Allergies: _____
Room number: _____	Diet: _____
Doctor: _____	Height/weight: _____
Age: _____	Vital signs: TPR/BP _____
Sex: _____	Name and phone no. of significant other: _____
Race: _____	
Dominant language: _____	City of residence: _____
Marital status: _____	Diagnosis (admitting & current): _____
Chief complaint: _____ _____	_____ _____

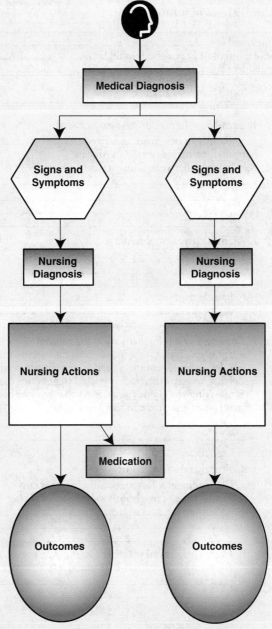

Figure 1-2: Example of a format for a concept map care plan.

II. Conditions of admission

Date: _____ Time: _____
Accompanied by: _____
Route of admission (wheelchair; ambulatory; cart): _____
Admitted from: _____

III. Predisposing Factors

A. *Genetic Influences*

1. Family configuration (use genograms):
   Family of origin: _____ Present family: _____
   Family dynamics (describe significant
   relationships between family members):

   _____
   _____
   _____
   _____

2. Medical/psychiatric history:
   a. Client:

   _____
   _____

   b. Family member _____

   _____
   _____

3. Other genetic influences affecting present
   adaptation. This might include effects specific to
   gender, race, appearance, such as genetic physical
   defects, or any other factor related to genetics that
   is affecting the client's adaptation that has not been
   mentioned elsewhere in this assessment.

   _____
   _____

B. *Past Experiences*

1. Cultural and social history:
   a. Environmental factors (family living arrange-
      ments, type of neighborhood, special working
      conditions): _____

      _____
      _____

   b. Health beliefs and practices (personal responsibility
      for health; special self-care practices):

      _____
      _____

    c. Religious beliefs and practices: _____

    d. Educational background: _____

    e. Significant losses/changes (include dates): _____

    f. Peer/friendship relationships: _____

    g. Occupational history: _____

    h. Previous pattern of coping with stress: _____

    i. Other lifestyle factors contributing to present
       adaptation: _____

C. *Existing Conditions*
  1. Stage of development (Erikson):
    a. Theoretically: _____
    b. Behaviorally: _____
    c. Rationale: _____

  2. Support systems: _____

  3. Economic security: _____

  4. Avenues of productivity/contribution:
    a. Current job status: _____

    b. Role contributions and responsibility for others:
    _____

IV. Precipitating Event

Describe the situation or events that precipitated this illness/
hospitalization: _____
_____
_____
_____

V. Client's Perception of the Stressor

Client's or family member's understanding or description of
stressor/illness and expectations of hospitalization: _____
_____
_____
_____

VI. Adaptation Responses

A. Psychosocial

1. Anxiety level (circle level, and check the
   behaviors that apply):

   Mild   Moderate   Severe   Panic
   Calm _____ Friendly _____ Passive _____
   Alert _____ Perceives environment correctly _____
   Cooperative _____ Impaired attention _____
   "Jittery" _____ Unable to concentrate _____
   Hypervigilant ____ Tremors ____ Rapid speech _____
   Withdrawn _____ Confused _____
   Disoriented ____ Fearful ____ Hyperventilating _____
   Misinterpreting the environment
   (hallucinations or delusions) _____
   Depersonalization _____ Obsessions _____
   Compulsions _____ Somatic complaints _____
   Excessive hyperactivity _____ Other _____

2. Mood/affect (circle as many as apply):

   Happiness   Sadness   Dejection   Despair
   Elation   Euphoria   Suspiciousness
   Apathy (little emotional tone)   Anger/hostility

3. Ego defense mechanisms (describe how used
   by client):

   Projection _____
   Suppression _____
   Undoing _____
   Displacement_____
   Intellectualization _____
   Rationalization _____
   Denial _____
   Repression _____

Isolation _____

Regression _____

Reaction formation _____

Splitting _____

Religiosity _____

Sublimation _____

Compensation _____

4. Level of self-esteem (circle one):

   low   moderate   high

   Things client likes about self _____

   _____

   Things client would like to change about self

   _____

   Nurse's objective assessment of self-esteem:

   Eye contact _____

   General appearance _____

   _____

   _____

   Personal hygiene _____

   Participation in group activities and interactions
   with others _____

   _____

5. Stage and manifestations of grief (circle one):

   Denial Anger Bargaining Depression
   Acceptance

   Describe the client's behaviors that are associated
   with this stage of grieving in response to loss or
   change. _____

   _____

6. Thought processes (circle as many as apply):

Clear	Logical	Easy to follow	Relevant
Confused	Blocking	Delusional	Rapid flow of thoughts

   Slowness in thought association   Suspicious

   Recent memory: Loss   Intact

   Remote memory: Loss   Intact

   Other: _____

   _____

7. Communication patterns (circle as many as
   apply):

Clear	Coherent	Slurred speech	Incoherent
Neologisms	Loose associations	Flight of ideas	

Aphasic   Perseveration   Rumination
Tangential   Loquaciousness
speech
Slow, impoverished speech
Speech impediment (describe) _____
Other _____
_____

8. Interaction patterns (describe client's pattern of interpersonal interactions with staff and peers on the unit, e.g., manipulative, withdrawn, isolated, verbally or physically hostile, argumentative, passive, assertive, aggressive, passive-aggressive, other):

_____
_____
_____

9. Reality orientation (check those that apply):
   Oriented to: Time _____ Person _____
                    Place _____ Situation _____

10. Ideas of destruction to self/others? Yes No
    If yes, consider plan; available means _____
    _____
    _____
    _____

B. Physiological

1. Psychosomatic manifestations (describe any somatic complaints that may be stress-related):

   _____
   _____
   _____

2. Drug history and assessment:
   Use of prescribed drugs:

NAME	DOSAGE	PRESCRIBED FOR	RESULTS

   Use of over-the-counter drugs:

NAME	DOSAGE	USED FOR	RESULTS

Use of street drugs or alcohol:

NAME	AMOUNT USED	HOW OFTEN USED	WHEN LAST USED	EFFECTS PRODUCED

3. Pertinent physical assessments:
   a. Respirations: Normal _____ Labored _____
      Rate _____ Rhythm _____
   b. Skin: Warm _____ Dry _____ Moist _____
      Cool _____ Clammy _____ Pink _____
      Cyanotic _____ Poor turgor _____ Edematous _____
      Evidence of: Rash _____ Bruising _____
      Needle tracks ___ Hirsutism ___ Loss of hair ___
      Other _____
   c. Musculoskeletal status: Weakness _____
      Tremors _____
      Degree of range of motion (describe limitations)
      _____
      Pain (describe) _____
      Skeletal deformities (describe) _____
      Coordination (describe limitations) _____
   d. Neurological status:
      History of (check all that apply): _____
      Seizures (describe method of control) _____
      _____
      Headaches (describe location and frequency) _____
      Fainting spells _____ Dizziness _____
      Tingling/numbness (describe location) _____
   e. Cardiovascular: B/P _____ Pulse _____
      History of (check all that apply):
      Hypertension _____ Palpitations _____
      Heart murmur _____ Chest pain _____
      Shortness of breath _____ Pain in legs _____
      Phlebitis _____ Ankle/leg edema _____
      Numbness/tingling in extremities _____
      Varicose veins _____
   f. Gastrointestinal:
      Usual diet pattern: _____
      Food allergies: _____
      Dentures? Upper _____ Lower _____
      Any problems with chewing or
      swallowing? _____
      Any recent change in weight? _____

Any problems with:

Indigestion/heartburn? _____

Relieved by _____

Nausea/vomiting? _____

Relieved by _____

History of ulcers? _____

Usual bowel pattern _____

Constipation? _____ Diarrhea? _____

Type of self-care assistance provided for either of the above problems _____

_____

g. Genitourinary/Reproductive:

Usual voiding pattern _____

Urinary hesitancy? _____

Frequency? _____

Nocturia? _____ Pain/burning? _____

Incontinence? _____

Any genital lesions? _____

Discharge? _____ Odor? _____

History of sexually transmitted disease? _____

If yes, please explain: _____

_____

Any concerns about sexuality/sexual activity?

_____

Method of birth control used _____

Females:

Date of last menstrual cycle _____

Length of cycle _____

Problems associated with menstruation? _____

_____

Breasts: Pain/tenderness? _____

Swelling? _____ Discharge?_____

Lumps? _____ Dimpling? _____

Practice breast self-examination? _____

Frequency? _____

Males:

Penile discharge? _____

Prostate problems?_____

h. Eyes:

	Yes	No	Explain
Glasses?	____	____	_____
Contacts?	____	____	_____
Swelling?	____	____	_____
Discharge?	____	____	_____
Itching?	____	____	_____
Blurring?	____	____	_____
Double vision?	____	____	_____

  i. Ears:

	Yes	No	Explain
Pain?	____	____	_____
Drainage?	____	____	_____
Difficulty hearing?	____	____	_____
Hearing aid?	____	____	_____
Tinnitus?	____	____	_____

  j. Medication side effects:
     What symptoms is the client experiencing that
     may be attributed to current medication usage?

     _____

     _____

  k. Altered lab values and possible significance: _____

     _____

     _____

  l. Activity/rest patterns:
     Exercise (amount, type, frequency) _____

     _____

     Leisure time activities: _____

     _____

     Patterns of sleep: Number of hours per night ____
     Use of sleep aids? _____
     Pattern of awakening during the night? _____
     Feel rested upon awakening? _____

  m. Personal hygiene/activities of daily living:
     Patterns of self-care: Independent _____
     Requires assistance with:

                              Mobility _____
                              Hygiene _____
                              Toileting _____
                              Feeding _____
                              Dressing _____
                              Other _____
     Statement describing personal hygiene and
     general appearance _____

     _____

  n. Other pertinent physical assessments: _____

     _____

     _____

VII. Summary of Initial Psychosocial/ Physical Assessment:

Knowledge Deficits Identified: _____

Nursing Diagnoses Indicated: _____

ALTERATIONS IN PSYCHOSOCIAL ADAPTATION

CHAPTER **2**

Disorders Usually First Diagnosed in Infancy, Childhood, or Adolescence

● **BACKGROUND ASSESSMENT DATA**

Several common psychiatric disorders may arise or become evident during infancy, childhood, or adolescence. Essential features of many disorders are identical, regardless of the age of the individual. Examples include the following:

Cognitive disorders	Personality disorders
Schizophrenia	Substance-related disorders
Schizophreniform disorder	Mood disorders
Adjustment disorder	Somatoform disorders
Sexual disorders	Psychological factors affecting medical condition

There are, however, several disorders that appear during the early developmental years and are identified according to the child's ability or inability to perform age-appropriate tasks or intellectual functions. Selected disorders are presented here. It is essential that the nurse working with these clients understand normal behavior patterns characteristic of the infant, childhood, and adolescent years.

● MENTAL RETARDATION

Defined

Mental retardation is defined by deficits in general intellectual functioning and adaptive functioning and measured by an individual's performance on intelligence quotient (IQ) tests (American Psychiatric Association [APA], 2000). Mental retardation is coded on Axis II in the APA (2000) *Diagnostic and Statistical Manual of Mental Disorders, Fourth Edition, Text Revision (DSM-IV-TR)* Classification (see Appendix L). Mental retardation is further categorized (by IQ level) as follows:

Mild (IQ of 50–70)
Moderate (IQ of 35–49)
Severe (IQ of 20–34)
Profound (IQ below 20)

Predisposing Factors

1. **Physiological**
   a. About 5% of cases of mental retardation are caused by hereditary factors, such as Tay-Sachs disease, phenylketonuria, and hyperglycinemia. Chromosomal disorders, such as Down syndrome and Klinefelter syndrome, have also been implicated.
   b. Events that occur during the prenatal period (e.g., fetal malnutrition, viral and other infections, maternal ingestion of alcohol or other drugs, and uncontrolled diabetes) and the perinatal period (e.g., birth trauma or premature separation of the placenta) can result in mental retardation.
   c. Mental retardation can occur as an outcome of childhood illnesses, such as encephalitis or meningitis, or be the result of poisoning or physical trauma in childhood.
2. **Psychosocial**
   a. From 15% to 20% of cases of mental retardation are attributed to deprivation of nurturance and social, linguistic, and other stimulation and to severe mental disorders, such as autistic disorder (APA, 2000).

Symptomatology (Subjective and Objective Data)

1. At the mild level (IQ of 50–70), the individual can live independently but with some assistance. He or she is capable of sixth-grade–level work and can learn a vocational skill. Social skills are possible, but the individual functions best in

a structured, sheltered setting. Coordination may be slightly affected.

2. At the moderate level (IQ of 35–49), the individual can perform some activities independently but requires supervision. Academic skill can be achieved to about the second-grade level. The individual may experience some limitation in speech communication and in interactions with others. Motor development may be limited to gross motor ability.

3. The severe level of mental retardation (IQ of 20–34) is characterized by the need for complete supervision. Systematic habit training may be accomplished, but the individual does not have the ability for academic or vocational training. Verbal skills are minimal and psychomotor development is poor.

4. The profoundly mentally retarded individual (IQ of less than 20) has no capacity for independent living. Constant aid and supervision are required. No ability exists for academic or vocational training. There is a lack of ability for speech development, socialization skills, or fine or gross motor movements. The individual requires constant supervision and care.

Common Nursing Diagnoses and Interventions for the Client with Mental Retardation

(Interventions are applicable to various health care settings, such as inpatient and partial hospitalization, community outpatient clinic, home health, and private practice.)

● RISK FOR INJURY

Definition: At risk of injury as a result of environmental conditions interacting with the individual's adaptive and defensive resources

Related/Risk Factors ("related to")

Altered physical mobility
[Aggressive behavior]

Goals/Objectives

Short-/Long-term Goal

Client will not experience injury.

Interventions with *Selected Rationales*

1. *To ensure client safety:*
   a. Create a safe environment for client. Remove small items from the area where client will be ambulating and move sharp items out of his or her reach.

b. Store items that client uses frequently within easy reach.
c. Pad side rails and headboard of client with history of seizures.
d. Prevent physical aggression and acting out behaviors by learning to recognize signs that client is becoming agitated.

Outcome Criteria

1. Client has experienced no physical harm.
2. Client responds to attempts to inhibit agitated behavior.

● SELF-CARE DEFICIT

Definition: Impaired ability to perform or complete [activities of daily living] for self

Possible Etiologies ("related to")

Musculoskeletal impairment
Cognitive impairment

Defining Characteristics ("evidenced by")

Inability to wash body
Inability to put on clothing
Inability to bring food from receptacle to mouth
[Inability to toilet self without assistance]

Goals/Objectives

Short-term Goal

Client will be able to participate in aspects of self-care.

Long-term Goal

Client will have all self-care needs met.

Interventions with *Selected Rationales*

1. Identify aspects of self-care that may be within client's capabilities. Work on one aspect of self-care at a time. Provide simple, concrete explanations. *Because clients' capabilities vary so widely, it is important to know each client individually and to ensure that no client is set up to fail.*
2. Offer positive feedback for efforts at assisting with own self-care. *Positive reinforcement enhances self-esteem and encourages repetition of desirable behaviors.*
3. When one aspect of self-care has been mastered to the best of client's ability, move on to another. Encourage independence but intervene when client is unable to perform. *Client comfort and safety are nursing priorities.*

Outcome Criteria

1. Client assists with self-care activities to the best of his or her ability.
2. Client's self-care needs are being met.

● IMPAIRED VERBAL COMMUNICATION

Definition: Decreased, delayed, or absent ability to receive, process, transmit, and use a system of symbols [to communicate]

Possible Etiologies ("related to")
[Developmental alteration]

Defining Characteristics ("evidenced by")
Speaks or verbalizes with difficulty
Difficulty forming words or sentences
Difficulty expressing thought verbally
Inappropriate verbalization
Does not or cannot speak

Goals/Objectives
Short-term Goal
Client will establish trust with caregiver and a means of communicating needs.

Long-term Goals
1. Client's needs are being met through established means of communication.
2. If client cannot speak or communicate by other means, needs are met by caregiver's anticipation of client's needs.

Interventions with *Selected Rationales*

1. Maintain consistency of staff assignment over time. *This facilitates trust and the ability to understand client's actions and communication.*
2. Anticipate and fulfill client's needs until satisfactory communication patterns are established. Learn (from family, if possible) special words client uses that are different from the norm.
3. Identify nonverbal gestures or signals that client may use to convey needs if verbal communication is absent. Practice these communication skills repeatedly. *Some children with mental retardation, particularly at the severe level, can only learn by systematic habit training.*

Outcome Criteria

1. Client is able to communicate with consistent caregiver.
2. (For client who is unable to communicate): Client's needs, as anticipated by caregiver, are being met.

● IMPAIRED SOCIAL INTERACTION

Definition: Insufficient or excessive quantity or ineffective quality of social exchange

Possible Etiologies ("related to")

[Speech deficiencies]
[Difficulty adhering to conventional social behavior (because of delayed maturational development)]

Defining Characteristics ("evidenced by")

Use of unsuccessful social interaction behaviors
Dysfunctional interaction with others
[Observed] discomfort in social situations

Goals/Objectives

Short-term Goal

Client will attempt to interact with others in the presence of trusted caregiver.

Long-term Goal

Client will be able to interact with others using behaviors that are socially acceptable and appropriate to developmental level.

Interventions with *Selected Rationales*

1. Remain with client during initial interactions with others. *The presence of a trusted individual provides a feeling of security.*
2. Explain to other clients the meaning of some of client's nonverbal gestures and signals. *Others may be more accepting of client's differentness if they have a better understanding of his or her behavior.*
3. Use simple language to explain to client which behaviors are acceptable and which are not. Establish a procedure for behavior modification that offers rewards for appropriate behaviors and renders an aversive reinforcement in response to the use of inappropriate behaviors. *Positive, negative, and aversive reinforcements can contribute to desired changes in behavior. The privileges and penalties are individually determined as caregiver learns the likes and dislikes of client.*

Outcome Criterion

1. Client interacts with others in a socially appropriate manner.

● AUTISTIC DISORDER

Defined

Autistic disorder is characterized by a withdrawal of the child into the self and into a fantasy world of his or her own creation. Activities and interests are restricted and may be considered somewhat bizarre. In 2009, the Centers for Disease Control and Prevention reported that in the United States 1.1% of children aged 3 to 17 years had an autism spectrum disorder (ASD). ASD includes several disorders with similar symptoms based on level of severity. These include autistic disorder, Rett's disorder, childhood disintegrative disorder, pervasive developmental disorder not otherwise specified, and Asperger's disorder. Autistic disorder occurs about four times more often in boys than in girls. Onset of the disorder occurs before age 3, and in most cases it runs a chronic course, with symptoms persisting into adulthood.

Predisposing Factors

1. **Physiological**
   a. **Genetics.** An increased risk of autistic disorder exists among siblings of individuals with the disorder (APA, 2000). Studies with both monozygotic and dizygotic twins have also provided evidence of a genetic involvement.
   b. **Neurological Factors.** Abnormalities in brain structures or functions have been correlated with autistic disorder (National Institute of Mental Health [NIMH], 2009). Certain developmental problems, such as postnatal neurological infections, congenital rubella, phenylketonuria, and fragile X syndrome, also have been implicated.

Symptomatology (Subjective and Objective Data)

1. Failure to form interpersonal relationships, characterized by unresponsiveness to people; lack of eye contact and facial responsiveness; indifference or aversion to affection and physical contact. In early childhood, there is a failure to develop cooperative play and friendships.
2. Impairment in communication (verbal and nonverbal) characterized by absence of language or, if developed, often an immature grammatical structure, incorrect use of words, echolalia, or inability to use abstract terms. Accompanying nonverbal expressions may be inappropriate or absent.
3. Bizarre responses to the environment, characterized by resistance or extreme behavioral reactions to minor occurrences; abnormal, obsessive attachment to peculiar objects; ritualistic behaviors.

4. Extreme fascination for objects that move (e.g., fans, trains). Special interest in music, playing with water, buttons, or parts of the body.
5. Unreasonable insistence on following routines in precise detail (e.g., insisting that exactly the same route always be followed when shopping).
6. Marked distress over changes in trivial aspects of environment (e.g., when a vase is moved from its usual position).
7. Stereotyped body movements (e.g., hand flicking or twisting, spinning, head banging, complex whole-body movements).

Common Nursing Diagnoses and Interventions for the Client with Autistic Disorder

(Interventions are applicable to various health care settings, such as inpatient and partial hospitalization, community outpatient clinic, home health, and private practice.)

● RISK FOR SELF-MUTILATION

Definition: At risk for deliberate self-injurious behavior causing tissue damage with the intent of causing nonfatal injury to attain relief of tension

Related/Risk Factors ("related to")

[Neurological alterations]
[History of self-mutilative behaviors in response to increasing anxiety]
[Obvious indifference to environment or hysterical reactions to changes in the environment]

Goals/Objectives

Short-term Goal

Client will demonstrate alternative behavior (e.g., initiating interaction between self and nurse) in response to anxiety within specified time. (Length of time required for this objective will depend on severity and chronicity of the disorder.)

Long-term Goal

Client will not inflict harm on self.

Interventions with *Selected Rationales*

1. Intervene to protect child when self-mutilative behaviors, such as head banging or other hysterical behaviors, become evident. *The nurse is responsible for ensuring client safety.*

2. A helmet may be used to protect against head banging, hand mitts to prevent hair pulling, and appropriate padding to protect extremities from injury during hysterical movements.
3. Try to determine if self-mutilative behaviors occur in response to increasing anxiety and, if so, to what the anxiety may be attributed. *Mutilative behaviors may be averted if the cause can be determined.*
4. Work on one-to-one basis with child *to establish trust.*
5. Offer self to child during times of increasing anxiety, *in order to decrease need for self-mutilative behaviors and provide feelings of security.*

Outcome Criteria
1. Anxiety is maintained at a level at which client feels no need for self-mutilation.
2. When feeling anxious, client initiates interaction between self and nurse.

• IMPAIRED SOCIAL INTERACTION

Definition: Insufficient or excessive quantity or ineffective quality of social exchange

Possible Etiologies ("related to")
Self-concept disturbance
Absence of [available] significant others
[Unfulfilled tasks of trust versus mistrust]
[Neurological alterations]

Defining Characteristics ("evidenced by")
[Lack of responsiveness to, or interest in, people]
[Failure to cuddle]
[Lack of eye contact and facial responsiveness]
[Indifference or aversion to affection and physical contact]
[Failure to develop cooperative play and peer friendships]

Goals/Objectives
Short-term Goal
Client will demonstrate trust in one caregiver (as evidenced by facial responsiveness and eye contact) within specified time (depending on severity and chronicity of disorder).

Long-term Goal

Client will initiate social interactions (physical, verbal, nonverbal) with caregiver by discharge from treatment.

Interventions with *Selected Rationales*

1. Function in a one-to-one relationship with child. *Consistency of staff–client interaction enhances the establishment of trust.*
2. Provide child with familiar objects (favorite toys, blanket). *These items will offer security during times when child feels distressed.*
3. Convey a manner of warmth, acceptance, and availability as client attempts to fulfill basic needs. *These characteristics enhance establishment and maintenance of a trusting relationship.*
4. Go slowly. Do not force interactions. Begin with positive reinforcement for eye contact. Gradually introduce touch, smiling, hugging. *The autistic client may feel threatened by an onslaught of stimuli to which he or she is unaccustomed.*
5. Support client with your presence as he or she endeavors to relate to others in the environment. *The presence of an individual with whom a trusting relationship has been established provides a feeling of security.*

Outcome Criteria

1. Client initiates interactions between self and others.
2. Client uses eye contact, facial responsiveness, and other nonverbal behaviors in interactions with others.
3. Client does not withdraw from physical contact.

• IMPAIRED VERBAL COMMUNICATION

Definition: Decreased, delayed, or absent ability to receive, process, transmit, and use a system of symbols [to communicate]

Possible Etiologies ("related to")

[Inability to trust]
[Withdrawal into the self]
[Neurological alterations]

Defining Characteristics ("evidenced by")

Does not or cannot speak.
[Immature grammatical structure]

[Echolalia]
[Pronoun reversal]
[Inability to name objects]
[Inability to use abstract terms]
[Absence of nonverbal expression (e.g., eye contact, facial responsiveness, gestures)]

Goals/Objectives
Short-term Goal
Client will establish trust with one caregiver (as evidenced by facial responsiveness and eye contact) by specified time (depending on severity and chronicity of disorder).

Long-term Goal
Client will have established a means for communicating (verbally or nonverbally) needs and desires to staff by time of discharge from treatment.

Interventions with *Selected Rationales*

1. Maintain consistency in assignment of caregivers. *Consistency facilitates trust and enhances caregiver's ability to understand child's attempts to communicate.*
2. Anticipate and fulfill client's needs until satisfactory communication patterns are established. *Anticipating needs helps to minimize frustration while child is learning communication skills.*
3. Use the techniques of consensual *validation* and *seeking clarification* to decode communication patterns. (Examples: "I think you must have meant..." or "Did you mean to say that...?") (see Appendix E). *These techniques work to verify the accuracy of the message received, or to clarify any hidden meanings within the message. Take caution not to "put words into client's mouth."*
4. Use "en face" approach (face-to-face, eye-to-eye) to convey correct nonverbal expressions by example. *Eye contact expresses genuine interest in, and respect for, the individual.*

Outcome Criteria

1. Client is able to communicate in a manner that is understood by others.
2. Client's nonverbal messages are congruent with verbalizations.
3. Client initiates verbal and nonverbal interaction with others.

● DISTURBED PERSONAL IDENTITY

Definition: Inability to maintain an integrated and complete perception of self

Possible Etiologies ("related to")
[Unfulfilled tasks of trust versus mistrust]
[Neurological alterations]
[Inadequate sensory stimulation]

Defining Characteristics ("evidenced by")
[Inability to separate own physiological and emotional needs from those of others]
[Increased levels of anxiety resulting from contact with others]
[Inability to differentiate own body boundaries from those of others]
[Repeating words he or she hears others say or mimicking movements of others]

Goals/Objectives
Short-term Goal
Client will name own body parts and body parts of caregiver within specified time (depending on severity and chronicity of disorder).

Long-term Goal
Client will develop ego identity (evidenced by ability to recognize physical and emotional self as separate from others) by time of discharge from treatment.

Interventions with *Selected Rationales*
1. Function in a one-to-one relationship with child. *Consistency of staff–client interaction enhances the establishment of trust.*
2. Assist child to recognize separateness during self-care activities, such as dressing and feeding. *These activities increase child's awareness of self as separate from others.*
3. Point out and assist child in naming own body parts. *This activity may increase child's awareness of self as separate from others.*
4. Gradually increase amount of physical contact, using touch to point out differences between client and nurse. Be cautious with touch until trust is established, *because this gesture may be interpreted by client as threatening.*
5. Use mirrors and drawings or pictures of child to reinforce child's learning of body parts and boundaries.

Outcome Criteria
1. Client is able to differentiate own body parts from those of others.
2. Client communicates ability to separate self from environment by discontinuing use of echolalia (repeating words heard) and echopraxia (imitating movements seen).

● DISRUPTIVE BEHAVIOR DISORDERS

Attention-Deficit/Hyperactivity Disorder

Defined

Attention-deficit/hyperactivity disorder (ADHD) is character-ized by a "persistent pattern of inattention and/or hyperactivity-impulsivity that is more frequent and severe than is typically observed in individuals at a comparable level of development" (APA, 2000). The disorder is frequently not diagnosed until the child begins school because, prior to that time, childhood behavior is much more variable than that of older children. ADHD is 4 to 9 times more common in boys than in girls and may occur in as many as 3% to 7% of school-age children. The course can be chronic, persisting into adulthood. The *DSM-IV-TR* further categorizes the disorder into the following subtypes: com-bined type, predominantly inattentive type, and predominantly hyperactive-impulsive type.

Predisposing Factors

1. **Physiological**
   a. *Genetics.* A number of studies have indicated that heredi-tary factors may be implicated in the predisposition to ADHD. Siblings of hyperactive children are more likely than normal children to have the disorder.
   b. *Biochemical.* Abnormal levels of the neurotransmitters dopamine, norepinephrine, and possibly serotonin have been suggested as a causative factor.
   c. *Prenatal, Perinatal, and Postnatal Factors.* Maternal smoking during pregnancy has been linked to ADHD in offspring (Linnet et al., 2005). Intrauterine exposure to toxic substances, including alcohol, can produce effects on behavior. Premature birth, fetal distress, precipitated or prolonged labor, and perinatal asphyxia have also been im-plicated. Postnatal factors include cerebral palsy, epilepsy, and other central nervous system abnormalities resulting from trauma, infections, or other neurological disorders.
2. **Psychosocial**
   a. *Environmental Influences.* Disorganized or chaotic en-vironments or a disruption in family equilibrium may predispose some individuals to ADHD. A high degree of psychosocial stress, maternal mental disorder, paternal criminality, low socioeconomic status, poverty, growing up in an institution, and unstable foster care are factors that have been implicated (Dopheide, 2001; Voeller, 2004).

Symptomatology (Subjective and Objective Data)

1. Difficulties in performing age-appropriate tasks.
2. Highly distractible.

3. Extremely limited attention span.
4. Shifts from one uncompleted activity to another.
5. Impulsivity, or deficit in inhibitory control, is common.
6. Difficulty forming satisfactory interpersonal relationships.
7. Disruptive and intrusive behaviors inhibit acceptable social interaction.
8. Difficulty complying with social norms.
9. Some children with ADHD are very aggressive or oppositional. Others exhibit more regressive and immature behaviors.
10. Low frustration tolerance and outbursts of temper are common.
11. Boundless energy, exhibiting excessive levels of activity, restlessness, and fidgeting
12. Often described as "perpetual motion machines," continuously running, jumping, wiggling, or squirming
13. They experience a greater than average number of accidents, from minor mishaps to more serious incidents that may lead to physical injury or the destruction of property.

Conduct Disorder

Defined

The *DSM-IV-TR* describes the essential feature of this disorder as a "repetitive and persistent pattern of conduct in which the basic rights of others or major age-appropriate societal norms or rules are violated" (APA, 2000). The conduct is more serious than the ordinary mischief and pranks of children and adolescents. The disorder is more common in boys than in girls, and the behaviors may continue into adulthood, often meeting the criteria for antisocial personality disorder. Conduct disorder is divided into two subtypes based on the age at onset: childhood-onset type (onset of symptoms before age 10 years) and adolescent-onset type (absence of symptoms before age 10 years).

Predisposing Factors
1. **Physiological**
   a. ***Birth Temperament.*** The term *temperament* refers to personality traits that become evident very early in life and may be present at birth. Evidence suggests a genetic component in temperament and an association between temperament and behavioral problems later in life.
   b. ***Genetics.*** Twin studies have revealed a significantly higher number of conduct disorders among those who have family members with the disorder.

2. **Psychosocial**
   a. *Peer Relationships.* Social groups have a significant impact on a child's development. Peers play an essential role in the socialization of interpersonal competence, and skills acquired in this manner affect the child's long-term adjustment. Studies have shown that poor peer relations during childhood were consistently implicated in the etiology of later deviance (Ladd, 1999). Aggression was found to be the principal cause of peer rejection, thus contributing to a cycle of maladaptive behavior.
   b. *Theory of Family Dynamics.* The following factors related to family dynamics have been implicated as contributors in the predisposition to this disorder (Foley et al., 2004; Popper et al., 2003; Sadock & Sadock, 2007):
      • Parental rejection
      • Inconsistent management with harsh discipline
      • Early institutional living
      • Frequent shifting of parental figures
      • Large family size
      • Absent father
      • Parents with antisocial personality disorder and/or alcohol dependence
      • Association with a delinquent subgroup
      • Marital conflict and divorce
      • Inadequate communication patterns
      • Parental permissiveness

Symptomatology (Subjective and Objective Data)

1. Uses physical aggression in the violation of the rights of others.
2. The behavior pattern manifests itself in virtually all areas of the child's life (home, school, with peers, and in the community).
3. Stealing, fighting, lying, and truancy are common problems.
4. There is an absence of feelings of guilt or remorse.
5. The use of tobacco, liquor, or nonprescribed drugs, as well as the participation in sexual activities, occurs earlier than the peer group's expected age.
6. Projection is a common defense mechanism.
7. Low self-esteem is manifested by a "tough guy" image. Often threatens and intimidates others.
8. Characteristics include poor frustration tolerance, irritability, and frequent temper outbursts.
9. Symptoms of anxiety and depression are not uncommon.
10. Level of academic achievement may be low in relation to age and IQ.

11. Manifestations associated with ADHD (e.g., attention difficulties, impulsiveness, and hyperactivity) are very common in children with conduct disorder.

Oppositional Defiant Disorder

Defined

The *DSM-IV-TR* defines this disorder as a pattern of negativistic, defiant, disobedient, and hostile behavior toward authority figures that occurs more frequently than is typically observed in individuals of comparable age and developmental level (APA, 2000). The disorder typically begins by 8 years of age and usually not later than early adolescence. The disorder is more prevalent in boys than in girls and is often a developmental antecedent to conduct disorder.

Predisposing Factors

1. **Physiological**
   a. Refer to this section under Conduct Disorder.
2. **Psychosocial**
   a. ***Theory of Family Dynamics.*** It is thought that some parents interpret average or increased levels of developmental oppositionalism as hostility and a deliberate effort on the part of the child to be in control. If power and control are issues for parents, or if they exercise authority for their own needs, a power struggle can be established between the parents and the child that sets the stage for the development of oppositional defiant disorder.

Symptomatology *(Subjective and Objective Data)*

1. Characterized by passive-aggressive behaviors such as stubbornness, procrastination, disobedience, carelessness, negativism, testing of limits, resistance to directions, deliberately ignoring the communication of others, and unwillingness to compromise.
2. Other symptoms that may be evident are running away, school avoidance, school underachievement, temper tantrums, fighting, and argumentativeness.
3. In severe cases, there may be elective mutism, enuresis, encopresis, or eating and sleeping problems.
4. Blames others for mistakes and misbehavior.
5. Has poor peer relationships.

Common Nursing Diagnoses and Interventions for Clients with Disruptive Behavior Disorders

(Interventions are applicable to various health care settings, such as inpatient and partial hospitalization, community outpatient clinic, home health, and private practice.)

● RISK FOR SELF-DIRECTED OR OTHER-DIRECTED VIOLENCE

Definition: At risk for behaviors in which an individual demonstrates that he or she can be physically, emotionally, and/or sexually harmful [either to self or to others]

Related/Risk Factors ("related to")

[Unsatisfactory parent–child relationship]
[Neurological alteration related to premature birth, fetal distress, precipitated or prolonged labor]
[Dysfunctional family system]
[Disorganized or chaotic environments]
[Child abuse or neglect]
[Birth temperament]
Body language (e.g., rigid posture, clenching of fists and jaw, hyperactivity, pacing, breathlessness, threatening stances)
[History or threats of violence toward self or others or of destruction to the property of others]
Impulsivity
[History of] cruelty to animals
Suicidal ideation, plan [available means]

Goals/Objectives

Short-term Goals

1. Client will seek out staff at any time if thoughts of harming self or others should occur.
2. Client will not harm self or others.

Long-term Goal

Client will not harm self or others.

Interventions with *Selected Rationales*

1. Observe client's behavior frequently. Do this through routine activities and interactions to avoid appearing watchful and suspicious. *Clients at high risk for violence require close observation to prevent harm to self or others.*
2. Observe for suicidal behaviors: verbal statements, such as "I'm going to kill myself" or "Very soon my mother won't have to worry herself about me any longer," or nonverbal behaviors, such as giving away cherished items or mood swings. *Most clients who attempt suicide have communicated their intent, either verbally or nonverbally.*
3. Determine suicidal intent and available means. Ask, "Do you plan to kill yourself?" and "How do you plan to do it?"

Direct, closed-ended questions are appropriate in this instance. The client who has a usable plan is at higher risk than one who does not.

4. Obtain verbal or written contract from client agreeing not to harm self and agreeing to seek out staff in the event that such ideation occurs. *Discussion of suicidal feelings with a trusted individual provides a degree of relief to client. A contract gets the subject out in the open and places some of the responsibility for his or her safety with client. An attitude of acceptance of client as a worthwhile individual is conveyed.*

5. Help client to recognize when anger occurs and to accept those feelings as his or her own. Have client keep an "anger notebook," in which a record of anger experienced on a 24-hour basis is kept. Information regarding source of anger, behavioral response, and client's perception of the situation should also be noted. Discuss entries with client, suggesting alternative behavioral responses for those identified as maladaptive.

6. Act as a role model for appropriate expression of angry feelings, and give positive reinforcement to client for attempting to conform. *It is vital that client express angry feelings, because suicide and other self-destructive behaviors are often viewed as a result of anger turned inward on the self.*

7. Remove all dangerous objects from client's environment. *Client's physical safety is a nursing priority.*

8. Try to redirect violent behavior with physical outlets for client's anxiety (e.g., punching bag, jogging, volleyball). *Anxiety and tension can be relieved safely and with benefit to client in this manner.*

9. Be available to stay with client as anxiety level and tensions begin to rise. *The presence of a trusted individual provides a feeling of security.*

10. Staff should maintain and convey a calm attitude to client. Anxiety is contagious and can be communicated from staff to client and vice versa. *A calm attitude conveys a sense of control and a feeling of security to client.*

11. Have sufficient staff available to indicate a show of strength to client if it becomes necessary. *This conveys to client an evidence of control over the situation and provides some physical security for staff.*

12. Administer tranquilizing medications as ordered by physician, or obtain an order if necessary. Monitor medication for effectiveness and for adverse side effects. *Short-term use of antianxiety medications (e.g., chlordiazepoxide, alprazolam, lorazepam) provides relief from the immobilizing effects of anxiety and facilitates client's cooperation with therapy.*

13. Mechanical restraints or isolation room may be required if less restrictive interventions are unsuccessful. *It is client's right to expect the use of techniques that ensure the safety of client and others by the least restrictive means.*

Outcome Criteria

1. Anxiety is maintained at a level at which client feels no need for aggression.
2. Client seeks out staff to discuss true feelings.
3. Client recognizes, verbalizes, and accepts possible consequences of own maladaptive behaviors.
4. Client does not harm self or others.

● DEFENSIVE COPING

Definition: Repeated projection of falsely positive self-evaluation based on a self-protective pattern that defends against underlying perceived threats to positive self-regard

Possible Etiologies ("related to")

[Low self-esteem]
[Negative role models]
[Lack of positive feedback]
[Repeated negative feedback, resulting in feelings of diminished self-worth]
[Unsatisfactory parent–child relationship]
[Disorganized or chaotic environments]
[Child abuse or neglect]
[Dysfunctional family system]
[Neurological alteration related to premature birth, fetal distress, precipitated or prolonged labor]

Defining Characteristics ("evidenced by")

Denial of obvious problems or weaknesses
Projection of blame or responsibility
Rationalization of failures
Hypersensitivity to criticism
Grandiosity
Superior attitude toward others
Difficulty establishing or maintaining relationships
Hostile laughter or ridicule of others
Difficulty in perception of reality testing
Lack of follow-through or participation in treatment or therapy

Goals/Objectives

Short-term Goal

Client will verbalize personal responsibility for difficulties experienced in interpersonal relationships.

Long-term Goal

Client will demonstrate ability to interact with others without becoming defensive, rationalizing behaviors, or expressing grandiose ideas.

Interventions with Selected Rationales

1. Recognize and support basic ego strengths. *Focusing on positive aspects of the personality may help to improve self-concept.*
2. Encourage client to recognize and verbalize feelings of inadequacy and need for acceptance from others and to recognize how these feelings provoke defensive behaviors, such as blaming others for own behaviors. *Recognition of the problem is the first step in the change process toward resolution.*
3. Provide immediate, matter-of-fact, nonthreatening feedback for unacceptable behaviors. *Client may lack knowledge about how he or she is being perceived by others. Providing this information in a nonthreatening manner may help to eliminate these undesirable behaviors.*

> **CLINICAL PEARL** 🗨 Say to the client, "When you say those things to people, they don't like it, and they don't want to be around you. Try to think how you would feel if someone said those things to you."

4. Help client identify situations that provoke defensiveness and practice through role-play more appropriate responses. *Role-playing provides confidence to deal with difficult situations when they actually occur.*
5. Provide immediate positive feedback for acceptable behaviors. *Positive feedback enhances self-esteem and encourages repetition of desirable behaviors.*
6. Help client set realistic, concrete goals and determine appropriate actions to meet those goals. *Success increases self-esteem.*
7. With client, evaluate the effectiveness of the new behaviors and discuss any modifications for improvement. *Because of limited problem-solving ability, assistance may be required to reassess and develop new strategies in the event that some new coping methods prove ineffective.*

Outcome Criteria
1. Client verbalizes and accepts responsibility for own behavior.

2. Client verbalizes correlation between feelings of inadequacy and the need to defend the ego through rationalization and grandiosity.
3. Client does not ridicule or criticize others.
4. Client interacts with others in group situations without taking a defensive stance.

● IMPAIRED SOCIAL INTERACTION

Definition: Insufficient or excessive quantity or ineffective quality of social exchange

Possible Etiologies ("related to")
Self-concept disturbance
  [Neurological alterations related to premature birth, fetal distress, precipitated or prolonged labor]
[Dysfunctional family system]
[Disorganized or chaotic environments]
[Child abuse or neglect]
[Unsatisfactory parent–child relationship]
[Negative role models]

Defining Characteristics ("evidenced by")
[Verbalized or observed] discomfort in social situations
[Verbalized or observed] inability to receive or communicate a satisfying sense of belonging, caring, interest, or shared history
[Observed] use of unsuccessful social interaction behaviors
Dysfunctional interaction with others
[Behavior unacceptable for appropriate age by dominant cultural group]

Goals/Objectives
Short-term Goal
Client will interact in age-appropriate manner with nurse in one-to-one relationship within 1 week.

Long-term Goal
Client will be able to interact with staff and peers, by the time of discharge from treatment, with no indication of discomfort.

Interventions with *Selected Rationales*
1. Develop trusting relationship with client. Be honest; keep all promises; convey acceptance of the person, separate from

unacceptable behaviors ("It is not *you*, but *your behavior*, that is unacceptable.") *Acceptance of client increases his or her feelings of self-worth.*
2. Offer to remain with client during initial interactions with others. *Presence of a trusted individual provides a feeling of security.*
3. Provide constructive criticism and positive reinforcement for client's efforts. *Positive feedback enhances self-esteem and encourages repetition of desirable behaviors.*
4. Confront client and withdraw attention when interactions with others are manipulative or exploitative. *Attention to the unacceptable behavior may reinforce it.*
5. Act as a role model for client through appropriate interactions with other clients and staff members.
6. Provide group situations for client. *It is through these group interactions that client will learn socially acceptable behavior, with positive and negative feedback from his or her peers.*

Outcome Criteria

1. Client seeks out staff member for social, as well as therapeutic, interaction.
2. Client has formed and satisfactorily maintained one inter-personal relationship with another client.
3. Client willingly and appropriately participates in group activities.
4. Client verbalizes reasons for past inability to form close interpersonal relationships.

● INEFFECTIVE COPING

Definition: Inability to form a valid appraisal of the stressors, inadequate choices of practiced responses, and/or inability to use available resources

Possible Etiologies ("related to")

Situational crisis
Maturational crisis
[Inadequate support systems]
[Inadequate coping strategies]
[Negative role models]
[Neurological alteration related to premature birth, fetal distress, precipitated or prolonged labor]
[Low self-esteem]
[Dysfunctional family system]
[Disorganized or chaotic environments]
[Child abuse or neglect]

Defining Characteristics ("evidenced by")

Inability to meet [age-appropriate] role expectations
Inadequate problem solving
Poor concentration
Risk taking
[Manipulation of others in the environment for purposes of fulfilling own desires]
[Verbal hostility toward staff and peers]
[Hyperactivity, evidenced by excessive motor activity, easily distracted, short attention span]
[Unable to delay gratification]
[Oppositional and defiant responses to adult requests or rules]

Goals/Objectives

Short-term Goal

Within 7 days, client will demonstrate ability and willingness to follow rules of the treatment setting.

Long-term Goal

By discharge from treatment, client will develop, and use, age-appropriate, socially acceptable coping skills.

Interventions with *Selected Rationales*

1. If client is hyperactive, make environment safe for continuous large-muscle movement. Rearrange furniture and other objects to prevent injury. *Client physical safety is a nursing priority.*
2. Provide large motor activities in which client may participate. Nurse may join in some of these activities *to facilitate relationship development. Tension is released safely and with benefit to client through physical activities.*
3. Provide frequent, nutritious snacks that client may "eat on the run," *to ensure adequate calories to offset client's excessive use of energy.*

CLINICAL PEARL 🐚 Set limits on manipulative behavior. Say, "I understand why you are saying these things (or doing these things) and I will not tolerate these behaviors from you." Take caution not to reinforce manipulative behaviors by providing desired attention.

---

4. Identify for client the consequences of manipulative behavior. All staff must follow through and be consistent. *Client may try to play one staff member against another, so consistency is vital if intervention is to be successful. Aversive reinforcement may work to decrease unacceptable behaviors.*
5. Do not debate, argue, rationalize, or bargain with client. *Ignoring these attempts may work to decrease manipulative behaviors.*

6. Caution should be taken to avoid reinforcing manipulative behaviors by providing desired attention. *Attention provides positive reinforcement and encourages repetition of the undesirable behavior.*
7. Confront client's use of manipulative behaviors and explore their damaging effects on interpersonal relationships. *Manipulative clients often deny responsibility for their behaviors.*
8. Encourage discussion of angry feelings. Help client identify the true object of the hostility. *Dealing with the feelings honestly and directly will discourage displacement of the anger onto others.*
9. Explore with client alternative ways of handling frustration that would be most suited to his or her lifestyle. Provide support and positive feedback to client as new coping strategies are tried. *Positive feedback encourages use of the acceptable behaviors.*

Outcome Criteria

1. Client is able to delay gratification, without resorting to manipulation of others.
2. Client is able to express anger in a socially acceptable manner.
3. Client is able to verbalize alternative, socially acceptable, and lifestyle-appropriate coping skills he or she plans to use in response to frustration.

● LOW SELF-ESTEEM

Definition: Negative self-evaluating/feelings about self or self-capabilities

Possible Etiologies ("related to")

[Negative role models]
Lack of approval
Repeated negative reinforcement
[Unsatisfactory parent–child relationship]
[Disorganized or chaotic environments]
[Child abuse or neglect]
[Dysfunctional family system]

Defining Characteristics ("evidenced by")

Lack of eye contact
Exaggerates negative feedback about self
Expressions of shame or guilt
Evaluation of self as unable to deal with events
Rejects positive feedback about self

Hesitant to try new things or situations
[Denial of problems obvious to others]
[Projection of blame or responsibility for problems]
[Rationalization of personal failures]
[Hypersensitivity to criticism]
[Grandiosity]

Goals/Objectives
Short-term Goal
Client will independently direct own care and activities of daily living within 1 week.
Long-term Goal
By time of discharge from treatment, client will exhibit increased feelings of self-worth as evidenced by verbal expression of positive aspects about self, past accomplishments, and future prospects.

Interventions with *Selected Rationales*
1. Ensure that goals are realistic. It is important for client to achieve something, so plan for activities in which the possibility for success is likely. *Success enhances self-esteem.*
2. Convey unconditional positive regard for client. *Communication of your acceptance of him or her as a worthwhile human being increases self-esteem.*
3. Spend time with client, both on a one-to-one basis and in group activities. *This conveys to client that you feel he or she is worth your time.*
4. Assist client in identifying positive aspects of self and in developing plans for changing the characteristics he or she views as negative.
5. Help client decrease use of denial as a defense mechanism. Give positive reinforcement for problem identification and development of more adaptive coping behaviors. *Positive reinforcement enhances self-esteem and increases client's use of acceptable behaviors.*
6. Encourage and support client in confronting the fear of failure by having client attend therapy activities and undertake new tasks. Offer recognition of successful endeavors and positive reinforcement for attempts made. *Recognition and positive reinforcement enhance self-esteem.*

Outcome Criteria
1. Client verbalizes positive perception of self.
2. Client participates in new activities without exhibiting extreme fear of failure.

● ANXIETY (MODERATE TO SEVERE)

Definition: Vague uneasy feeling of discomfort or dread accompanied by an autonomic response (the source often nonspecific or unknown to the individual); a feeling of apprehension caused by anticipation of danger. It is an alerting signal that warns of impending danger and enables the individual to take measures to deal with threat.

Possible Etiologies ("related to")
Situational and maturational crises
Threat to self-concept [perceived or real]
Threat of death
Unmet needs
[Fear of failure]
[Dysfunctional family system]
[Unsatisfactory parent–child relationship]
[Innately, easily agitated temperament since birth]

Defining Characteristics ("evidenced by")
Overexcited
Fearful
Feelings of inadequacy
Fear of unspecified consequences
Restlessness
Insomnia
Poor eye contact
Focus on self
[Continuous attention-seeking behaviors]
Difficulty concentrating
Impaired attention
Increased respiration and pulse

Goals/Objectives
Short-term Goals
1. Within 7 days, client will be able to verbalize behaviors that become evident as anxiety starts to rise.
2. Within 7 days, client will be able to verbalize strategies to interrupt escalation of anxiety.

Long-term Goal
By time of discharge from treatment, client will be able to maintain anxiety below the moderate level as evidenced by absence of disabling behaviors in response to stress.

Interventions with *Selected Rationales*

1. Establish a trusting relationship with client. Be honest, consistent in responses, and available. Show genuine positive regard. *Honesty, availability, and acceptance promote trust in the nurse–client relationship.*

2. Provide activities geared toward reduction of tension and decreasing anxiety (walking or jogging, volleyball, musical exercises, housekeeping chores, group games). *Tension and anxiety are released safely and with benefit to client through physical activities.*

3. Encourage client to identify true feelings, and to acknowledge ownership of those feelings. *Anxious clients often deny a relationship between emotional problems and their anxiety. Use of the defense mechanisms of projection and displacement is exaggerated.*

4. Nurse must maintain an atmosphere of calmness; *anxiety is easily transmitted from one person to another.*

5. Offer support during times of elevated anxiety. Reassure client of physical and psychological safety. *Client safety is a nursing priority.*

6. Use of touch is comforting to some clients. However, nurse must be cautious with its use, *because anxiety may foster suspicion in some individuals who might misinterpret touch as aggression.*

7. As anxiety diminishes, assist client to recognize specific events that preceded its onset. Work on alternative responses to future occurrences. *A plan of action provides client with a feeling of security for handling a difficult situation more successfully, should it recur.*

8. Help client recognize signs of escalating anxiety, and explore ways client may intervene before behaviors become disabling.

9. Administer tranquilizing medication, as ordered. Assess for effectiveness, and instruct client regarding possible adverse side effects. *Short-term use of antianxiety medications (e.g., lorazepam, chlordiazepoxide, alprazolam) provides relief from the immobilizing effects of anxiety and facilitates client's cooperation with therapy.*

Outcome Criteria

1. Client is able to verbalize behaviors that become evident when anxiety starts to rise, and takes appropriate action to interrupt progression of the condition.

2. Client is able to maintain anxiety at a manageable level.

● **NONCOMPLIANCE**

Definition: Behavior of person and/or caregiver that fails to coincide with a health-promoting or therapeutic plan agreed on by the person [or caregiver] and health care professional. In the presence of an agreed-on, health-promoting or therapeutic plan, person's or caregiver's behavior is fully or partially nonadherent and may lead to clinically ineffective or partially ineffective outcomes.

Possible Etiologies ("related to")

[Biochemical alteration]
[Neurological alteration related to premature birth, fetal distress, precipitated or prolonged labor]
[Negative temperament]
[Dysfunctional family system]
[Negative role models]
[Retarded ego development]
[Low frustration tolerance and short attention span]
[Denial of problems]

Defining Characteristics ("evidenced by")

Behavior indicative of failure to adhere [to treatment regimen]
[Inability to sit still long enough to complete a task]
[Expression of opposition to requests for participation]
[Refusal to follow directions or suggestions of treatment team]

Goals/Objectives

Short-term Goal

Client will participate in and cooperate during therapeutic activities.

Long-term Goal

Client will complete assigned tasks willingly and independently or with a minimum of assistance.

Interventions with *Selected Rationales*

For the client with inattention and hyperactivity:

1. Provide an environment for task efforts that is as free of distractions as possible. *Client is highly distractible and is unable to perform in the presence of even minimal stimulation.*
2. Provide assistance on a one-to-one basis, beginning with simple, concrete instructions. *Client lacks the ability to assimilate information that is complicated or has abstract meaning.*
3. Ask that instructions be repeated *to determine client's level of comprehension.*
4. Establish goals that allow client to complete a part of the task, rewarding completion of each step with a break for physical activity. *Short-term goals are not so overwhelming to client with such a short attention span. The positive reinforcement*

(physical activity) increases self-esteem and provides incentive for client to pursue the task to completion.

5. Gradually decrease the amount of assistance given to task performance, while assuring client that assistance is still available if deemed necessary. *This encourages client to perform independently while providing a feeling of security with the presence of a trusted individual.*

For the client with oppositional tendencies:

6. Set forth a structured plan of therapeutic activities. Start with minimum expectations and increase as client begins to manifest evidence of compliance. *Structure provides security, and one or two activities may not seem as overwhelming as the whole schedule of activities presented at one time.*

7. Establish a system of rewards for compliance with therapy and consequences for noncompliance. Ensure that the rewards and consequences are concepts of value to client. *Positive and negative reinforcements can contribute to desired changes in behavior.*

8. Convey acceptance of client separate from the undesirable behaviors being exhibited. ("It is not *you*, but *your behavior*, that is unacceptable.") *Unconditional acceptance enhances self-worth and may contribute to a decrease in the need for passive-aggressive behavior toward others.*

Outcome Criteria

1. Client cooperates with staff in an effort to complete assigned tasks.
2. Client complies with treatment by participating in therapies without negativism.
3. Client takes direction from staff without becoming defensive.

● TOURETTE'S DISORDER

Defined

Tourette's disorder is characterized by the presence of multiple motor tics and one or more vocal tics that may appear simultaneously or at different periods during the illness (APA, 2000). Onset of the disorder can be as early as 2 years, but it occurs most commonly during childhood (around age 6 to 7 years). Tourette's disorder is more common in boys than in girls. The duration of the disorder may be lifelong, although there may be periods of remission that last from weeks to years (APA, 2000). The symptoms usually diminish during adolescence and adulthood and, in some cases, disappear altogether by early adulthood.

Predisposing Factors

1. *Physiological*
   a. *Genetics.* Family studies have shown that Tourette's disorder is more common in relatives of individuals with the disorder than in the general population. It may be transmitted in an autosomal pattern intermediate between dominant and recessive (Sadock & Sadock, 2007).
   b. *Brain Alterations.* Altered levels of neurotransmitters and dysfunction in the area of the basal ganglia have been implicated in the etiology of Tourette's disorder.
   c. *Biochemical Factors.* Abnormalities in levels of dopamine, serotonin, dynorphin, gamma-aminobutyric acid (GABA), acetylcholine, and norepinephrine have been associated with Tourette's disorder (Popper et al., 2003).
2. *Psychosocial*
   a. The genetic predisposition to Tourette's disorder may be reinforced by certain factors in the environment, such as complications of pregnancy (e.g., severe nausea and vomiting or excessive stress), low birth weight, head trauma, carbon monoxide poisoning, and encephalitis.

Symptomatology (Subjective and Objective Data)

Signs and symptoms of Tourette's disorder are as follows (APA, 2000; Popper et al., 2003):

1. The disorder may begin with a single motor tic, such as eye blinking, neck jerking, shoulder shrugging, facial grimacing, or coughing.
2. Complex motor tics may follow and include touching, squatting, hopping, skipping, deep knee bends, retracing steps, and twirling when walking.
3. Vocal tics include various words or sounds such as clicks, grunts, yelps, barks, sniffs, snorts, coughs; in about 10% of cases, a complex vocal tic involves uttering obscenities.
4. Vocal tics may include repeating certain words or phrases out of context, repeating one's own sounds or words (palilalia), or repeating what others say (echolalia).
5. The movements and vocalizations are experienced as compulsive and irresistible, but they can be suppressed for varying lengths of time.
6. Tics are exacerbated by stress and attenuated during periods in which the individual becomes totally absorbed by an activity.
7. Tics are markedly diminished during sleep.

Common Nursing Diagnoses and Interventions for the Client with Tourette's Disorder

(Interventions are applicable to various health care settings, such as inpatient and partial hospitalization, community outpatient clinic, home health, and private practice.)

● RISK FOR SELF-DIRECTED OR OTHER-DIRECTED VIOLENCE

Definition: At risk for behaviors in which an individual demonstrates that he or she can be physically, emotionally, and/or sexually harmful [either to self or to others]

Related/Risk Factors ("related to")

[Low tolerance for frustration]

[Abnormalities in brain neurotransmitters]

Body language (e.g., rigid posture, clenching of fists and jaw, hyperactivity, pacing, breathlessness, and threatening stances)

[History or threats of violence toward self or others or of destruction to the property of others]

Impulsivity

Suicidal ideation, plan, [available means]

Goals/Objectives

Short-term Goals

1. Client will seek out staff or support person at any time if thoughts of harming self or others should occur.
2. Client will not harm self or others.

Long-term Goal

Client will not harm self or others.

Interventions with *Selected Rationales*

1. Observe client's behavior frequently through routine activities and interactions. Become aware of behaviors that indicate a rise in agitation. *Stress commonly increases tic behaviors. Recognition of behaviors that precede the onset of aggression may provide the opportunity to intervene before violence occurs.*
2. Monitor for self-destructive behavior and impulses. A staff member may need to stay with client to prevent self-mutilation. *Client safety is a nursing priority.*
3. Provide hand coverings and other restraints that prevent client from self-mutilative behaviors. *Provide immediate external controls against self-aggressive behaviors.*
4. Redirect violent behavior with physical outlets for frustration. *Excess energy is released through physical activities and a feeling of relaxation is induced.*

5. Administer medication as ordered by physician. Several medications have been used to treat Tourette's disorder. The most common ones include the following:

  a. **Haloperidol (Haldol).** Haloperidol has been the drug of choice for Tourette's disorder. Children on this medication must be monitored for adverse effects associated with most antipsychotic medications (see Chapter 28). Because of the potential for adverse effects, haloperidol should be reserved for children with severe symptoms or with symptoms that interfere with their ability to function. Usual dosage for children 3 to 12 years of age is 0.05 to 0.075 mg/kg/day in two or three divided doses.

  b. **Pimozide (Orap).** The response rate and side effect profile of pimozide are similar to those of haloperidol. It is used in the management of severe motor or vocal tics that have failed to respond to more conventional treatment. It is not recommended for children younger than age 12 years. Dosage is initiated at 0.05 mg/kg at bedtime; dosage may be increased every third day to a maximum of 0.2 mg/kg, not to exceed 10 mg/day.

  c. **Clonidine (Catapres).** Clonidine is an antihypertensive medication, the efficacy of which in the treatment of Tourette's disorder has been mixed. Some physicians like it and use it as a drug of first choice because of its relative safety and few side effects. Recommended dosage is 150 to 200 mcg/day.

  d. **Atypical Antipsychotics.** Atypical antipsychotics are less likely to cause extrapyramidal side effects than are the older antipsychotics (e.g., haloperidol and pimozide). Risperidone, the most studied atypical antipsychotic in Tourette's disorder, has been shown to reduce symptoms by 21% to 61% compared with placebo (results that are similar to those of pimozide and clonidine) (Dion et al., 2002). Both olanzapine and ziprasidone have demonstrated effectiveness in decreasing tic symptoms of Tourette's disorder. However, weight gain and abnormal glucose tolerance may be troublesome side effects, and ziprasidone has been associated with increased risk of QTc interval prolongation (Zinner, 2004).

Outcome Criteria

1. Anxiety is maintained at a level at which client feels no need for aggression.
2. Client seeks out staff or support person for expression of true feelings.
3. Client has not harmed self or others.

• IMPAIRED SOCIAL INTERACTION

Definition: Insufficient or excessive quantity or ineffective quality of social exchange

Possible Etiologies ("related to")

Self-concept disturbance
[Low tolerance for frustration]
[Impulsiveness]
[Oppositional behavior]
[Aggressive behavior]

Defining Characteristics ("evidenced by")

[Verbalized or observed] discomfort in social situations
[Verbalized or observed] inability to receive or communicate a satisfying sense of belonging, caring, interest, or shared history
[Observed] use of unsuccessful social interaction behaviors
Dysfunctional interaction with others

Goals/Objectives

Short-term Goal

Client will develop a one-to-one relationship with nurse or support person within 1 week.

Long-term Goal

Client will be able to interact with staff and peers using age-appropriate, acceptable behaviors.

Interventions with *Selected Rationales*

1. Develop a trusting relationship with client. Convey acceptance of the person separate from the unacceptable behavior. ***Unconditional acceptance increases feelings of self-worth.***
2. Discuss with client which behaviors are and are not acceptable. Describe in matter-of-fact manner the consequences of unacceptable behavior. Follow through. ***Aversive reinforcement can alter undesirable behaviors.***
3. Provide group situations for client. ***Appropriate social behavior is often learned from the positive and negative feedback of peers.***
4. Act as a role model for client through appropriate interactions with others. ***Role modeling of a respected individual is one of the strongest forms of learning.***

Outcome Criteria

1. Client seeks out staff or support person for social, as well as for therapeutic, interaction.
2. Client verbalizes reasons for past inability to form close interpersonal relationships.
3. Client interacts with others using age-appropriate, acceptable behaviors.

● LOW SELF-ESTEEM

Definition: Negative self-evaluating/feelings about self or self-capabilities

Possible Etiologies ("related to")
[Shame associated with tic behaviors]

Defining Characteristics ("evidenced by")
Lack of eye contact
Self-negating verbalizations
Expressions of shame or guilt
Hesitant to try new things or situations
[Manipulation of others]

Goals/Objectives

Short-term Goal
Client will verbalize positive aspects about self not associated with tic behaviors.

Long-term Goal
Client will exhibit increased feeling of self-worth as evidenced by verbal expression of positive aspects about self, past accomplishments, and future prospects.

Interventions with *Selected Rationales*

1. Convey unconditional acceptance and positive regard. *Communication of client as worthwhile human being may increase self-esteem.*
2. Set limits on manipulative behavior. Take caution not to re-inforce manipulative behaviors by providing desired attention. Identify the consequences of manipulation. Administer consequences matter-of-factly when manipulation occurs. *Aversive reinforcement may work to decrease unacceptable behaviors.*

3. Help client understand that he or she uses this behavior in order to try to increase own self-esteem. Interventions should reflect other actions to accomplish this goal. *When client feels better about self, the need to manipulate others will diminish.*
4. If client chooses to suppress tics in the presence of others, provide a specified "tic time," during which client "vents" tics, feelings, and behaviors (alone or with staff). *Allows for release of tics and assists in sense of control and management of symptoms.*
5. Ensure that client has regular one-to-one time with staff or support person. *One-to-one time gives nurse the opportunity to provide client with information about the illness and healthy ways to manage it. Exploring feelings about the illness helps client incorporate the illness into a healthy sense of self.*

Outcome Criteria
1. Client verbalizes positive perception of self.
2. Client willingly participates in new activities and situations.

● SEPARATION ANXIETY DISORDER
Defined
The APA (2000) defines separation anxiety disorder as "excessive anxiety concerning separation from the home or from those to whom the person is attached." Onset may occur as early as preschool age, rarely as late as adolescence, but always before age 18, and is more common in girls than in boys.

Predisposing Factors
1. **Physiological**
   a. *Genetics.* The results of studies indicate that a greater number of children with relatives who manifest anxiety problems develop anxiety disorders themselves than do children with no such family patterns.
   b. *Temperament.* Studies have shown that differences in temperamental characteristics at birth may be correlated to the acquisition of fear and anxiety disorders in childhood. This may denote an inherited vulnerability or predisposition toward developing these disorders.
2. **Psychosocial**
   a. *Stressful Life Events.* Studies indicate that children who are predisposed to anxiety disorders may be affected significantly by stressful life events.
   b. *Family Influences.* Several theories exist that relate the development of separation anxiety to the following dynamics within the family:
      → An overattachment to the mother (primary caregiver)
      → Separation conflicts between parent and child

→ Enmeshment of members within a family
→ Overprotection of the child by the parents
→ Transfer of parents' fears and anxieties to the children through role modeling

Symptomatology (Subjective and Objective Data)

Symptoms of separation anxiety disorder include the following:

1. In most cases the child has difficulty separating from the mother, although occasionally the separation reluctance is directed toward the father, siblings, or other significant individual to whom the child is attached.
2. Anticipation of separation may result in tantrums, crying, screaming, complaints of physical problems, and clinging behaviors.
3. Reluctance or refusal to attend school is especially common in adolescence.
4. Younger children may "shadow" or follow around the person from whom they are afraid to be separated.
5. During middle childhood or adolescence he or she may refuse to sleep away from home (e.g., at a friend's house or at camp).
6. Worrying is common and relates to the possibility of harm coming to self or to the attachment figure. Younger children may have nightmares to this effect.
7. Specific phobias may be present.
8. Depressed mood is frequently present and often precedes the onset of the anxiety symptoms, which commonly occur following a major stressor.

Common Nursing Diagnoses and Interventions for the Client with Separation Anxiety Disorder

(Interventions are applicable to various health care settings, such as inpatient and partial hospitalization, community outpatient clinic, home health, and private practice.)

● ANXIETY (SEVERE)

Definition: Vague uneasy feeling of discomfort or dread accompanied by an autonomic response (the source is often nonspecific or unknown to the individual); a feeling of apprehension caused by anticipation of danger. It is an alerting signal that warns of impending danger and enables the individual to take measures to deal with threat.

Possible Etiologies ("related to")

Heredity
[Birth temperament]
[Overattachment to parent]
[Negative role modeling]

Defining Characteristics ("evidenced by")

[Excessive distress when separated from attachment figure]
[Fear of anticipation of separation from attachment figure]
[Fear of being alone or without attachment figure]
[Reluctance or refusal to go to school or anywhere else without attachment figure]
[Nightmares about being separated from attachment figure]
[Somatic symptoms occurring as a result of fear of separation]

Goals/Objectives

Short-term Goal

Client will discuss fears of separation with trusted individual.

Long-term Goal

Client will maintain anxiety at no higher than moderate level in the face of events that formerly have precipitated panic.

Interventions with *Selected Rationales*

1. Establish an atmosphere of calmness, trust, and genuine positive regard. *Trust and unconditional acceptance are necessary for satisfactory nurse–client relationship. Calmness is important because anxiety is easily transmitted from one person to another.*
2. Assure client of his or her safety and security. *Symptoms of panic anxiety are very frightening.*
3. Explore child's or adolescent's fears of separating from parents. Explore with parents possible fears they may have of separation from child. *Some parents may have an underlying fear of separation from child, of which they are unaware and which they are unconsciously transferring to child.*
4. Help parents and child initiate realistic goals (e.g., child to stay with sitter for 2 hours with minimal anxiety or child to stay at friend's house without parents until 9:00 PM without experiencing panic anxiety). *Parents may be so frustrated with child's clinging and demanding behaviors that assistance with problem solving may be required.*
5. Give, and encourage parents to give, positive reinforcement for desired behaviors. *Positive reinforcement encourages repetition of desirable behaviors.*

Outcome Criteria

1. Client and parents are able to discuss their fears regarding separation.
2. Client experiences no somatic symptoms from fear of separation.
3. Client maintains anxiety at moderate level when separation occurs or is anticipated.

● INEFFECTIVE COPING

Definition: Inability to form a valid appraisal of the stressors, inadequate choices of practiced responses, and/or inability to use available resources

Possible Etiologies ("related to")

[Unresolved separation conflicts]
[Inadequate coping skills]

Defining Characteristics ("evidenced by")

[Somatic complaints in response to occurrence or anticipation of separation from attachment figure]

Goals/Objectives

Short-term Goal

Client will verbalize correlation of somatic symptoms to fear of separation.

Long-term Goal

Client will demonstrate use of more adaptive coping strategies (than physical symptoms) in response to stressful situations.

Interventions with *Selected Rationales*

1. Encourage child or adolescent to discuss specific situations in life that produce the most distress and describe his or her response to these situations. Include parents in the discussion. *Client and family may be unaware of the correlation between stressful situations and the exacerbation of physical symptoms.*
2. Help child or adolescent who is perfectionistic to recognize that self-expectations may be unrealistic. Connect times of unmet self-expectations to the exacerbation of physical symptoms. *Recognition of maladaptive patterns is the first step in the change process.*
3. Encourage parents and child to identify more adaptive coping strategies that child could use in the face of anxiety that

feels overwhelming. Practice through role-play. *Practice facilitates the use of the desired behavior when individual is actually faced with the stressful situation.*

Outcome Criteria
1. Client and family verbalize the correlation between separation anxiety and somatic symptoms.
2. Client verbalizes the correlation between unmet self-expectations and somatic symptoms.
3. Client responds to stressful situations without exhibiting physical symptoms.

● IMPAIRED SOCIAL INTERACTION

Definition: Insufficient or excessive quantity or ineffective quality of social exchange

Possible Etiologies ("related to")
[Reluctance to be away from attachment figure]

Defining Characteristics ("evidenced by")
[Symptoms of severe anxiety]
[Verbalized or observed] discomfort in social situations
[Verbalized or observed] inability to receive or communicate a satisfying sense of belonging, caring, interest, or shared history
[Observed] use of unsuccessful social interaction behaviors
Dysfunctional interaction with others

Goals/Objectives
Short-term Goal
Client will spend time with staff or other support person, without presence of attachment figure, without excessive anxiety.

Long-term Goal
Client will be able to spend time with others (without presence of attachment figure) without excessive anxiety.

Interventions with *Selected Rationales*
1. Develop a trusting relationship with client. *This is the first step in helping client learn to interact with others.*
2. Attend groups with child and support efforts to interact with others. Give positive feedback. *Presence of a trusted individual provides security during times of distress. Positive feedback encourages repetition.*

3. Convey to the child the acceptability of his or her not participating in group in the beginning. Gradually encourage small contributions until client is able to participate more fully. ***Small successes will gradually increase self-confidence and decrease self-consciousness, so that client will feel less anxious in the group situation.***

4. Help client set small personal goals (e.g., "Today I will speak to one person I don't know."). ***Simple, realistic goals provide opportunities for success that increase self-confidence and may encourage client to attempt more difficult objectives in the future.***

Outcome Criteria

1. Client spends time with others using acceptable, age-appropriate behaviors.
2. Client is able to interact with others away from the attachment figure without excessive anxiety.

@ INTERNET REFERENCES

- Additional information about attention-deficit/hyperactivity disorder may be located at the following websites:
  a. http://www.chadd.org
  b. http://www.nimh.nih.gov/health/topics/attention-deficit-hyperactivity-disorder-adhd/index.shtml
- Additional information about autism may be located at the following websites:
  a. http://www.autism-society.org
  b. http://www.nimh.nih.gov/health/topics/autism-spectrum-disorders-pervasive-developmental-disorders/index.shtml
- Additional information about medications to treat attention-deficit/hyperactivity disorder may be located at the following websites:
  a. http://www.fadavis.com/townsend
  b. http://www.drugs.com/condition/attention-deficit-disorder.html
  c. http://www.nimh.nih.gov/health/publications/medications/complete-publication.shtml

Movie Connections

Bill (MR) • Bill: On His Own (MR) • Sling Blade (MR) • Forrest Gump (MR) • Rain Man (autistic disorder) • Mercury Rising (autistic disorder) • Niagara, Niagara (Tourette's disorder) • Toughlove (conduct disorder)

Delirium, Dementia, and Amnestic Disorders

● BACKGROUND ASSESSMENT DATA
Delirium
Defined

The American Psychiatric Association (APA, 2000) *Diagnostic and Statistical Manual of Mental Disorders, Fourth Edition, Text Revision (DSM-IV-TR)* defines "delirium" as a disturbance of consciousness and a change in cognition that develop rapidly over a short period. The symptoms of delirium usually begin quite abruptly, and the duration is usually brief (e.g., 1 week; rarely more than 1 month). The disorder subsides completely on recovery from the underlying determinant. If the underlying condition persists, the delirium may gradually shift to the syndrome of dementia or progress to coma. The individual then recovers, becomes chronically vegetative, or dies.

Predisposing Factors to Delirium

The *DSM-IV-TR* differentiates among the disorders of delirium by their etiology, although they share a common symptom presentation. Categories of delirium include the following:

1. **Delirium Due to a General Medical Condition**. Certain medical conditions, such as systemic infections, metabolic disorders, fluid and electrolyte imbalances, liver or kidney disease, thiamine deficiency, postoperative states, hypertensive encephalopathy, postictal states, and sequelae of head trauma, can cause the symptoms of delirium.
2. **Substance-Induced Delirium**. The symptoms of delirium can be induced by the exposure to a toxin or the ingestion of medications, such as anticonvulsants, neuroleptics, anxiolytics, antidepressants, cardiovascular medications, antineoplastics, analgesics, antiasthmatic agents, antihistamines, antiparkinsonian drugs, corticosteroids, and gastrointestinal medications.

3. **Substance-Intoxication Delirium**. Delirium symptoms can occur in response to taking high doses of cannabis, cocaine, hallucinogens, alcohol, anxiolytics, or narcotics.
4. **Substance-Withdrawal Delirium.** Reduction or termination of long-term, high-dose use of certain substances, such as alcohol, sedatives, hypnotics, or anxiolytics, can result in withdrawal delirium symptoms.
5. **Delirium Due to Multiple Etiologies**. Symptoms of delirium may be related to more than one general medical condition or to the combined effects of a general medical condition and substance use.

Symptomatology *(Subjective and Objective Data)*

The following symptoms have been identified with the syndrome of delirium:

1. Altered consciousness ranging from hypervigilance to stupor or semicoma.
2. Extreme distractibility with difficulty focusing attention.
3. Disorientation to time and place.
4. Impaired reasoning ability and goal-directed behavior.
5. Disturbance in the sleep-wake cycle.
6. Emotional instability as manifested by fear, anxiety, depression, irritability, anger, euphoria, or apathy.
7. Misperceptions of the environment, including illusions and hallucinations.
8. Autonomic manifestations, such as tachycardia, sweating, flushed face, dilated pupils, and elevated blood pressure.
9. Incoherent speech.
10. Impairment of recent memory.

Dementia

Defined

"Dementia" is defined by a loss of previous levels of cognitive, executive, and memory function in a state of full alertness (Bourgeois, Seaman, & Servis, 2008). The disease usually has a slow, insidious onset and is chronic, progressive, and irreversible.

Predisposing Factors to Dementia

Following are major etiologic categories for the syndrome of dementia:

1. **Dementia of the Alzheimer's Type.** The exact cause of Alzheimer's disease (AD) is unknown, but several theories have been proposed, such as reduction in brain acetylcholine, the formation of plaques and tangles, serious head trauma, and genetic factors. Pathologic changes in the brain include atrophy, enlarged ventricles, and the presence of numerous neurofibrillary plaques and tangles. Definitive diagnosis is

by biopsy or autopsy examination of brain tissue, although refinement of diagnostic criteria and new diagnostic tools now enable clinicians to use specific clinical features to identify the disease at an accuracy rate of 70% to 90% (Bourgeois, Seaman, & Servis, 2008).

2. **Vascular Dementia**. This type of dementia is caused by significant cerebrovascular disease. The client suffers the equivalent of small strokes caused by arterial hypertension or cerebral emboli or thrombi, which destroy many areas of the brain. The onset of symptoms is more abrupt than in AD and runs a highly variable course, progressing in steps rather than as a gradual deterioration.

3. **Dementia Due to HIV Disease**. The immune dysfunction associated with human immunodeficiency virus (HIV) disease can lead to brain infections by other organisms. HIV also appears to cause dementia directly.

4. **Dementia Due to Head Trauma**. The syndrome of symptoms associated with dementia can be brought on by a traumatic brain injury.

5. **Dementia Due to Lewy Body Disease.** Clinically, Lewy body disease is fairly similar to AD; however, it tends to progress more rapidly, and there is an earlier appearance of visual hallucinations and parkinsonian features (Rabins, et al., 2006). This disorder is distinctive by the presence of Lewy bodies—eosinophilic inclusion bodies—seen in the cerebral cortex and brainstem (Andreasen & Black, 2006).

6. **Dementia Due to Parkinson's Disease.** Parkinson's disease is caused by a loss of nerve cells in the substantia nigra of the basal ganglia. The symptoms of dementia associated with Parkinson's disease closely resemble those of AD.

7. **Dementia Due to Huntington's Disease.** This disease is transmitted as a Mendelian dominant gene, and damage occurs in the areas of the basal ganglia and the cerebral cortex. The average duration of the disease is based on age at onset. One study concluded that juvenile-onset and late-onset clients have the shortest duration (Foroud et al., 1999). In this study, the median duration of the disease was 21.4 years.

8. **Dementia Due to Pick's Disease.** Pathology occurs from atrophy in the frontal and temporal lobes of the brain. Symptoms are strikingly similar to those of AD, and Pick's disease is often misdiagnosed as AD.

9. **Dementia Due to Creutzfeldt-Jakob Disease.** This form of dementia is caused by a transmissible agent known as a "slow virus" or prion. The clinical presentation is typical of the syndrome of dementia, and the course is extremely rapid, with progressive deterioration and death within 1 year after onset.

10. **Dementia Due to Other General Medical Conditions.** A number of other general medical conditions can cause dementia. Some of these include endocrine conditions (e.g., hypoglycemia, hypothyroidism), pulmonary disease, hepatic or renal failure, cardiopulmonary insufficiency, fluid and electrolyte imbalances, nutritional deficiencies, frontal or temporal lobe lesions, central nervous system (CNS) or systemic infections, uncontrolled epilepsy, and other neurological conditions such as multiple sclerosis (APA, 2000).

11. **Substance-Induced Persisting Dementia.** This type of dementia is related to the persisting effects of substances such as alcohol, inhalants, sedatives, hypnotics, anxiolytics, other medications, and environmental toxins. The term "persisting" is used to indicate that the dementia persists long after the effects of substance intoxication or substance withdrawal have subsided.

Symptomatology *(Subjective and Objective Data)*

The following symptoms have been identified with the syndrome of dementia:

1. Memory impairment (impaired ability to learn new information or to recall previously learned information).
2. Impairment in abstract thinking, judgment, and impulse control.
3. Impairment in language ability, such as difficulty naming objects. In some instances, the individual may not speak at all (aphasia).
4. Personality changes are common.
5. Impaired ability to perform motor activities despite intact motor abilities (apraxia).
6. Disorientation.
7. Wandering.
8. Delusions are common (particularly delusions of persecution).

Amnestic Disorders

Defined

Amnestic disorders are characterized by an inability to learn new information (short-term memory deficit) despite normal attention and an inability to recall previously learned information (long-term memory deficit). No other cognitive deficits exist.

Predisposing Factors to Amnestic Disorders

The *DSM-IV-TR* identifies the following categories as etiologies for the syndrome of symptoms known as amnestic disorders:

1. **Amnestic Disorder Due to a General Medical Condition**. The symptoms may be associated with head trauma, cerebrovascular disease, cerebral neoplastic disease, cerebral

anoxia, herpes simplex encephalitis, poorly controlled insulin dependent diabetes, and surgical intervention to the brain (APA, 2000; Bourgeois, Seaman, & Servis, 2008). Transient amnestic syndromes can also occur from epileptic seizures, electroconvulsive therapy, severe migraine, and drug overdose.

2. **Substance-Induced Persisting Amnestic Disorder**. This type of amnestic disorder is related to the persisting effects of substances such as alcohol, sedatives, hypnotics, anxiolytics, other medications, and environmental toxins. The term "persisting" is used to indicate that the symptoms persist long after the effects of substance intoxication or substance withdrawal have subsided.

Symptomatology (Subjective and Objective Data)

The following symptoms have been identified with amnestic disorder:

1. Disorientation to place and time may occur with profound amnesia.
2. There is an inability to recall events from the recent past and events from the remote past. (Events from the very remote past are often more easily recalled than recently occurring ones.)
3. The individual is prone to confabulation. That is, the individual may create imaginary events to fill in the memory gaps.
4. Apathy, lack of initiative, and emotional blandness are common.

Common Nursing Diagnoses and Interventions for Delirium, Dementia, and Amnestic Disorders

(Interventions are applicable to various health-care settings, such as inpatient and partial hospitalization, community outpatient clinic, home health, and private practice.)

● RISK FOR TRAUMA

Definition: [The client has] accentuated risk of accidental tissue injury (e.g., wound, burn, fracture).

Related/Risk Factors ("related to")

[Chronic alteration in structure or function of brain tissue, secondary to the aging process, multiple infarcts, HIV disease, head trauma, chronic substance abuse, or progressively dysfunctional physical condition resulting in the following symptoms:

Disorientation; confusion
Weakness
Muscular incoordination
Seizures
Memory impairment
Poor vision
Extreme psychomotor agitation observed in the late stages of delirium]

[Frequent shuffling of feet and stumbling]
[Falls, caused by muscular incoordination or seizures]
[Bumping into furniture]
[Exposing self to frigid conditions with insufficient protective clothing]
[Cutting self when using sharp instruments]
[History of attempting to light burner or oven and leaving gas on in house]
[Smoking and leaving burning cigarettes in various places; smoking in bed; falling asleep sitting on couch or chair with lighted cigarette in hand]
[Purposeless, thrashing movements; hyperactivity that is out of touch with the environment]

Goals/Objectives

Short-term Goals

1. Client will accept assistance when ambulating or carrying out other activities.
2. Client will not experience physical injury.

Long-term Goal

Client will not experience physical injury.

Interventions with *Selected Rationales*

1. Assess client's level of disorientation and confusion to determine specific requirements for safety. *Knowledge of client's level of functioning is necessary to formulate appropriate plan of care.*
2. Institute appropriate safety measures, such as the following:
   a. Place furniture in room in an arrangement that best accommodates client's disabilities.
   b. Observe client behaviors frequently; assign staff on one-to-one basis if condition warrants; accompany and assist client when ambulating; use wheelchair for transporting long distances.

c. Store items that client uses frequently within easy access.
d. Remove potentially harmful articles from client's room: cigarettes, matches, lighters, sharp objects.
e. Remain with client while he or she smokes.
f. Pad side rails and headboard of client with seizure disorder. Institute seizure precautions as described in procedure manual of individual institution.
g. If client is prone to wander, provide an area within which wandering can be carried out safely.
3. Frequently orient client to reality and surroundings. *Disorientation may endanger client safety if he or she unknowingly wanders away from safe environment.*
4. Use tranquilizing medications and soft restraints, as prescribed by physician, for client's protection during periods of excessive hyperactivity. *Use restraints judiciously, because they can increase agitation. They may be required, however, to provide for client safety.*
5. Teach prospective caregivers methods that have been successful in preventing client injury. *These caregivers will be responsible for client's safety after discharge from the hospital. Sharing successful interventions may be helpful.*

Outcome Criteria
1. Client is able to accomplish daily activities within the environment without experiencing injury.
2. Prospective caregivers are able to verbalize means of providing safe environment for client.

● RISK FOR SELF-DIRECTED OR OTHER-DIRECTED VIOLENCE

Definition: At risk for behaviors in which an individual demonstrates that he or she can be physically, emotionally, and/or sexually harmful [either to self or to others].

Related/Risk Factors ("related to")
[Chronic alteration in structure or function of brain tissue, secondary to the aging process, multiple infarcts, HIV disease, head trauma, chronic substance abuse, or progressively dysfunctional physical condition resulting in the following symptoms:
    Delusional thinking
    Suspiciousness of others
    Hallucinations
    Illusions

Disorientation or confusion
Impairment of impulse control]
[Inaccurate perception of the environment]
Body language—rigid posture, clenching of fists and jaw, hyper-
   activity, pacing, breathlessness, and threatening stances
Suicidal ideation, plan, available means
Cognitive impairment
[Depressed mood]

Goals/Objectives
Short-term Goals
1. Client will maintain agitation at manageable level so as not to
   become violent.
2. Client will not harm self or others.

Long-term Goal
Client will not harm self or others.

Interventions with *Selected Rationales*
1. Assess client's level of anxiety and behaviors that indicate
   the anxiety is increasing. *Recognizing these behaviors, nurse
   may be able to intervene before violence occurs.*
2. Maintain low level of stimuli in client's environment (low
   lighting, few people, simple decor, low noise level). *Anxiety
   increases in a highly stimulating environment.*
3. Remove all potentially dangerous objects from client's environment. *In a disoriented, confused state, client may use
   these objects to harm self or others.*
4. Have sufficient staff available to execute a physical confrontation, if necessary. *Assistance may be required from others to
   provide for physical safety of client or primary nurse or both.*
5. Maintain a calm manner with client. Attempt to prevent
   frightening client unnecessarily. Provide continual reassurance and support. *Anxiety is contagious and can be
   transferred to client.*
6. Interrupt periods of unreality and reorient. *Client safety is
   jeopardized during periods of disorientation. Correcting
   misinterpretations of reality enhances client's feelings of
   self-worth and personal dignity.*
7. Use tranquilizing medications and soft restraints, as prescribed by physician, *for protection of client and others during
   periods of elevated anxiety.* Use restraints judiciously, *because
   agitation sometimes increases; however, they may be required
   to ensure client safety.*
8. Sit with client and provide one-to-one observation if assessed
   to be actively suicidal. *Client safety is a nursing priority,
   and one-to-one observation may be necessary to prevent a
   suicidal attempt.*

9. Teach relaxation exercises *to intervene in times of increasing anxiety.*
10. Teach prospective caregivers to recognize client behaviors that indicate anxiety is increasing and ways to intervene before violence occurs.

Outcome Criteria

1. Prospective caregivers are able to verbalize behaviors that indicate an increasing anxiety level and ways they may assist client to manage the anxiety before violence occurs.
2. With assistance from caregivers, client is able to control impulse to perform acts of violence against self or others.

● CHRONIC CONFUSION

Definition: Irreversible, long-standing, and/or progressive deterioration of intellect and personality characterized by decreased ability to interpret environmental stimuli; decreased capacity for intellectual thought processes; and manifested by disturbances of memory, orientation, and behavior.

Possible Etiologies ("related to")

[Alteration in structure/function of brain tissue, secondary to the following conditions:
   Advanced age
   Vascular disease
   Hypertension
   Cerebral hypoxia
   Long-term abuse of mood- or behavior-altering substances
   Exposure to environmental toxins
   Various other physical disorders that predispose to cerebral abnormalities (see Predisposing Factors)]

Defining Characteristics ("evidenced by")

Altered interpretation
Altered personality
Altered response to stimuli
Clinical evidence of organic impairment
Impaired long-term memory
Impaired short-term memory
Impaired socialization
Longstanding cognitive impairment
No change in level of consciousness
Progressive cognitive impairment

Goals/Objectives

Short-term Goal

Client will accept explanations of inaccurate interpretations within the environment.

Long-term Goal

With assistance from caregiver, client will be able to interrupt non–reality-based thinking.

Interventions with *Selected Rationales*

1. Frequently orient client to reality and surroundings. Allow client to have familiar objects around him or her. Use other items, such as a clock, a calendar, and daily schedules, to assist in maintaining reality orientation. *Client safety is jeopardized during periods of disorientation. Maintaining reality orientation enhances client's sense of self-worth and personal dignity.*

2. Teach prospective caregivers how to orient client to time, person, place, and circumstances, as required. *These caregivers will be responsible for client safety after discharge from the hospital. Sharing successful interventions may be helpful.*

3. Give positive feedback when thinking and behavior are appropriate, or when client verbalizes that certain ideas expressed are not based in reality. *Positive feedback increases self-esteem and enhances desire to repeat appropriate behaviors.*

4. Use simple explanations and face-to-face interaction when communicating with client. Do not shout message into client's ear. *Speaking slowly and in a face-to-face position is most effective when communicating with an elderly individual experiencing a hearing loss. Visual cues facilitate understanding. Shouting causes distortion of high-pitched sounds and in some instances creates a feeling of discomfort for client.*

5. Express reasonable doubt if client relays suspicious beliefs in response to delusional thinking. Discuss with client the potential personal negative effects of continued suspiciousness of others. Reinforce accurate perception of people and situations. *Expressions of doubt by a trusted individual may foster similar uncertainties about delusion on the part of client.*

6. Do not permit rumination of false ideas. When this begins, talk to client about real people and real events. *Reality orientation increases client's sense of self-worth and personal dignity.*

7. Close observation of client's behavior is indicated if delusional thinking reveals an intention for violence. *Client safety is a nursing priority.*

> **CLINICAL PEARL** 🐟 **Medications for Alzheimer's disease.** Cholinesterase inhibitors are used for mild to moderate cognitive impairment in clients with Alzheimer's disease. Examples include *tacrine (Cognex), donepezil (Aricept), rivastigmine (Exelon),* and *galantamine (Razadyne).* Common side effects include dizziness, headache, and gastrointestinal upset. *Memantine (Namenda),* an NMDA receptor antagonist, is used for treatment of moderate to severe cognitive impairment in clients with Alzheimer's disease. Common side effects of memantine include dizziness, headache, and constipation. These medications do not stop or reverse the disease process but may slow down the progression of the decline in functionality.

Outcome Criteria

1. With assistance from caregiver, client is able to distinguish between reality-based and non–reality-based thinking.
2. Prospective caregivers are able to verbalize ways in which to orient client to reality, as needed.

● SELF-CARE DEFICIT

Definition: Impaired ability to perform or complete [activities of daily living (ADLs)] for self.

Possible Etiologies ("related to")
Cognitive impairment

Defining Characteristics ("evidenced by")
Inability to wash body
Inability to put on clothing
Inability to bring food from receptacle to mouth
[Inability to toilet self without assistance]

Goals/Objectives
Short-term Goal
Client will participate in ADLs with assistance from caregiver.
Long-term Goal
Client will accomplish ADLs to the best of his or her ability. Unfulfilled needs will be met by caregiver.

Interventions with *Selected Rationales*

1. Provide a simple, structured environment *to minimize confusion:*
   a. Identify self-care deficits and provide assistance as required.
   b. Allow plenty of time for client to perform tasks.
   c. Provide guidance and support for independent actions by talking client through the task one step at a time.

    d. Provide a structured schedule of activities that does not change from day to day.

    e. Ensure that ADLs follow home routine as closely as possible.

    f. Provide for consistency in assignment of daily caregivers.

2. In planning for discharge:

    a. Perform ongoing assessment of client's ability to fulfill nutritional needs, ensure personal safety, follow medication regimen, and communicate need for assistance with those activities that he or she cannot accomplish independently. *Client safety and security are nursing priorities.*

    b. Assess prospective caregivers' ability to anticipate and fulfill client's unmet needs. Provide information to assist caregivers with this responsibility. Ensure that caregivers are aware of available community support systems from which they can seek assistance when required. *This will facilitate transition to discharge from treatment center.*

    c. National support organizations can provide information:

        National Parkinson Foundation, Inc.
        1501 NW 9th Ave.
        Miami, FL 33136-1494
        1-800-327-4545

        Alzheimer's Association
        225 N. Michigan Ave., Fl. 17
        Chicago, IL 60601-7633
        1-800-272-3900

Outcome Criteria

1. Client willingly participates in ADLs.
2. Client accomplishes ADLs to the best of his or her ability.
3. Client's unfulfilled needs are met by caregivers.

• DISTURBED SENSORY PERCEPTION (Specify)

Definition: Change in the amount or patterning of incoming stimuli [either internally or externally initiated] accompanied by a diminished, exaggerated, distorted, or impaired response to such stimuli.

Possible Etiologies ("related to")

[Alteration in structure/function of brain tissue, secondary to the following conditions:

    Advanced age

    Vascular disease

Hypertension
Cerebral hypoxia
Abuse of mood- or behavior-altering substances
Exposure to environmental toxins
Various other physical disorders that predispose to cerebral abnormalities (see Predisposing Factors)]

Defining Characteristics ("evidenced by")

Poor concentration
Sensory distortions
Hallucinations
[Disorientation to time, place, person, or circumstances]
[Inappropriate responses]
[Talking and laughing to self]
[Suspiciousness]

Goals/Objectives

Short-term Goal

With assistance from caregiver, client will maintain orientation to time, place, person, and circumstances for specified period of time.

Long-term Goal

Client will demonstrate accurate perception of the environment by responding appropriately to stimuli indigenous to the surroundings.

Interventions with *Selected Rationales*

1. Decrease the amount of stimuli in client's environment (e.g., low noise level, few people, simple decor). *This decreases the possibility of client's forming inaccurate sensory perceptions.*
2. Do not reinforce the hallucination. Let client know that you do not share the perception. Maintain reality through reorientation and focus on real situations and people. *Reality orientation decreases false sensory perceptions and enhances client's sense of self-worth and personal dignity.*
3. Provide reassurance of safety if client responds with fear to inaccurate sensory perception. *Client safety and security are nursing priorities.*
4. Correct client's description of inaccurate perception, and describe the situation as it exists in reality. *Explanation of and participation in real situations and real activities interfere with the ability to respond to hallucinations.*
5. Allow for care to be given by same personnel on a regular basis, if possible, *to provide a feeling of security and stability in client's environment.*

6. Teach prospective caregivers how to recognize signs and symptoms of client's inaccurate sensory perceptions. Explain techniques they may use to restore reality to the situation.

Outcome Criteria
1. With assistance from caregiver, client is able to recognize when perceptions within the environment are inaccurate.
2. Prospective caregivers are able to verbalize ways in which to correct inaccurate perceptions and restore reality to the situation.

• LOW SELF-ESTEEM

Definition: Negative self-evaluating/feelings about self or self-capabilities.

Possible Etiologies ("related to")
[Loss of independent functioning]
[Loss of capacity for remembering]
[Loss of capability for effective verbal communication]

Defining Characteristics ("evidenced by")
[Withdraws into social isolation]
Lack of eye contact
[Excessive crying alternating with expressions of anger]
[Refusal to participate in therapies]
[Refusal to participate in own self-care activities]
[Becomes increasingly dependent on others to perform ADLs]
Expressions of shame or guilt

Goals/Objectives
Short-term Goal
Client will voluntarily spend time with staff and peers in day-room activities (time dimension to be individually determined).

Long-term Goal
Client will exhibit increased feelings of self-worth as evidenced by voluntary participation in own self-care and interaction with others (time dimension to be individually determined).

Interventions with *Selected Rationales*
1. Encourage client to express honest feelings in relation to loss of prior level of functioning. Acknowledge pain of loss.

Support client through process of grieving. *Client may be fixed in anger stage of grieving process, which is turned inward on the self, resulting in diminished self-esteem.*

2. Devise methods for assisting client with memory deficit. *These aids may assist client to function more independently, thereby increasing self-esteem.* Examples follow:
   a. Name sign on door identifying client's room.
   b. Identifying sign on outside of dining room door.
   c. Identifying sign on outside of restroom door.
   d. Large clock, with oversized numbers and hands, appropriately placed.
   e. Large calendar, indicating one day at a time, with month, day, and year identified in bold print.
   f. Printed, structured daily schedule, with one copy for client and one posted on unit wall.
   g. "News board" on unit wall where current national and local events may be posted.

3. Encourage client's attempts to communicate. If verbalizations are not understandable, express to client what you think he or she intended to say. It may be necessary to reorient client frequently. *The ability to communicate effectively with others may enhance self-esteem.*

4. Encourage reminiscence and discussion of life review. Also discuss present-day events. Sharing picture albums, if possible, is especially good. *Reminiscence and life review help client resume progression through the grief process associated with disappointing life events and increase self-esteem as successes are reviewed.*

5. Encourage participation in group activities. Caregiver may need to accompany client at first, until he or she feels secure that group members will be accepting, regardless of limitations in verbal communication. *Positive feedback from group members will increase self-esteem.*

6. Offer support and empathy when client expresses embarrassment at inability to remember people, events, and places. Focus on accomplishments *to lift self-esteem.*

7. Encourage client to be as independent as possible in self-care activities. Provide written schedule of tasks to be performed. Intervene in areas where client requires assistance. *The ability to perform independently preserves self-esteem.*

Outcome Criteria

1. Client initiates own self-care according to written schedule and willingly accepts assistance as needed.
2. Client interacts with others in group activities, maintaining anxiety at minimal level in response to difficulties with verbal communication.

● CAREGIVER ROLE STRAIN

Definition: Difficulty in performing family caregiver role.

Possible Etiologies ("related to")

Severity of care receiver's illness
Chronicity of care receiver's illness
[Lack of respite and recreation for caregiver]
Caregiver's competing role commitments
Inadequate physical environment for providing care
Family or caregiver isolation
Complexity and amount of caregiving activities

Defining Characteristics ("evidenced by")

Apprehension about possible institutionalization of care receiver
Apprehension about future regarding care receiver's health and
    caregiver's ability to provide care
Difficulty performing and/or completing required tasks
Apprehension about care receiver's care if caregiver unable to
    provide care

Goals/Objectives

Short-term Goal

Caregivers will verbalize understanding of ways to facilitate the
caregiver role.

Long-term Goal

Caregivers will demonstrate effective problem-solving skills and
develop adaptive coping mechanisms to regain equilibrium.

Interventions with *Selected Rationales*

1. Assess caregivers' ability to anticipate and fulfill client's unmet needs. Provide information to assist caregivers with this
   responsibility. *Caregivers may be unaware of what client will
   realistically be able to accomplish. They may be unaware of
   the progressive nature of the illness.*
2. Ensure that caregivers are aware of available community
   support systems from which they can seek assistance when
   required. Examples include adult day-care centers, housekeeping and homemaker services, respite-care services,
   and a local chapter of the Alzheimer's Association. This
   organization sponsors a nationwide 24-hour hot line to
   provide information and link families who need assistance
   with nearby chapters and affiliates. The hotline number is
   1-800-272-3900. *Caregivers require relief from the pressures
   and strain of providing 24-hour care for their loved ones.*

Studies show that elder abuse arises out of caregiving situations that place overwhelming stress on caregivers.
3. Encourage caregivers to express feelings, particularly anger. *Release of these emotions can serve to prevent psychopathology, such as depression or psychophysiological disorders, from occurring.*
4. Encourage participation in support groups composed of members with similar life situations. *Hearing others who are experiencing the same problems discuss ways in which they have coped may help caregiver adopt more adaptive strategies. Individuals who are experiencing similar life situations provide empathy and support for each other.*

Outcome Criteria

1. Caregivers are able to problem solve effectively regarding care of elderly client.
2. Caregivers demonstrate adaptive coping strategies for dealing with stress of caregiver role.
3. Caregivers express feelings openly.
4. Caregivers express desire to join support group of other caregivers.

@ INTERNET REFERENCES

- Additional information about Alzheimer's disease may be located at the following websites:
  a. http://www.alz.org
  b. http://www.nia.nih.gov/
  c. http://www.ninds.nih.gov/disorders/alzheimersdisease/alzheimersdisease.htm
- Information on caregiving can be located at the following website:
  a. http://www.aarp.org
- Additional information about medications to treat Alzheimer's disease may be located at the following websites:
  a. http://www.fadavis.com/townsend
  b. http://www.nimh.nih.gov/publicat/medicate.cfm
  c. http://www.drugs.com/condition/alzheimer-s-disease html.
  d. http://www.nlm.nih.gov/medlineplus/druginformation html.

Movie Connections

The Notebook (Alzheimer's disease) • *Away from Her (Alzheimer's disease)* • *Iris (Alzheimer's disease)*

Substance-Related Disorders

● BACKGROUND ASSESSMENT DATA

The substance-related disorders are composed of two groups: the substance-use disorders (dependence and abuse) and the substance-induced disorders (intoxication and withdrawal). Other substance-induced disorders (delirium, dementia, amnesia, psychosis, mood disorder, anxiety disorder, and sexual dysfunction) are included in the chapters with which they share symptomatology (e.g., substance-induced anxiety disorder is included in Chapter 8; substance-induced sexual dysfunction is included in Chapter 11, etc.).

● SUBSTANCE-USE DISORDERS

Substance Abuse

Defined

The American Psychiatric Association (APA, 2000) *Diagnostic and Statistical Manual of Mental Disorders, Fourth Edition, Text Revision (DSM-IV-TR)* defines "substance abuse" as "a maladaptive pattern of substance use manifested by recurrent and significant adverse consequences related to repeated use of the substance." Symptoms include use of substances in physically harmful circumstances, impaired role performance (school, work, or home), repeated encounters with the legal system for substance-related conduct, and experiencing personal problems related to substance use.

Substance Dependence

Defined

"Dependence" is defined as a compulsive or chronic requirement. The need is so strong as to generate distress (either physical or psychological) if left unfulfilled (Townsend, 2009). Dependence on substances is identified by the appearance of unpleasant effects characteristic of a withdrawal syndrome when a drug is discontinued. Dependence on substances can also be associated with *tolerance*, in which there is a need for increasingly larger or more frequent doses of a substance to obtain the desired effects originally produced by a lower dose. The individual who is dependent on substances continues to increase the amount consumed to achieve the desired effect and to relieve or avoid withdrawal symptoms.

● SUBSTANCE-INDUCED DISORDERS
Substance Intoxication
Defined
"Intoxication" is defined as a physical and mental state of exhilaration and emotional frenzy or lethargy and stupor (Townsend, 2009). With substance intoxication, the individual experiences a reversible syndrome of symptoms that occur with ingestion of a substance and that are specific to the substance ingested. The behavior changes can be attributed to the physiological effects of the substance on the central nervous system (CNS).

Substance Withdrawal
Defined
"Withdrawal" is defined as the physiological and mental readjustment that accompanies the discontinuation of an addictive substance (Townsend, 2009). The symptoms of withdrawal are specific to the substance that has been ingested and occur after prolonged or heavy use of the substance. The effects are of sufficient significance to interfere with usual role performance.

● CLASSIFICATION OF SUBSTANCES
Alcohol
Although alcohol is a CNS depressant, it is considered separately because of the complex effects and widespread nature of its use. Low to moderate consumption produces a feeling of well-being and reduced inhibitions. At higher concentrations, motor and intellectual functioning are impaired, mood becomes very labile, and behaviors characteristic of depression, euphoria, and aggression are exhibited. The only medical use for alcohol (with the exception of its inclusion in a number of pharmacological concentrates) is as an antidote for methanol consumption.

EXAMPLES: Beer, wine, bourbon, scotch, gin, vodka, rum, tequila, liqueurs.

Common substances containing alcohol and used by some dependent individuals to satisfy their need include liquid cough medications, liquid cold preparations, mouthwashes, isopropyl rubbing alcohol, nail polish removers, colognes, and aftershave and preshave preparations.

Opioids

Opioids have a medical use as analgesics, antitussives, and antidiarrheals. They produce the effects of analgesia and euphoria by stimulating the opiate receptors in the brain, thereby mimicking the naturally occurring endorphins.

EXAMPLES: Opium, morphine, codeine, heroin, hydrocodone, oxycodone, meperidine, methadone.

COMMON STREET NAMES: Horse, junk, H (heroin); black stuff, poppy, big O (opium); M, morph (morphine); dollies (methadone); terp (terpin hydrate or cough syrup with codeine); oxy, O.C. (oxycodone); Vike (hydrocodone).

CNS Depressants

CNS depressants have a medical use as antianxiety agents, sedatives, hypnotics, anticonvulsants, and anesthetics. They depress the action of the CNS, resulting in an overall calming, relaxing effect on the individual. At higher dosages they can induce sleep.

EXAMPLES: Benzodiazepines, barbiturates, chloral hydrate, meprobamate, flunitrazepam.

COMMON STREET NAMES: Peter, Mickey (chloral hydrate); green and whites, roaches (Librium); blues (Valium, 10 mg); yellows (Valium, 5 mg); candy, tranks (other benzodiazepines); red birds, red devils (secobarbital); downers (barbiturates; tranquilizers); rophies, forget-me pill, R2 (flunitrazepam [Rohypnol]).

CNS Stimulants

CNS stimulants have a medical use in the management of hyperkinesia, narcolepsy, and weight control. They stimulate the action of the CNS, resulting in increased alertness, excitation, euphoria, increased pulse rate and blood pressure, insomnia, and loss of appetite.

EXAMPLES: Amphetamines, methylphenidate (Ritalin), phendimetrazine (Bontril), cocaine, hydrochloride cocaine, caffeine, tobacco, methylenedioxymethamphetamine (MDMA).

COMMON STREET NAMES: Bennies, wake-ups, uppers, speed (amphetamines); coke, snow, gold dust, girl (cocaine); crack, rock (hydrochloride cocaine); speedball (mixture of heroin and cocaine); Adam, ecstasy, XTC (MDMA).

Hallucinogens

Hallucinogens act as sympathomimetic agents, producing effects resembling those resulting from stimulation of the sympathetic nervous system (e.g., excitation, increased energy, distortion of the senses). Therapeutic medical uses for lysergic acid diethylamide (LSD) have been proposed in the treatment of chronic alcoholism and in the reduction of intractable pain, such as terminal malignant disease and phantom limb sensations. At this time there is no real evidence of the safety and efficacy of the drug in humans.

Examples: LSD, mescaline, phencyclidine (PCP), psilocybin.

Common Street Names: Acid, cube, big D, California sunshine (LSD); angel dust, hog, peace pill, crystal (PCP); cactus, mescal, mesc (mescaline); magic mushroom, shrooms (psilocybin).

Cannabinols

Cannabinols depress higher centers in the brain and consequently release lower centers from inhibitory influence. They produce an anxiety-free state of relaxation characterized by a feeling of extreme well-being. Large doses of the drug can produce hallucinations. Marijuana has been used therapeutically in the relief of nausea and vomiting associated with antineoplastic chemotherapy.

Examples: Marijuana, hashish.

Common Street Names: Joints, reefers, pot, grass, Mary Jane (marijuana); hash (hashish).

Inhalants

Inhalant disorders are induced by inhaling the aliphatic and aromatic hydrocarbons found in substances such as fuels, solvents, adhesives, aerosol propellants, and paint thinners. Inhalants are absorbed through the lungs and reach the CNS very rapidly. Inhalants generally act as a CNS depressant. The effects are relatively brief, lasting from several minutes to a few hours, depending on the specific substance and amount consumed.

Examples: Gasoline, varnish remover, lighter fluid, airplane glue, rubber cement, cleaning fluid, spray paint, shoe conditioner, typewriter correction fluid.

A profile summary of these psychoactive substances is presented in Table 4-1.

● PREDISPOSING FACTORS FOR SUBSTANCE-RELATED DISORDERS

1. *Physiological*
   a. *Genetics.* A genetic link may be involved in the development of substance-related disorders. This is especially evident with alcoholism, and less so with other substances. Children of alcoholics are three times more likely than are other children to become alcoholics (Harvard Medical School, 2001). Studies with monozygotic and dizygotic twins have also supported the genetic hypothesis.

TABLE 4–1 Psychoactive Substances: A Profile Summary

Class of Drugs	Symptoms of Use	Therapeutic Uses	Symptoms of Overdose	Trade Names	Common Names
CNS Depressants					
Alcohol	Relaxation, loss of inhibitions, lack of concentration, drowsiness, slurred speech, sleep	Antidote for methanol consumption; ingredient in many pharmacological concentrates	Nausea, vomiting; shallow respirations; cold, clammy skin; weak, rapid pulse; coma; possible death	Ethyl alcohol, beer, gin, rum, vodka, bourbon, whiskey, liqueurs, wine, brandy, sherry, champagne	Booze, alcohol, liquor, drinks, cocktails, highballs, nightcaps, moonshine, white lightning, firewater
Other (barbiturates and nonbarbiturates)	Same as alcohol	Relief from anxiety and insomnia; as anticonvulsants and anesthetics	Anxiety, fever, agitation, hallucinations, disorientation, tremors, delirium, convulsions, possible death	Seconal, Nembutal, Amytal Valium Librium Noctec Miltown Rohypnol	Red birds, yellow birds, blue birds Blues/yellows Green and whites Mickies Downers Rophies, forget-me pill, R2
CNS Stimulants					
Amphetamines and related drugs	Hyperactivity, agitation, euphoria, insomnia, loss of appetite	Management of narcolepsy, hyperkinesia, and weight control	Cardiac arrhythmias, headache, convulsions, hypertension, rapid heart rate, coma, possible death	Dexedrine, Didrex, Tenuate, Bontril, Ritalin, Focalin, Meridia, Provigil, Methylenedioxymethamphetamine (MDMA)	Uppers, pep pills, wakeups, bennies, eye-openers, speed, black beauties, sweet A's ecstasy, Adam, XTC

Continued

Table 4–1 Psychoactive Substances: A Profile Summary—cont'd

Class of Drugs	Symptoms of Use	Therapeutic Uses	Symptoms of Overdose	Trade Names	Common Names
Cocaine	Euphoria, hyperactivity, restlessness, talkativeness, increased pulse, dilated pupils, rhinitis		Hallucinations, convulsions, pulmonary edema, respiratory failure, coma, cardiac arrest, possible death	Cocaine hydrochloride	Coke, flake, snow, dust, happy dust, gold dust, girl, cecil, C, toot, blow, crack
Opioids	Euphoria, lethargy, drowsiness, lack of motivation, constricted pupils	As analgesics; methadone in substitution therapy; heroin has no therapeutic use	Shallow breathing, slowed pulse, clammy skin, pulmonary edema, respiratory arrest, convulsions, coma, possible death	Heroin Morphine Codeine Dilaudid Demerol Dolophine Percodan Talwin Opium	Snow, stuff, H, harry, horse, M, morph, Miss Emma Schoolboy Lords Doctors Dollies Perkies Ts Big O, black stuff
Hallucinogens	Visual hallucinations, disorientation, confusion, paranoid delusions, euphoria, anxiety, panic, increased pulse	LSD has been proposed in the treatment of chronic alcoholism, and in the reduction of intractable pain.	Agitation, extreme hyperactivity, violence, hallucinations, psychosis, convulsions, possible death	LSD PCP Mescaline DMT STP	Acid, cube, big D Angel dust, hog, peace pill Mesc Businessman's trip Serenity and peace

	Effects	Therapeutic Use	Overdose/Adverse Effects	Examples	Street Names
Cannabinols	Relaxation, talkativeness, lowered inhibitions, euphoria, mood swings	No therapeutic use at this time. Marijuana has been used for relief of nausea and vomiting associated with antineoplastic chemotherapy and to reduce eye pressure in glaucoma	Fatigue, paranoia, delusions, hallucinations, possible psychosis	Cannabis Hashish	Marijuana, pot, grass, joint, Mary Jane, MJ Hash, rope, Sweet Lucy
Inhalants	Dizziness, weakness, tremor, euphoria, slurred speech, unsteady gait, lethargy, nystagmus, blurred vision, diplopia		Can proceed to coma and death	Gasoline Solvents Adhesives Paint thinner Lighter fluid Glue Cleaning fluid	

b. ***Biochemical.*** A second physiological hypothesis relates to the possibility that alcohol may produce morphine-like substances in the brain that are responsible for alcohol addiction. This occurs when the products of alcohol metabolism react with biologically active amines.

2. **Psychosocial**

   a. ***Psychodynamic Theory.*** The psychodynamic approach to the etiology of substance abuse focuses on a punitive superego and fixation at the oral stage of psychosexual development (Sadock & Sadock, 2007). Individuals with punitive superegos turn to alcohol to diminish unconscious anxiety and increase feelings of power and self-worth. Sadock and Sadock (2007) stated, "As a form of self-medication, alcohol may be used to control panic, opioids to diminish anger, and amphetamines to alleviate depression" (p. 386).

   b. ***Social Learning Theory.*** The effects of modeling, imitation, and identification on behavior can be observed from early childhood onward. In relation to drug consumption, the family appears to be an important influence. Various studies have shown that children and adolescents are more likely to use substances if they have parents who provide a model for substance use. Peers often exert a great deal of influence in the life of the child or adolescent who is being encouraged to use substances for the first time. Modeling may continue to be a factor in the use of substances once the individual enters the work force. This is particularly true in the work setting that provides plenty of leisure time with coworkers and where drinking is valued and is used to express group cohesiveness.

● **COMMON PATTERNS OF USE IN SUBSTANCE-RELATED DISORDERS**

Symptomatology (Subjective and Objective Data)

Alcohol Abuse/Dependence

1. Begins with social drinking that provides feeling of relaxation and well-being. Soon requires more and more to produce the same effects.
2. Drinks in secret; hides bottles of alcohol; drinks first thing in the morning (to "steady my nerves") and at any other opportunity that arises during the day.
3. As the disease progresses, the individual may drink in binges. During a binge, drinking continues until the individual is too intoxicated or too sick to consume any more. Behavior borders on the psychotic, with the individual wavering in and out of reality.

4. Begins to have blackouts. Periods of amnesia occur (in the absence of intoxication or loss of consciousness) during which the individual is unable to remember periods of time or events that have occurred.
5. Experiences multisystem physiological impairments from chronic use that include (but are not limited to) the following:
   a. *Peripheral Neuropathy:* Numbness, tingling, pain in extremities (caused by thiamine deficiency).
   b. *Wernicke-Korsakoff Syndrome:* Mental confusion, agitation, diplopia (caused by thiamine deficiency). Without immediate thiamine replacement, rapid deterioration to coma and death will occur.
   c. *Alcoholic Cardiomyopathy:* Enlargement of the heart caused by an accumulation of excess lipids in myocardial cells. Symptoms of tachycardia, dyspnea, and arrhythmias may be evident.
   d. *Esophagitis:* Inflammation of, and pain in, the esophagus.
   e. *Esophageal Varices:* Distended veins in the esophagus, with risk of rupture and subsequent hemorrhage.
   f. *Gastritis:* Inflammation of lining of stomach caused by irritation from the alcohol, resulting in pain, nausea, vomiting, and possibility of bleeding because of erosion of blood vessels.
   g. *Pancreatitis:* Inflammation of the pancreas, resulting in pain, nausea and vomiting, and abdominal distention. With progressive destruction to the gland, symptoms of diabetes mellitus could occur.
   h. *Alcoholic Hepatitis:* Inflammation of the liver, resulting in enlargement, jaundice, right upper quadrant pain, and fever.
   i. *Cirrhosis of the Liver:* Fibrous and degenerative changes occurring in response to chronic accumulation of large amounts of fatty acids in the liver. In cirrhosis, symptoms of alcoholic hepatitis progress to include the following:
      • **Portal Hypertension:** Elevation of blood pressure through the portal circulation resulting from defective blood flow through the cirrhotic liver.
      • **Ascites**: An accumulation of serous fluid in the peritoneal cavity.
      • **Hepatic Encephalopathy:** Liver disorder caused by inability of the liver to convert ammonia to urea (the body's natural method of discarding excess ammonia); as serum ammonia levels rise, confusion occurs, accompanied by restlessness, slurred speech, fever, and, without intervention, an eventual progression to coma and death.

Alcohol Intoxication

1. Symptoms of alcohol intoxication include disinhibition of sexual or aggressive impulses, mood lability, impaired judgment, impaired social or occupational functioning, slurred speech, incoordination, unsteady gait, nystagmus, and flushed face.
2. Physical and behavioral impairment based on blood alcohol concentrations differ according to gender, body size, physical condition, and level of tolerance.
3. The legal definition of intoxication in most states in the United States is a blood alcohol concentration of 80 or 100 mg ethanol per deciliter of blood (mg/dL), which is also measured as 0.08 to 0.10 g/dL.
4. Nontolerant individuals with blood alcohol concentrations greater than 300 mg/dL are at risk for respiratory failure, coma, and death (Sadock & Sadock, 2007).

Alcohol Withdrawal

1. Occurs within 4 to 12 hours of cessation of, or reduction in, heavy and prolonged alcohol use.
2. Symptoms include coarse tremor of hands, tongue, or eyelids; nausea or vomiting; malaise or weakness; tachycardia; sweating; elevated blood pressure; anxiety; depressed mood or irritability; transient hallucinations or illusions; headache; seizures; and insomnia.
3. Without aggressive intervention, the individual may progress to *alcohol withdrawal delirium* about the second or third day following cessation of, or reduction in, prolonged, heavy alcohol use. Symptoms include those described under the syndrome of delirium (see Chapter 3).

Amphetamine (or Amphetamine-like) Dependence/Abuse

1. The use of amphetamines is often initiated for their appetite-suppressant effect in an attempt to lose or control weight.
2. Amphetamines are also taken for the initial feeling of well-being and confidence.
3. They are typically taken orally, intravenously, or by nasal inhalation.
4. Chronic daily (or almost daily) use usually results in an increase in dosage over time to produce the desired effect.
5. Episodic use often takes the form of binges, followed by an intense and unpleasant "crash" in which the individual experiences anxiety, irritability, and feelings of fatigue and depression.
6. Continued use appears to be related to a "craving" for the substance, rather than to prevention or alleviation of withdrawal symptoms.

Amphetamine (or Amphetamine-like) Intoxication

1. Amphetamine intoxication usually begins with a "high" feeling, followed by the development of symptoms such as euphoria with enhanced vigor, gregariousness, hyperactivity, restlessness, hypervigilance, interpersonal sensitivity, talkativeness, anxiety, tension, alertness, grandiosity, stereotypical and repetitive behavior, anger, fighting, and impaired judgment (APA, 2000).
2. Physical signs and symptoms that occur with amphetamine intoxication include tachycardia or bradycardia, pupillary dilation, elevated or lowered blood pressure, perspiration or chills, nausea or vomiting, psychomotor retardation or agitation, muscular weakness, respiratory depression, chest pain or cardiac arrhythmias, confusion, seizures, dyskinesias, dystonias, or coma (APA, 2000).

Amphetamine (or Amphetamine-like) Withdrawal

1. Amphetamine withdrawal symptoms occur after cessation of (or reduction in) amphetamine (or a related substance) use that has been heavy and prolonged.
2. Symptoms of amphetamine withdrawal develop within a few hours to several days and include fatigue; vivid, unpleasant dreams; insomnia or hypersomnia; increased appetite; and psychomotor retardation or agitation.

Cannabis Dependence/Abuse/

1. Cannabis preparations are almost always smoked but may also be taken orally.
2. It is commonly regarded incorrectly to be a substance without potential for dependence.
3. Tolerance to the substance may result in increased frequency of its use.
4. Abuse is evidenced by participation in hazardous activities while motor coordination is impaired from cannabis use.

Cannabis Intoxication

1. Cannabis intoxication is characterized by impaired motor coordination, euphoria, anxiety, sensation of slowed time, impaired judgment, and social withdrawal that develop during or shortly after cannabis use (APA, 2000).
2. Physical symptoms of cannabis intoxication include conjunctival injection, increased appetite, dry mouth, and tachycardia.
3. The impairment of motor skills lasts for 8 to 12 hours.

Cocaine Dependence/Abuse

1. Various forms are smoked, inhaled, injected, or taken orally.
2. Chronic daily (or almost daily) use usually results in an increase in dosage over time to produce the desired effect.

3. Episodic use often takes the form of binges, followed by an intense and unpleasant "crash" in which the individual experiences anxiety, irritability, and feelings of fatigue and depression.
4. The drug user often abuses, or is dependent on, a CNS depressant to relieve the residual effects of cocaine.
5. Cocaine abuse and dependence lead to tolerance of the substance and subsequent use of increasing doses.
6. Continued use appears to be related to a "craving" for the substance, rather than to prevention or alleviation of withdrawal symptoms.

Cocaine Intoxication

1. Symptoms of cocaine intoxication develop during, or shortly after, use of cocaine.
2. Symptoms of cocaine intoxication include euphoria or affective blunting, changes in sociability, hypervigilance, interpersonal sensitivity, anxiety, tension, anger, stereotyped behaviors, impaired judgment, and impaired social or occupational functioning.
3. Physical symptoms of cocaine intoxication include tachycardia or bradycardia, pupillary dilation, elevated or lowered blood pressure, perspiration or chills, nausea or vomiting, psychomotor agitation or retardation, muscular weakness, respiratory depression, chest pain, cardiac arrhythmias, confusion, seizures, dyskinesias, dystonias, or coma.

Cocaine Withdrawal

1. Symptoms of withdrawal occur after cessation of, or reduction in, cocaine use that has been heavy and prolonged.
2. Symptoms of cocaine withdrawal include dysphoric mood; fatigue; vivid, unpleasant dreams; insomnia or hypersomnia; increased appetite; psychomotor retardation or agitation.

Hallucinogen Dependence/Abuse

1. Hallucinogenic substances are taken orally.
2. The cognitive and perceptual impairment may last for up to 12 hours, so use is generally episodic, because the individual must organize time during the daily schedule for its use.
3. Frequent use results in tolerance to the effects of the substance.
4. Dependence is rare, and most people are able to resume their previous lifestyle, following a period of hallucinogen use, without much difficulty.
5. Flashbacks may occur following cessation of hallucinogen use. These episodes consist of visual or auditory misperceptions usually lasting only a few seconds but sometimes lasting up to several hours.

6. Hallucinogens are highly unpredictable in the effects they may induce each time they are used.

Hallucinogen Intoxication

1. Symptoms of intoxication develop during or shortly after hallucinogen use.
2. Symptoms include marked anxiety or depression, ideas of reference, fear of losing one's mind, paranoid ideation, and impaired judgment.
3. Other symptoms include subjective intensification of perceptions, depersonalization, derealization, illusions, hallucinations, and synesthesias.
4. Physical symptoms include pupillar dilation, tachycardia, sweating, palpitations, blurring of vision, tremors, and incoordination (APA, 2000).

Inhalant Dependence/Abuse

1. Effects are induced by inhaling the vapors of volatile substances through the nose or mouth.
2. Examples of substances include glue, gasoline, paint, paint thinners, various cleaning chemicals, and typewriter correction fluid.
3. Use of inhalants often begins in childhood, and considerable family dysfunction is characteristic.
4. Use may be daily or episodic, and chronic use may continue into adulthood.
5. Tolerance has been reported among individuals with heavy use, but a withdrawal syndrome from these substances has not been well documented.

Inhalant Intoxication

1. Symptoms of intoxication develop during, or shortly after, use of, or exposure to, volatile inhalants.
2. Symptoms of inhalant intoxication include belligerence, assaultiveness, apathy, impaired judgment, and impaired social or occupational functioning.
3. Physical symptoms of inhalant intoxication include dizziness, nystagmus, incoordination, slurred speech, unsteady gait, lethargy, depressed reflexes, psychomotor retardation, tremor, generalized muscle weakness, blurred vision or diplopia, stupor or coma, and euphoria (APA, 2000).

Nicotine Dependence

1. The effects of nicotine are induced through inhaling the smoke of cigarettes, cigars, or pipe tobacco and orally through the use of snuff or chewing tobacco.
2. Continued use results in a "craving" for the substance.

3. Nicotine is commonly used to relieve or to avoid withdrawal symptoms that occur when the individual has been in a situation where use is restricted.
4. Continued use despite knowledge of medical problems related to smoking is a particularly important health problem.

Nicotine Withdrawal

1. Symptoms of withdrawal develop within 24 hours after abrupt cessation of (or reduction in) prolonged nicotine use.
2. Symptoms of nicotine withdrawal include dysphoric or depressed mood, insomnia, irritability, frustration, anger, anxiety, difficulty concentrating, restlessness, decreased heart rate, and increased appetite.

Opioid Dependence/Abuse

1. Various forms are taken orally, intravenously, by nasal inhalation, and by smoking.
2. Dependence occurs after recreational use of the substance "on the street" or after prescribed use of the substance for relief of pain or cough.
3. Chronic use leads to remarkably high levels of tolerance.
4. Once abuse or dependence is established, substance procurement often comes to dominate the person's life.
5. Cessation or decreased consumption results in a "craving" for the substance and produces a specific syndrome of withdrawal.

Opioid Intoxication

1. Symptoms of intoxication develop during or shortly after opioid use.
2. Symptoms of opioid intoxication include euphoria (initially) followed by apathy, dysphoria, psychomotor agitation or retardation, impaired judgment, and impaired social or occupational functioning.
3. Physical symptoms of opioid intoxication include pupillary constriction, drowsiness or coma, slurred speech, and impairment in attention or memory (APA, 2000).

Opioid Withdrawal

1. Symptoms of opioid withdrawal occur after cessation of (or reduction in) heavy and prolonged opioid use. Symptoms of withdrawal can also occur after administration of an opioid antagonist after a period of opioid use.
2. Symptoms of opioid withdrawal can occur within minutes to several days following use (or antagonist), and include dysphoric mood, nausea or vomiting, muscle aches, lacrimation or rhinorrhea, pupillary dilation, piloerection, sweating, abdominal cramping, diarrhea, yawning, fever, and insomnia.

Phencyclidine Dependence/Abuse

1. Phencyclidine (PCP) is taken orally, intravenously, or by smoking or inhaling.
2. Use can be on a chronic daily basis but more often is taken episodically in binges that can last several days.
3. Physical dependence does not occur with PCP; however, psychological dependence characterized by craving for the drug has been reported in chronic users, as has the development of tolerance.
4. Tolerance apparently develops quickly with frequent use.

Phencyclidine Intoxication

1. Symptoms of intoxication develop during or shortly after PCP use.
2. Symptoms of PCP intoxication include belligerence, assaultiveness, impulsiveness, unpredictability, psychomotor agitation, and impaired judgment.
3. Physical symptoms occur within 1 hour of PCP use and include vertical or horizontal nystagmus, hypertension or tachycardia, numbness or diminished responsiveness to pain, ataxia, dysarthria, muscle rigidity, seizures or coma, and hyperacusis (APA, 2000).

Sedative, Hypnotic, or Anxiolytic Dependence/ Abuse

1. Effects are produced through oral intake of these substances.
2. Dependence can occur following recreational use of the substance "on the street" or after prescribed use of the substance for relief of anxiety or insomnia.
3. Chronic use leads to remarkably high levels of tolerance.
4. Once dependence develops, there is evidence of strong substance-seeking behaviors (obtaining prescriptions from several physicians or resorting to illegal sources to maintain adequate supplies of the substance).
5. Abrupt cessation of these substances can result in life-threatening withdrawal symptoms.

Sedative, Hypnotic, or Anxiolytic Intoxication

1. Symptoms of intoxication develop during or shortly after intake of sedatives, hypnotics, or anxiolytics.
2. Symptoms of intoxication include inappropriate sexual or aggressive behavior, mood lability, impaired judgment, and impaired social or occupational functioning.
3. Physical symptoms of sedative, hypnotic, or anxiolytic intoxication include slurred speech, incoordination, unsteady gait, nystagmus, impairment in attention or memory, stupor, or coma (APA, 2000).

Sedative, Hypnotic, or Anxiolytic Withdrawal

1. Withdrawal symptoms occur after cessation of (or reduction in) heavy and prolonged use of sedatives, hypnotics, or anxiolytics.
2. Symptoms of withdrawal occur within several hours to a few days after abrupt cessation or reduction in use of the drug.
3. Symptoms of withdrawal include autonomic hyperactivity (e.g., sweating or pulse rate greater than 100); increased hand tremor; insomnia; nausea or vomiting; transient visual, tactile, or auditory hallucinations or illusions; psychomotor agitation; anxiety; or grand mal seizures.

   A summary of symptoms associated with the syndromes of intoxication and withdrawal is presented in Table 4–2.

Common Nursing Diagnoses and Interventions for Clients with Substance-Related Disorders

(Interventions are applicable to various health-care settings, such as inpatient and partial hospitalization, community outpatient clinic, home health, and private practice.)

● RISK FOR INJURY

Definition: At risk for injury as a result of [internal or external] environmental conditions interacting with the individual's adaptive and defensive resources.

Related/Risk Factors ("related to")

[Substance intoxication]
[Substance withdrawal]
[Disorientation]
[Seizures]
[Hallucinations]
[Psychomotor agitation]
[Unstable vital signs]
[Delirium]
[Flashbacks]
[Panic level of anxiety]

Goals/Objectives
Short-term Goal
Client's condition will stabilize within 72 hours.
Long-term Goal
Client will not experience physical injury.

TABLE 4–2 Summary of Symptoms Associated with the Syndromes of Intoxication and Withdrawal

Class of Drugs	Intoxication	Withdrawal	Comments
Alcohol	Aggressiveness, impaired judgment, impaired attention, irritability, euphoria, depression, emotional lability, slurred speech, incoordination, unsteady gait, nystagmus, flushed face	Tremors, nausea/vomiting, malaise, weakness, tachycardia, sweating, elevated blood pressure, anxiety, depressed mood, irritability, hallucinations, headache, insomnia, seizures	Alcohol withdrawal begins within 4 to 6 hr after last drink. May progress to delirium tremens on second or third day. Use of Librium or Serax is common for substitution therapy.
Amphetamines and related substances	Fighting, grandiosity, hypervigilance, psychomotor agitation, impaired judgment, tachycardia, pupillary dilation, elevated blood pressure, perspiration or chills, nausea and vomiting	Anxiety, depressed mood, irritability, craving for the substance, fatigue, insomnia or hypersomnia, psychomotor agitation, paranoid and suicidal ideation	Withdrawal symptoms usually peak within 2 to 4 days, although depression and irritability may persist for months. Antidepressants may be used.
Caffeine	Restlessness, nervousness, excitement, insomnia, flushed face, diuresis, gastrointestinal complaints, muscle twitching, rambling flow of thought and speech, cardiac arrhythmia, periods of inexhaustibility, psychomotor agitation	Headache, fatigue, anxiety, irritability, depression, nausea, vomiting, muscle pain and stiffness.	Caffeine is contained in coffee, tea, colas, cocoa, chocolate, some over-the-counter analgesics, "cold" preparations, and stimulants.
Cannabis	Euphoria, anxiety, suspiciousness, sensation of slowed time, impaired judgment, social withdrawal, tachycardia, conjunctival redness, increased appetite, hallucinations	Restlessness, irritability, insomnia, loss of appetite	Intoxication occurs immediately and lasts about 3 hours. Oral ingestion is more slowly absorbed and has longer-lasting effects.

Continued

TABLE 4-2 Summary of Symptoms Associated with the Syndromes of Intoxication and Withdrawal—cont'd

Class of Drugs	Intoxication	Withdrawal	Comments
Cocaine	Euphoria, fighting, grandiosity, hypervigilance, psychomotor agitation, impaired judgment, tachycardia, pupillary dilation, elevated blood pressure, perspiration or chills, nausea/vomiting, hallucinations, delirium	Depression, anxiety, irritability, fatigue, insomnia or hypersomnia, psychomotor agitation, paranoid or suicidal ideation, apathy, social withdrawal	Large doses of the drug can result in convulsions or death from cardiac arrhythmias or respiratory paralysis.
Inhalants	Belligerence, assaultiveness, apathy, impaired judgment, dizziness, nystagmus, slurred speech, unsteady gait, lethargy, depressed reflexes, tremor, blurred vision, stupor or coma, euphoria, irritation around eyes, throat, and nose		Intoxication occurs within 5 min of inhalation. Symptoms last 60 to 90 min. Large doses can result in death from CNS depression or cardiac arrhythmia.
Nicotine		Craving for the drug, irritability, anger, frustration, anxiety, difficulty concentrating, restlessness, decreased heart rate, increased appetite, weight gain, tremor, headaches, insomnia	Symptoms of withdrawal begin within 24 hr of last drug use and decrease in intensity over days, weeks, or sometimes longer.

Opioids	Euphoria, lethargy, somnolence, apathy, dysphoria, impaired judgment, pupillary constriction, drowsiness, slurred speech, constipation, nausea, decreased respiratory rate and blood pressure	Craving for the drug, nausea/vomiting, muscle aches, lacrimation or rhinorrhea, pupillary dilation, piloerection or sweating, diarrhea, yawning, fever, insomnia	Withdrawal symptoms appear within 6 to 8 hr after last dose, reach a peak in the second or third day, and disappear in 7 to 10 days. Times are shorter with meperidine and longer with methadone.
Phencyclidine and related substances	Belligerence, assaultiveness, impulsiveness, psychomotor agitation, impaired judgment, nystagmus, increased heart rate and blood pressure, diminished pain response, ataxia, dysarthria, muscle rigidity, seizures, hyperacusis, delirium		Delirium can occur within 24 hr after use of phencyclidine, or may occur up to 1 week following recovery from an overdose of the drug.
Sedatives, hypnotics, and anxiolytics	Disinhibition of sexual or aggressive impulses, mood lability, impaired judgment, slurred speech, incoordination, unsteady gait, impairment in attention or memory, disorientation, confusion	Nausea/vomiting, malaise, weakness, tachycardia, sweating, anxiety, irritability, orthostatic hypotension, tremor, insomnia, seizures	Withdrawal may progress to delirium, usually within 1 week of last use. Long-acting barbiturates or benzodiazepines may be used in withdrawal substitution therapy.

Interventions with *Selected Rationales*

1. Assess client's level of disorientation to determine specific requirements for safety. *Knowledge of client's level of functioning is necessary to formulate appropriate plan of care.*

2. Obtain a drug history, if possible, to determine the following:
   a. Type of substance(s) used.
   b. Time of last ingestion and amount consumed.
   c. Length and frequency of consumption.
   d. Amount consumed on a daily basis.

3. Obtain urine sample for laboratory analysis of substance content. *Subjective history is often not accurate. Knowledge regarding substance ingestion is important for accurate assessment of client condition.*

4. Place client in quiet, private room. *Excessive stimuli increase client agitation.*

5. Institute necessary safety precautions *(CLIENT safety is a nursing priority.):*
   a. Observe client behaviors frequently; assign staff on one-to-one basis if condition is warranted; accompany and assist client when ambulating; use wheelchair for transporting long distances.
   b. Be sure that side rails are up when client is in bed.
   c. Pad headboard and side rails of bed with thick towels to protect client in case of seizure.
   d. Use mechanical restraints as necessary to protect client if excessive hyperactivity accompanies the disorientation.

6. Ensure that smoking materials and other potentially harmful objects are stored away from client's access. *Client may harm self or others in disoriented, confused state.*

7. Frequently orient client to reality and surroundings. *Disorientation may endanger client safety if he or she unknowingly wanders away from safe environment.*

8. Monitor client's vital signs every 15 minutes initially and less frequently as acute symptoms subside. *Vital signs provide the most reliable information about client condition and need for medication during acute detoxification period.*

9. Follow medication regimen, as ordered by physician. Common medical intervention for detoxification from the following substances includes:
   a. **Alcohol.** Benzodiazepines are the most widely used group of drugs for substitution therapy in alcohol withdrawal. They are administered in decreasing doses until withdrawal is complete. Commonly used agents include chlordiazepoxide (Librium), oxazepam (Serax), diazepam (Valium), and alprazolam (Xanax). In clients with liver disease, accumulation of the longer-acting agents, such as chlordiazepoxide (Librium), may be problematic, and the

use of shorter-acting benzodiazepines, such as oxazepam (Serax), is more appropriate. Some physicians may order anticonvulsant medication to be used prophylactically; however, this is not a universal intervention. Multivitamin therapy, in combination with daily thiamine (either orally or by injection), is common protocol.

b. **Narcotics**. Narcotic antagonists, such as naloxone (Narcan), naltrexone (ReVia), or nalmefene (Revex), are administered intravenously for narcotic overdose. Withdrawal is managed with rest and nutritional therapy. Substitution therapy may be instituted to decrease withdrawal symptoms using propoxyphene (Darvon), methadone (Dolophine), or buprenorphine (Subutex).

c. **Depressants**. Substitution therapy may be instituted to decrease withdrawal symptoms using a long-acting barbiturate, such as phenobarbital (Luminal). The dosage required to suppress withdrawal symptoms is given. When stabilization has been achieved, the dose is gradually decreased by 30 mg/day until withdrawal is complete. Long-acting benzodiazepines are commonly used for substitution therapy when the abused substance is a nonbarbiturate CNS depressant.

d. **Stimulants**. Treatment of stimulant intoxication usually begins with minor tranquilizers such as chlordiazepoxide (Librium) and progresses to major tranquilizers such as haloperidol (Haldol). Antipsychotics should be administered with caution because of their propensity to lower seizure threshold. Repeated seizures are treated with intravenous diazepam. Withdrawal treatment is usually aimed at reducing drug craving and managing severe depression. The client is placed in a quiet atmosphere and allowed to sleep and eat as much as is needed or desired. Suicide precautions may need to be instituted. Antidepressant therapy may be helpful in treating symptoms of depression. Desipramine has been especially successful with symptoms of cocaine withdrawal and abstinence (Mack, Franklin, & Frances, 2003).

e. **Hallucinogens and Cannabinols.** Substitution therapy is not required with these drugs. When adverse reactions, such as anxiety or panic, occur, benzodiazepines (e.g., diazepam or chlordiazepoxide) may be prescribed to prevent harm to the client or others. Psychotic reactions may be treated with antipsychotic medications.

Outcome Criteria

1. Client is no longer exhibiting any signs or symptoms of substance intoxication or withdrawal.

2. Client shows no evidence of physical injury obtained during substance intoxication or withdrawal.

● INEFFECTIVE DENIAL

Definition: Conscious or unconscious attempt to disavow the knowledge or meaning of an event to reduce anxiety/fear, but leading to the detriment of health.

Possible Etiologies ("related to")
[Weak, underdeveloped ego]
[Underlying fears and anxieties]
[Low self-esteem]
[Fixation in early level of development]

Defining Characteristics ("evidenced by")
[Denies substance abuse or dependence]
[Denies that substance use creates problems in his or her life]
[Continues to use substance, knowing it contributes to impairment in functioning or exacerbation of physical symptoms]
[Uses substance(s) in physically hazardous situations]
[Use of rationalization and projection to explain maladaptive behaviors]
Unable to admit impact of disease on life pattern

Goals/Objectives
Short-term Goal
Client will divert attention away from external issues and focus on behavioral outcomes associated with substance use.
Long-term Goal
Client will verbalize acceptance of responsibility for own behavior and acknowledge association between substance use and personal problems.

Interventions with *Selected Rationales*
1. Begin by working to develop a trusting nurse-client relationship. Be honest. Keep all promises. *Trust is the basis of a therapeutic relationship.*
2. Convey an attitude of acceptance to client. Ensure that he or she understands, "It is not *you* but your *behavior* that is unacceptable." *An attitude of acceptance promotes feelings of dignity and self-worth.*
3. Provide information to correct misconceptions about substance abuse. Client may rationalize his or her behavior with

statements such as, "I'm not an alcoholic. I can stop drink-ing any time I want. Besides, I only drink beer." or "I only smoke pot to relax before class. So what? I know lots of people who do. Besides, you can't get hooked on pot." *Many myths abound regarding use of specific substances. Factual information presented in a matter-of-fact, nonjudgmental way explaining what behaviors constitute substance-related disorders may help client focus on his or her own behaviors as an illness that requires help.*

4. Identify recent maladaptive behaviors or situations that have occurred in client's life, and discuss how use of substances may have been a contributing factor. *The first step in decreas-ing use of denial is for client to see the relationship between substance use and personal problems.*

5. Use confrontation with caring. Do not allow client to fanta-size about his or her lifestyle. *Confrontation interferes with client's ability to use denial; a caring attitude preserves self-esteem and avoids putting client on the defensive.*

> **CLINICAL PEARL** It is important to speak objectively and nonjudgmentally to a person in denial. Examples: "It is my understanding that the last time you drank alcohol, you . . ." or "The lab report shows that your blood alcohol level was 250 when you were involved in that automobile accident."

6. Do not accept the use of rationalization or projection as client attempts to make excuses for or blame his or her be-havior on other people or situations. *Rationalization and projection prolong the stage of denial that problems exist in client's life because of substance use.*

7. Encourage participation in group activities. *Peer feedback is often more accepted than feedback from authority figures. Peer pressure can be a strong factor as well as the association with individuals who are experiencing or who have experi-enced similar problems.*

8. Offer immediate positive recognition of client's expres-sions of insight gained regarding illness and acceptance of responsibility for own behavior. *Positive reinforcement en-hances self-esteem and encourages repetition of desirable behaviors.*

Outcome Criteria

1. Client verbalizes understanding of the relationship between personal problems and the use of substances.
2. Client verbalizes acceptance of responsibility for own behavior.
3. Client verbalizes understanding of substance dependence and abuse as an illness requiring ongoing support and treatment.

● INEFFECTIVE COPING

Definition: Inability to form a valid appraisal of the stressors, inadequate choices of practiced responses, and/or inability to use available resources.

Possible Etiologies ("related to")

[Inadequate support systems]
[Inadequate coping skills]
[Underdeveloped ego]
[Possible hereditary factor]
[Dysfunctional family system]
[Negative role modeling]
[Personal vulnerability]

Defining Characteristics ("evidenced by")

[Low self-esteem]
[Chronic anxiety]
[Chronic depression]
Inability to meet role expectations
[Alteration in societal participation]
Inability to meet basic needs
[Inappropriate use of defense mechanisms]
Abuse of chemical agents
[Low frustration tolerance]
[Need for immediate gratification]
[Manipulative behavior]

Goals/Objectives

Short-term Goal

Client will express true feelings associated with use of substances as a method of coping with stress.

Long-term Goal

Client will be able to verbalize adaptive coping mechanisms to use, instead of substance abuse, in response to stress.

Interventions with *Selected Rationales*

1. Establish trusting relationship with client (be honest; keep appointments; be available to spend time). *The therapeutic nurse-client relationship is built on trust.*
2. Set limits on manipulative behavior. Be sure that client knows what is acceptable, what is not, and the consequences for violating the limits set. Ensure that all staff maintain consistency with this intervention. *Client is unable to*

establish own limits, so limits must be set for him or her. Unless administration of consequences for violation of limits is consistent, manipulative behavior will not be eliminated.

3. Encourage client to verbalize feelings, fears, and anxieties. Answer any questions he or she may have regarding the disorder. *Verbalization of feelings in a nonthreatening environment may help client come to terms with long-unresolved issues.*

4. Explain the effects of substance abuse on the body. Emphasize that prognosis is closely related to abstinence. *Many clients lack knowledge regarding the deleterious effects of substance abuse on the body.*

5. Explore with client the options available to assist with stressful situations rather than resorting to substance abuse (e.g., contacting various members of Alcoholics Anonymous or Narcotics Anonymous; physical exercise; relaxation techniques; meditation). *Client may have persistently resorted to chemical abuse and thus may possess little or no knowledge of adaptive responses to stress.*

6. Provide positive reinforcement for evidence of gratification delayed appropriately. *Positive reinforcement enhances self-esteem and encourages client to repeat acceptable behaviors.*

7. Encourage client to be as independent as possible in own self-care. Provide positive feedback for independent decision-making and effective use of problem-solving skills.

Outcome Criteria

1. Client is able to verbalize adaptive coping strategies as alternatives to substance use in response to stress.

2. Client is able to verbalize the names of support people from whom he or she may seek help when the desire for substance use is intense.

● IMBALANCED NUTRITION: LESS THAN BODY REQUIREMENTS

Definition: Intake of nutrients insufficient to meet metabolic needs.

Possible Etiologies ("related to")

[Drinking alcohol instead of eating nourishing food]
[Eating only "junk food"]
[Eating nothing (or very little) while on a "binge"]

[No money for food (having spent what is available on substances)]
[Problems with malabsorption caused by chronic alcohol abuse]

Defining Characteristics ("evidenced by")

Loss of weight
Pale conjunctiva and mucous membranes
Poor muscle tone
[Poor skin turgor]
[Edema of extremities]
[Electrolyte imbalances]
[Cheilosis (cracks at corners of mouth)]
[Scaly dermatitis]
[Weakness]
[Neuropathies]
[Anemias]
[Ascites]

Goals/Objectives

Short-term Goals

1. Client will gain 2 lb during next 7 days.
2. Client's electrolytes will be restored to normal within 1 week.

Long-term Goal

Client will exhibit no signs or symptoms of malnutrition by discharge. (This is not a realistic goal for a chronic alcoholic in the end stages of the disease. For such a client, it is more appropriate to establish short-term goals, as realistic step objectives, to use in the evaluation of care given.)

Interventions with *Selected Rationales*

1. In collaboration with dietitian, determine number of calories required to provide adequate nutrition and realistic (according to body structure and height) weight gain.
2. Strict documentation of intake, output, and calorie count. *This information is necessary to make an accurate nutritional assessment and maintain client safety.*
3. Weigh daily. *Weight loss or gain is important assessment information.*
4. Determine client's likes and dislikes and collaborate with dietitian to provide favorite foods. *Client is more likely to eat foods that he or she particularly enjoys.*
5. Ensure that client receives small, frequent feedings, including a bedtime snack, rather than three larger meals. *Large amounts of food may be objectionable, or even intolerable, to client.*
6. Administer vitamin and mineral supplements, as ordered by physician, *to improve nutritional state.*

7. If appropriate, ask family members or significant others to bring in special foods that client particularly enjoys.
8. Monitor laboratory work, and report significant changes to physician.
9. Explain the importance of adequate nutrition. *Client may have inadequate or inaccurate knowledge regarding the contribution of good nutrition to overall wellness.*

Outcome Criteria
1. Client has achieved and maintained at least 90% of normal body weight.
2. Client's vital signs, blood pressure, and laboratory serum studies are within normal limits.
3. Client is able to verbalize importance of adequate nutrition.

● CHRONIC LOW SELF-ESTEEM

Definition: Long-standing negative self-evaluating/feelings about self or self-capabilities.

Possible Etiologies ("related to")
[Retarded ego development]
[Dysfunctional family system]
[Lack of positive feedback]
[Perceived failures]

Defining Characteristics ("evidenced by")
[Difficulty accepting positive reinforcement]
[Failure to take responsibility for self-care]
[Self-destructive behavior (substance abuse)]
Lack of eye contact
[Withdraws into social isolation]
[Highly critical and judgmental of self and others]
[Sense of worthlessness]
[Fear of failure]
[Unable to recognize own accomplishments]
[Setting self up for failure by establishing unrealistic goals]
[Unsatisfactory interpersonal relationships]
[Negative or pessimistic outlook]
[Denial of problems obvious to others]
[Projection of blame or responsibility for problems]
[Rationalizing personal failures]
[Hypersensitivity to slight criticism]
[Grandiosity]

Goals/Objectives

Short-term Goal

Client will accept responsibility for personal failures and verbalize the role substances played in those failures.

Long-term Goal

By time of discharge, client will exhibit increased feelings of self-worth as evidenced by verbal expression of positive aspects about self, past accomplishments, and future prospects.

Interventions with Selected Rationales

1. Be accepting of client and his or her negativism. *An attitude of acceptance enhances feelings of self-worth.*
2. Spend time with client *to convey acceptance and contribute toward feelings of self-worth.*
3. Help client to recognize and focus on strengths and accomplishments. Discuss past (real or perceived) failures, but minimize amount of attention devoted to them beyond client's need to accept responsibility for them. *Client must accept responsibility for own behavior before change in behavior can occur. Minimizing attention to past failures may help to eliminate negative ruminations and increase client's sense of self-worth.*
4. Encourage participation in group activities *from which client may receive positive feedback and support from peers.*
5. Help client identify areas he or she would like to change about self and assist with problem solving toward this effort. *Low self-worth may interfere with client's perception of own problem-solving ability. Assistance may be required.*
6. Ensure that client is not becoming increasingly dependent and that he or she is accepting responsibility for own behaviors. *Client must be able to function independently if he or she is to be successful within the less-structured community environment.*
7. Ensure that therapy groups offer client simple methods of achievement. Offer recognition and positive feedback for actual accomplishments. *Successes and recognition increase self-esteem.*
8. Provide instruction in assertiveness techniques: the ability to recognize the difference among passive, assertive, and aggressive behaviors and the importance of respecting the human rights of others while protecting one's own basic human rights. *Self-esteem is enhanced by the ability to interact with others in an assertive manner.*
9. Teach effective communication techniques, such as the use of "I" messages and placing emphasis on ways to avoid making judgmental statements.

Outcome Criteria
1. Client is able to verbalize positive aspects about self.
2. Client is able to communicate assertively with others.
3. Client expresses an optimistic outlook for the future.

● DEFICIENT KNOWLEDGE (Effects of Substance Abuse on the Body)

Definition: Absence or deficiency of cognitive information related to [the effects of substance abuse on the body and its interference with achievement and maintenance of optimal wellness].

Possible Etiologies ("related to")
Lack of interest in learning
[Low self-esteem]
[Denial of need for information]
[Denial of risks involved with substance abuse]
Unfamiliarity with information resources

Defining Characteristics ("evidenced by")
[Abuse of substances]
[Statement of lack of knowledge]
[Statement of misconception]
[Request for information]
Verbalization of the problem

Goals/Objectives
Short-term Goal
Client will be able to verbalize effects of [substance used] on the body following implementation of teaching plan.

Long-term Goal
Client will verbalize the importance of abstaining from use of [substance] to maintain optimal wellness.

Interventions with *Selected Rationales*
1. Assess client's level of knowledge regarding effects of [substance] on body. *Baseline assessment of knowledge is required to develop appropriate teaching plan for client.*
2. Assess client's level of anxiety and readiness to learn. *Learning does not take place beyond moderate level of anxiety.*
3. Determine method of learning most appropriate for client (e.g., discussion, question and answer, use of audio or visual

aids, oral or written method). *Level of education and development are important considerations as to methodology selected.*

4. Develop teaching plan, including measurable objectives for the learner. *Measurable objectives provide criteria on which to base evaluation of the teaching experience.*

5. Include significant others, if possible. *Lifestyle changes often affect all family members.*

6. Implement teaching plan at a time that facilitates and in a place that is conducive to optimal learning (e.g., in the evening when family members visit, in an empty, quiet classroom or group therapy room). *Learning is enhanced by an environment with few distractions.*

7. Begin with simple concepts and progress to the more complex. *Retention is increased if introductory material presented is easy to understand.*

8. Include information on physical effects of [substance]: substance's capacity for physiological and psychological dependence, its effects on family functioning, its effects on a fetus (and the importance of contraceptive use until abstinence has been achieved), and the importance of regular participation in an appropriate treatment program.

9. Provide activities for client and significant others in which to participate actively during the learning exercise. *Active participation increases retention.*

10. Ask client and significant others to demonstrate knowledge gained by verbalizing information presented. *Verbalization of knowledge gained is a measurable method of evaluating the teaching experience.*

11. Provide positive feedback for participation as well as for accurate demonstration of knowledge gained. *Positive feedback enhances self-esteem and encourages repetition of acceptable behaviors.*

12. Evaluate teaching plan. Identify strengths and weaknesses, as well as any changes that may enhance the effectiveness of the plan.

Outcome Criteria

1. Client is able to verbalize effects of [substance] on the body.

2. Client verbalizes understanding of risks involved in use of [substance].

3. Client is able to verbalize community resources for obtaining knowledge and support with substance-related problems.

● DYSFUNCTIONAL FAMILY PROCESSES

Definition: Psychosocial, spiritual, and physiological functions of the family unit are chronically disorganized, which leads to conflict, denial of problems, resistance to change, ineffective problem solving, and a series of self-perpetuating crises.

Possible Etiologies ("related to")

Abuse of alcohol
Genetic predisposition
Lack of problem-solving skills
Inadequate coping skills
Family history of alcoholism, resistance to treatment
Biochemical influences
Addictive personality

Defining Characteristics ("evidenced by")

Anxiety, anger/suppressed rage; shame and embarrassment
Emotional isolation/loneliness; vulnerability; repressed emotions
Disturbed family dynamics; closed communication systems, ineffective spousal communication, and marital problems
Altered role function/disruption of family roles
Manipulation; dependency; blaming/criticizing; rationalization/denial of problems
Enabling to maintain drinking; refusal to get help/inability to accept and receive help appropriately

Goals/Objectives

Short-term Goals

1. Family members will participate in individual family programs and support groups.
2. Family members will identify ineffective coping behaviors and consequences.
3. Family members will initiate and plan for necessary lifestyle changes.

Long-term Goal

Family members will take action to change self-destructive behaviors and alter behaviors that contribute to client's addiction.

Interventions with *Selected Rationales*

1. Review family history; explore roles of family members, circumstances involving alcohol use, strengths, areas of growth. *This information determines areas for focus and potential for change.*

2. Explore how family members have coped with the client's addiction (e.g., denial, repression, rationalization, hurt, loneliness, projection). *Persons who enable also suffer from the same feelings as the client and use ineffective methods for dealing with the situation, necessitating help in learning new and effective coping skills.*

3. Determine understanding of current situation and previous methods of coping with life's problems. *Provides information on which to base present plan of care.*

4. Assess current level of functioning of family members. *Affects individual's ability to cope with the situation.*

5. Determine extent of enabling behaviors being evidenced by family members; explore with each individual and client. *Enabling is doing for the client what he or she needs to do for self (rescuing). People want to be helpful and do not want to feel powerless to help their loved one to stop substance use and change the behavior that is so destructive. However, the substance abuser often relies on others to cover up own inability to cope with daily responsibilities.*

6. Provide information about enabling behavior and addictive disease characteristics for both the user and nonuser. *Awareness and knowledge of behaviors (e.g., avoiding and shielding, taking over responsibilities, rationalizing, and subserving) provide opportunity for individuals to begin the process of change.*

7. Identify and discuss sabotage behaviors of family members. *Even though family member(s) may verbalize a desire for the individual to become substance-free, the reality of interactive dynamics is that they may unconsciously not want the individual to recover, as this would affect the family members' own role in the relationship. Additionally, they may receive sympathy or attention from others (secondary gain).*

8. Encourage participation in therapeutic writing, e.g., journaling (narrative), guided or focused. *Serves as a release for feelings (e.g., anger, grief, stress); helps move individual(s) forward in treatment process.*

9. Provide factual information to client and family about the effects of addictive behaviors on the family and what to expect after discharge. *Many people are unaware of the nature of addiction. If client is using legally obtained drugs, he or she may believe this does not constitute abuse.*

10. Encourage family members to be aware of their own feelings, to look at the situation with perspective and objectivity. They can ask themselves: "Am I being conned? Am I acting out of fear, shame, guilt, or anger? Do I have a need to control?" *When the enabling family members become*

aware of their own actions that perpetuate the client's problems, they need to decide to change themselves. If they change, the client can then face the consequences of own actions and may choose to get well.

11. Provide support for enabling family members. *For change to occur, families need support as much as the person who has the problem with alcohol.*

12. Assist the client's partner to become aware that client's abstinence and drug use are not the partner's responsibility. *Partners need to learn that the client's use of substances may or may not change despite partner's involvement in treatment.*

13. Help a recovering (former user) partner who is enabling to distinguish between destructive aspects of own behavior and genuine motivation to aid the client. *Enabling behavior can be a recovering individual's attempts at personal survival.*

14. Note how the partner relates to the treatment team and staff. *Determines enabling style. A parallel exists between how partner relates to client and to staff, based on the partner's feelings about self and situation.*

15. Explore conflicting feelings the enabling partner may have about treatment (e.g., feelings similar to those of the substance abuser [blend of anger, guilt, fear, exhaustion, embarrassment, loneliness, distrust, grief, and possibly relief]). *This is useful in establishing the need for therapy for the partner. This individual's own identity may have been lost—he or she may fear self-disclosure to staff and may have difficulty giving up the dependent relationship.*

16. Involve family members in discharge referral plans. *Alcohol abuse is a family illness. Because the family has been so involved in dealing with the substance abuse behavior, family members need help adjusting to the new behavior of sobriety/abstinence. Incidence of recovery is almost doubled when the family is treated along with the client.*

17. Encourage involvement with self-help associations, such as Alcoholics Anonymous, Al-Anon, Alateen, and professional family therapy. *Puts client and family in direct contact with support systems necessary for continued sobriety and assists with problem resolution.*

Outcome Criteria

1. Family members verbalize understanding of dynamics of enabling behaviors.
2. Family members demonstrate patterns of effective communication.
3. Family members regularly participate in self-help support programs.

4. Family members demonstrate behaviors required to change destructive patterns of behavior that contribute to and enable dysfunctional family process.

@ INTERNET REFERENCES

- Additional information on addictions may be located at the following websites:
  a. http://www.samhsa.gov/index.aspx
  b. http://www.ccsa.ca/Pages/Splash.htm
  c. http://www.well.com/user/woa
  d. http://www.apa.org/about/division/div50.html
- Additional information on self-help organizations may be located at the following websites:
  a. http://www.ca.org (Cocaine Anonymous)
  b. http://www.aa.org (Alcoholics Anonymous)
  c. http://www.na.org (Narcotics Anonymous)
  d. http://www.al-anon.org
- Additional information about medications for treatment of alcohol and drug dependence may be located at the following websites:
  a. http://www.fadavis.com/townsend
  b. http://www.nlm.nih.gov/medlineplus/
  c. http://www.nimh.nih.gov/publicat/medicate.cfm

Movie Connections

Affliction (alcoholism) ● *Days of Wine and Roses (alcoholism)*
● *I'll Cry Tomorrow (alcoholism)* ● *When a Man Loves a Woman (alcoholism)* ● *Clean and Sober (addiction—cocaine)* ● *28 Days (alcoholism)* ● *Lady Sings the Blues (addiction—heroin)* ● *I'm Dancing as Fast as I Can (addiction—sedatives)* ● *The Rose (polysubstance addiction)*

Schizophrenia and Other Psychotic Disorders

● BACKGROUND ASSESSMENT DATA

The syndrome of symptoms associated with schizophrenia and other psychotic disorders reveals alterations in content and organization of thoughts, perception of sensory input, affect or emotional tone, sense of identity, volition, psychomotor behavior, and ability to establish satisfactory interpersonal relationships.

Categories

Paranoid Schizophrenia

Paranoid schizophrenia is characterized by extreme suspiciousness of others and by delusions and hallucinations of a persecutory or grandiose nature. The individual is often tense and guarded and may be argumentative, hostile, and aggressive.

Disorganized Schizophrenia

In disorganized schizophrenia, behavior is typically regressive and primitive. Affect is inappropriate, with common characteristics being silliness, incongruous giggling, facial grimaces, and extreme social withdrawal. Communication is consistently incoherent.

Catatonic Schizophrenia

Catatonic schizophrenia manifests itself in the form of *stupor* (marked psychomotor retardation, mutism, waxy flexibility [posturing], negativism, and rigidity) or *excitement* (extreme psychomotor agitation, leading to exhaustion or the possibility of hurting self or others if not curtailed).

Undifferentiated Schizophrenia

Undifferentiated schizophrenia is characterized by disorganiz behaviors and psychotic symptoms (e.g., delusions, halluc' tions, incoherence, and grossly disorganized behavior) tha' appear in more than one category.

Residual Schizophrenia

Behavior in residual schizophrenia is eccentric, but psychotic symptoms, if present at all, are not prominent. Social withdrawal and inappropriate affect are characteristic. The patient has a history of at least one episode of schizophrenia in which psychotic symptoms were prominent.

Schizoaffective Disorder

Schizoaffective disorder refers to behaviors characteristic of schizophrenia, in addition to those indicative of disorders of mood, such as depression or mania.

Brief Psychotic Disorder

The essential features of brief psychotic disorder include a sudden onset of psychotic symptoms that last at least 1 day but less than 1 month and in which there is a virtual return to the premorbid level of functioning. The diagnosis is further specified by whether it follows a severe identifiable stressor or whether the onset occurs within 4 weeks postpartum.

Schizophreniform Disorder

The essential features of schizophreniform disorder are identical to those of schizophrenia, with the exception that the duration is at least 1 month but less than 6 months. The diagnosis is termed "provisional" if a diagnosis must be made prior to recovery.

Delusional Disorder

Delusional disorder is characterized by the presence of one or more nonbizarre delusions that last for at least 1 month. Hallucinatory activity is not prominent. Apart from the delusions, behavior and functioning are not impaired. The following types are based on the predominant delusional theme (American Medical Association [AMA], 2000):

1. **Persecutory Type**. Delusions that one is being malevolently treated in some way.
2. **Jealous Type**. Delusions that one's sexual partner is unfaithful.
3. **Erotomanic Type**. Delusions that another person of higher status is in love with him or her.
4. **Somatic Type**. Delusions that the person has some physical defect, disorder, or disease.
5. **Grandiose Type**. Delusions of inflated worth, power, knowledge, special identity, or special relationship to a deity or famous person.

Shared Psychotic Disorder (Folie à Deux)

In shared psychotic disorder, a delusional system develops in the context of a close relationship with another person who already has a psychotic disorder with prominent delusions.

Psychotic Disorder Due to a General Medical Condition

The American Psychiatric Association (APA, 2000) *Diagnostic and Statistical Manual of Mental Disorders, Fourth Edition, Text Revision (DSM-IV-TR)* identifies the essential features of this disorder as prominent hallucinations and delusions that can be directly attributed to a general medical condition. Examples of general medical conditions that may cause psychotic symptoms include neurologic conditions (e.g., neoplasms, Huntington's disease, central nervous system [CNS] infections); endocrine conditions (e.g., hyperthyroidism, hypothyroidism, hypoadrenocorticism); metabolic conditions (e.g., hypoxia, hypercarbia, hypoglycemia); autoimmune disorders (e.g., systemic lupus erythematosus); and others (e.g., fluid or electrolyte imbalances, hepatic or renal diseases) (APA, 2000).

Substance-Induced Psychotic Disorder

The essential features of this disorder are the presence of prominent hallucinations and delusions that are judged to be directly attributable to the physiological effects of a substance (i.e., a drug of abuse, a medication, or toxin exposure) (APA, 2000).

Predisposing Factors

1. **Physiological**
   a. *Genetics.* Studies show that relatives of individuals with schizophrenia have a much higher probability of developing the disease than does the general population. Whereas the lifetime risk for developing schizophrenia is about 1% in most population studies, the siblings or offspring of an identified client have a 5% to 10% risk of developing schizophrenia (Andreasen & Black, 2006). Twin and adoption studies add additional evidence for the genetic basis of schizophrenia.
   b. *Histological Changes.* Jonsson and associates (1997) have suggested that schizophrenic disorders may in fact be a birth defect, occurring in the hippocampus region of the brain, and related to an influenza virus encountered by the mother during the second trimester of pregnancy. The studies have shown a "disordering" of the pyramidal cells in the brains of individuals with schizophrenia, but the cells in the brains of individuals without the disorder appeared to be arranged in an orderly fashion. Further research is required to determine the possible link between this birth defect and the development of schizophrenia.
   c. *The Dopamine Hypothesis.* This theory suggests that schizophrenia (or schizophrenia-like symptoms) may be caused by an excess of dopamine-dependent neuronal activity in the brain. This excess activity may be related to

increased production or release of the substance at nerve terminals, increased receptor sensitivity, too many dopamine receptors, or a combination of these mechanisms (Sadock & Sadock, 2007).

d. *Anatomical Abnormalities.* With the use of neuroimaging technologies, structural brain abnormalities have been observed in individuals with schizophrenia. Ventricular enlargement is the most consistent finding; however, sulci enlargement and cerebellar atrophy are also reported.

2. **Environmental**

a. *Sociocultural Factors.* Many studies have been conducted that have attempted to link schizophrenia to social class. Indeed, epidemiological statistics have shown that greater numbers of individuals from the lower socioeconomic classes experience symptoms associated with schizophrenia than do those from the higher socioeconomic groups (Ho, Black, & Andreasen, 2003). This may occur as a result of the conditions associated with living in poverty, such as congested housing accommodations, inadequate nutrition, absence of prenatal care, few resources for dealing with stressful situations, and feelings of hopelessness for changing one's lifestyle of poverty.

An alternative view is that of the *downward drift hypothesis.* This hypothesis suggests that, because of the characteristic symptoms of the disorder, individuals with schizophrenia have difficulty maintaining gainful employment and "drift down" to a lower socioeconomic level (or fail to rise out of a lower socioeconomic group). Proponents of this notion view poor social conditions as a consequence rather than a cause of schizophrenia.

b. *Stressful Life Events.* Studies have been conducted in an effort to determine whether psychotic episodes may be precipitated by stressful life events. There is no scientific evidence to indicate that stress causes schizophrenia. It is very probable, however, that stress contributes to the severity and course of the illness. It is known that extreme stress can precipitate psychotic episodes. Stress may indeed precipitate symptoms in an individual who possesses a genetic vulnerability to schizophrenia. Stressful life events may be associated with exacerbation of schizophrenic symptoms and increased rates of relapse.

Symptomatology (Subjective/Objective Data)

1. **Autism.** There is a focus inward. The individual with psychosis may create his or her own world. Words and events may take on special meaning of a highly symbolic nature that only the individual can understand.

2. **Emotional Ambivalence.** Powerful emotions of love, hate, and fear produce much conflict within the individual. Each emotion tends to balance the other until an emotional neutralization occurs, and the individual experiences apathy or indifference.

3. **Inappropriate Affect.** The affect is blunted or flat, and often inappropriate (e.g., person who laughs when told of the death of a parent).

4. **Associative Looseness.** This term describes the very disorganized thoughts and verbalizations of the psychotic person. Ideas shift from one unrelated subject to another. When the condition is severe, speech may be incoherent.

5. **Echolalia.** The psychotic person often repeats words he or she hears.

6. **Echopraxia.** The psychotic person often repeats movements he or she sees in others. (Echolalia and echopraxia are products of the person's very weak ego boundaries.)

7. **Neologisms.** Words that are invented by the psychotic person that are meaningless to others but have symbolic meaning to the individual.

8. **Concrete Thinking.** The psychotic person has difficulty thinking on the abstract level and may use literal translations concerning aspects of the environment.

9. **Clang Associations.** The individual uses rhyming words in a nonsensical pattern.

10. **Word Salad.** The psychotic person may put together a random jumble of words.

11. **Mutism.** Psychotic individuals may refuse or be unable to speak.

12. **Circumstantiality.** Circumstantiality refers to a psychotic person's delay in reaching the point of a communication because of unnecessary and tedious details.

13. **Tangentiality.** Tangentiality differs from circumstantiality in that the psychotic person never really gets to the point of the communication. Unrelated topics are introduced, and the original discussion is lost.

14. **Perseveration.** The individual with psychosis may persistently repeat the same word or idea in response to different questions.

15. **Delusions.** These are false ideas or beliefs. Types of delusions include the following:

    a. *Grandeur.* The psychotic person has an exaggerated feeling of importance or power.

    b. *Persecution.* The psychotic person feels threatened and believes others intend harm or persecution toward him or her in some way.

    c. **Reference.** All events within the environment are referred by the psychotic person to himself or herself.

    d. **Control or Influence.** The psychotic individual believes certain objects or people have control over his or her behavior.

16. **Hallucinations.** Hallucinations are false sensory perceptions that may involve any of the five senses. Auditory and visual hallucinations are most common, although olfactory, tactile, and gustatory hallucinations can occur.

17. **Regression.** This is a primary ego defense mechanism used in psychoses. Childlike mannerisms and comfort techniques are employed. Socially inappropriate behavior may be evident.

18. **Religiosity.** The psychotic person becomes preoccupied with religious ideas, a defense mechanism thought to be used in an attempt to provide stability and structure to disorganized thoughts and behaviors.

Common Nursing Diagnoses and Interventions for Individuals with Schizophrenia and Other Psychotic Disorders

(Interventions are applicable to various health-care settings, such as inpatient and partial hospitalization, community outpatient clinic, home health, and private practice.)

● RISK FOR SELF-DIRECTED OR OTHER-DIRECTED VIOLENCE

Definition: At risk for behaviors in which an individual demonstrates that he or she can be physically, emotionally, and/or sexually harmful [either to self or to others.]

Related/Risk Factors ("related to")

[Lack of trust (suspiciousness of others)]
[Panic level of anxiety]
[Catatonic excitement]
[Negative role modeling]
[Rage reactions]
[Command hallucinations]
[Delusional thinking]
Body language—rigid posture, clenching of fists and jaw, hyperactivity, pacing, breathlessness, and threatening stances.
[History or threats of violence toward self or others or of destruction to the property of others]
Impulsivity

Suicidal ideation, plan, available means

[Perception of the environment as threatening]

[Receiving auditory or visual commands of a threatening nature]

Goals/Objectives

Short-term Goals

1. Within [a specified time], client will recognize signs of increasing anxiety and agitation and report to staff for assistance with intervention.
2. Client will not harm self or others

Long-term Goal

Client will not harm self or others.

Interventions with *Selected Rationales*

1. Maintain low level of stimuli in client's environment (low lighting, few people, simple decor, low noise level). *Anxiety level rises in a stimulating environment. A suspicious, agitated client may perceive individuals as threatening.*
2. Observe client's behavior frequently (every 15 minutes). Do this while carrying out routine activities *so as to avoid creating suspiciousness in the individual. Close observation is necessary so that intervention can occur if required to ensure client's (and others') safety.*
3. Remove all dangerous objects from client's environment *so that in his or her agitated, confused state client may not use them to harm self or others.*
4. Try to redirect the violent behavior with physical outlets for the client's anxiety (e.g., punching bag). *Physical exercise is a safe and effective way of relieving pent-up tension.*
5. Staff should maintain and convey a calm attitude toward client. *Anxiety is contagious and can be transmitted from staff to client.*
6. Have sufficient staff available to indicate a show of strength to client if it becomes necessary. *This shows the client evidence of control over the situation and provides some physical security for staff.*
7. Administer tranquilizing medications as ordered by physician. Monitor medication for its effectiveness and for any adverse side effects. *The avenue of the "least restrictive alternative" must be selected when planning interventions for a psychiatric client.*
8. If client is not calmed by "talking down" or by medication, use of mechanical restraints may be necessary. Restraints should be used only as a last resort, after all other interventions have been unsuccessful, and the client is clearly at risk of harm

to self or others. Be sure to have sufficient staff available to assist.

Follow protocol established by the institution. The Joint Commission formerly the Joint Commission on Acreditation of Healthcare Organizations [JCAHO]) requires that an in-person evaluation (by a physician, clinical psychologist, or other licensed independent practitioner responsible for the care of the patient) be conducted within 1 hour of initiating restraint or seclusion (The Joint Commission, 2010). The physician must physician reissue a new order for restraints every 4 hours for adults and every 1 to 2 hours for children and adolescents.

9. Observe the client in restraints every 15 minutes (or according to institutional policy). Ensure that circulation to extremities is not compromised (check temperature, color, pulses). Assist client with needs related to nutrition, hydration, and elimination. Position client so that comfort is facilitated and aspiration can be prevented. Continuous one-to-one monitoring may be necessary for the client who is highly agitated or for whom there is a high risk of self- or accidental injury. *Client safety is a nursing priority.*

10. As agitation decreases, assess client's readiness for restraint removal or reduction. Remove one restraint at a time while assessing client's response. *This minimizes risk of injury to client and staff.*

Outcome Criteria

1. Anxiety is maintained at a level at which client feels no need for aggression.
2. Client demonstrates trust of others in his or her environment.
3. Client maintains reality orientation.
4. Client causes no harm to self or others.

● SOCIAL ISOLATION

Definition: Aloneness experienced by the individual and perceived as imposed by others and as a negative or threatening state.

Possible Etiologies ("related to")

[Lack of trust]
[Panic level of anxiety]
[Regression to earlier level of development]
[Delusional thinking]
[Past experiences of difficulty in interactions with others]
[Repressed fears]
Unaccepted social behavior

Defining Characteristics ("evidenced by")

[Staying alone in room]
Uncommunicative, withdrawn, no eye contact [mutism, autism]
Sad, dull affect
[Lying on bed in fetal position with back to door]
[Inappropriate or immature interests and activities for developmental age or stage]
Preoccupation with own thoughts; repetitive, meaningless actions
[Approaching staff for interaction, then refusing to respond to staff's acknowledgment]
Expression of feelings of rejection or of aloneness imposed by others

Goals/Objectives

Short-term Goal

Client will willingly attend therapy activities accompanied by trusted staff member within 1 week.

Long-term Goal

Client will voluntarily spend time with other clients and staff members in group activities.

Interventions with *Selected Rationales*

1. Convey an accepting attitude by making brief, frequent contacts. *An accepting attitude increases feelings of self-worth and facilitates trust.*
2. Show unconditional positive regard. *This conveys your belief in the client as a worthwhile human being.*
3. Be with the client to offer support during group activities that may be frightening or difficult for him or her. *The presence of a trusted individual provides emotional security for the client.*
4. Be honest and keep all promises. *Honesty and dependability promote a trusting relationship.*
5. Orient client to time, person, and place, as necessary.
6. Be cautious with touch. Allow client extra space and an avenue for exit if he or she becomes too anxious. *A suspicious client may perceive touch as a threatening gesture.*
7. Administer tranquilizing medications as ordered by physician. Monitor for effectiveness and for adverse side effects. *Antipsychotic medications help to reduce psychotic symptoms in some individuals, thereby facilitating interactions with others.*
8. Discuss with client the signs of increasing anxiety and techniques to interrupt the response (e.g., relaxation exercises, thought stopping). *Maladaptive behaviors such as withdrawal and suspiciousness are manifested during times of increased anxiety.*

9. Give recognition and positive reinforcement for client's voluntary interactions with others. *Positive reinforcement enhances self-esteem and encourages repetition of acceptable behaviors.*

Outcome Criteria
1. Client demonstrates willingness and desire to socialize with others.
2. Client voluntarily attends group activities.
3. Client approaches others in appropriate manner for one-to-one interaction.

● INEFFECTIVE COPING

Definition: Inability to form a valid appraisal of the stressors, inadequate choices of practiced responses, and/or inability to use available resources.

Possible Etiologies ("related to")
[Inability to trust]
[Panic level of anxiety]
[Personal vulnerability]
[Low self-esteem]
[Inadequate support systems]
[Negative role model]
[Repressed fears]
[Possible hereditary factor]
[Dysfunctional family system]

Defining Characteristics ("evidenced by")
[Suspiciousness of others, resulting in:
• Alteration in societal participation
• Inability to meet basic needs
• Inappropriate use of defense mechanisms]

Goals/Objectives
Short-term Goal
Client will develop trust in at least one staff member within 1 week.

Long-term Goal
Client will demonstrate use of more adaptive coping skills as evidenced by appropriateness of interactions and willingness to participate in the therapeutic community.

Interventions with *Selected Rationales*

1. Encourage same staff to work with client as much as possible *in order to promote development of trusting relationship.*
2. Avoid physical contact. *Suspicious clients may perceive touch as a threatening gesture.*
3. Avoid laughing, whispering, or talking quietly where client can see but not hear what is being said. *Suspicious clients often believe others are discussing them, and secretive behaviors reinforce the paranoid feelings.*
4. Be honest and keep all promises. *Honesty and dependability promote a trusting relationship.*
5. A creative approach may have to be used to encourage food intake (e.g., canned food and own can opener or family-style meals). *Suspicious clients may believe they are being poisoned and refuse to eat food from the individually prepared tray.*
6. Mouth checks may be necessary following medication administration *to verify whether client is swallowing the tablets or capsules. Suspicious clients may believe they are being poisoned with their medication and attempt to discard the pills.*
7. Activities should never include anything competitive. Activities that encourage a one-to-one relationship with the nurse or therapist are best. *Competitive activities are very threatening to suspicious clients.*
8. Encourage client to verbalize true feelings. The nurse should avoid becoming defensive when angry feelings are directed at him or her. *Verbalization of feelings in a nonthreatening environment may help client come to terms with long-unresolved issues.*
9. An assertive, matter-of-fact, yet genuine approach is least threatening and most therapeutic. *A suspicious person does not have the capacity to relate to an overly friendly, overly cheerful attitude.*

Outcome Criteria

1. Client is able to appraise situations realistically and refrain from projecting own feelings onto the environment.
2. Client is able to recognize and clarify possible misinterpretations of the behaviors and verbalizations of others.
3. Client eats food from tray and takes medications without evidence of mistrust.
4. Client appropriately interacts and cooperates with staff and peers in therapeutic community setting.

● DISTURBED SENSORY PERCEPTION: AUDITORY/VISUAL

Definition: Change in the amount or patterning of incoming stimuli [either internally or externally initiated] accompanied by a diminished, exaggerated, distorted, or impaired response to such stimuli.

Possible Etiologies ("related to")

[Panic level of anxiety]
[Withdrawal into the self]
[Stress sufficiently severe to threaten an already weak ego]

Defining Characteristics ("evidenced by")

[Talking and laughing to self]
[Listening pose (tilting head to one side as if listening)]
[Stops talking in middle of sentence to listen]
[Rapid mood swings]
[Disordered thought sequencing]
[Inappropriate responses]
Disorientation
Poor concentration
Sensory distortions

Goals/Objectives

Short-term Goal

Client will discuss content of hallucinations with nurse or therapist within 1 week.

Long-term Goal

Client will be able to define and test reality, eliminating the occurrence of hallucinations. (This goal may not be realistic for the individual with chronic illness who has experienced auditory hallucinations for many years.) A more realistic goal may be:

Client will verbalize understanding that the voices are a result of his or her illness and demonstrate ways to interrupt the hallucination.

Interventions with *Selected Rationales*

1. Observe client for signs of hallucinations (listening pose, laughing or talking to self, stopping in mid-sentence). *Early intervention may prevent aggressive responses to command hallucinations.*

2. Avoid touching the client before warning him or her that you are about to do so. *Client may perceive touch as threatening and respond in an aggressive manner.*
3. An attitude of acceptance will encourage the client to share the content of the hallucination with you. *This is important in order to prevent possible injury to the client or others from command hallucinations.*
4. Do not reinforce the hallucination. Use words such as "the voices" instead of "they" when referring to the hallucination. *Words like "they" validate that the voices are real.*

CLINICAL PEARL Let the client who is "hearing voices" know that you do not share the perception.
Say "Even though I realize that the voices are real to you, I do not hear any voices speaking." The nurse must be honest with the client so that he or she may realize that the hallucinations are not real.

---

5. Try to connect the times of the hallucinations to times of increased anxiety. Help the client to understand this connection. *If client can learn to interrupt escalating anxiety, hallucinations may be prevented.*
6. Try to distract the client away from the hallucination. *Involvement in interpersonal activities and explanation of the actual situation will help bring the client back to reality.*
7. For some clients, auditory hallucinations persist after the acute psychotic episode has subsided. Listening to the radio or watching television helps distract some clients from attention to the voices. Others have benefited from an intervention called *voice dismissal*. With this technique, the client is taught to say loudly, "Go away!" or "Leave me alone!", thereby exerting some conscious control over the behavior.

Outcome Criteria
1. Client is able to recognize that hallucinations occur at times of extreme anxiety.
2. Client is able to recognize signs of increasing anxiety and employ techniques to interrupt the response.

● DISTURBED THOUGHT PROCESSES

Definition: Disruption in cognitive operations and activities.

Possible Etiologies ("related to")

[Inability to trust]
[Panic level of anxiety]
[Repressed fears]
[Stress sufficiently severe to threaten an already weak ego]
[Possible hereditary factor]

Defining Characteristics ("evidenced by")

[Delusional thinking (false ideas)]
[Inability to concentrate]
Hypervigilance
[Altered attention span]—distractibility
Inaccurate interpretation of the environment
[Impaired ability to make decisions, problem-solve, reason, abstract or conceptualize, calculate]
[Inappropriate social behavior (reflecting inaccurate thinking)]
Inappropriate [non–reality-based] thinking

Goals/Objectives

Short-term Goal

[By specified time deemed appropriate], client will recognize and verbalize that false ideas occur at times of increased anxiety.

Long-term Goal

Depending on chronicity of disease process, choose the most realistic long-term goal for the client:
1. By time of discharge from treatment, client's speech will reflect reality-based thinking.
2. By time of discharge from treatment, client will be able to differentiate between delusional thinking and reality.

Interventions with *Selected Rationales*

1. Convey your acceptance of client's need for the false belief, while letting him or her know that you do not share the belief. *It is important to communicate to the client that you do not accept the delusion as reality.*
2. Do not argue or deny the belief. Use *reasonable doubt* as a therapeutic technique: "I understand that you believe this is true, but I personally find it hard to accept." *Arguing with the client or denying the belief serves no useful purpose, because delusional ideas are not eliminated by this approach, and the development of a trusting relationship may be impeded.*
3. Help client trye to connect the false beliefs to times of increased anxiety. Discuss techniques that could be used to

control anxiety (e.g., deep-breathing exercises, other re-laxation exercises, thought stopping techniques). *If the client can learn to interrupt escalating anxiety, delusional thinking may be prevented.*

4. Reinforce and focus on reality. Discourage long ruminations about the irrational thinking. Talk about real events and real people. *Discussions that focus on the false ideas are purposeless and useless, and may even aggravate the psychosis.*

5. Assist and support client in his or her attempt to verbalize feelings of anxiety, fear, or insecurity. *Verbalization of feelings in a nonthreatening environment may help client come to terms with long-unresolved issues.*

Outcome Criteria

1. Verbalizations reflect thinking processes oriented in reality.
2. Client is able to maintain activities of daily living (ADLs) to his or her maximal ability.
3. Client is able to refrain from responding to delusional thoughts, should they occur.

• IMPAIRED VERBAL COMMUNICATION

Definition: Decreased, delayed, or absent ability to receive, process, transmit, and use a system of symbols [to communicate].

Possible Etiologies ("related to")

Altered perceptions
[Inability to trust]
[Panic level of anxiety]
[Regression to earlier level of development]
[Withdrawal into the self]
[Disordered, unrealistic thinking]

Defining Characteristics ("evidenced by")

[Loose association of ideas]
[Use of words that are symbolic to the individual (neologisms)]
[Use of words in a meaningless, disconnected manner (word salad)]
[Use of words that rhyme in a nonsensical fashion (clang association)]
[Repetition of words that are heard (echolalia)]
[Does not speak (mutism)]

[Verbalizations reflect concrete thinking (inability to think in abstract terms)]

[Poor eye contact (either no eye contact or continuous staring into the other person's eyes)]

Goals/Objectives

Short-term Goal

Client will demonstrate ability to remain on one topic, using appropriate, intermittent eye contact for 5 minutes with nurse or therapist.

Long-term Goal

By time of discharge from treatment, client will demonstrate ability to carry on a verbal communication in a socially acceptable manner with staff and peers.

Interventions with *Selected Rationales*

1. Use the techniques of *consensual validation* and *seeking clarification* to decode communication patterns. (*Examples:* "Is it that you mean...?" or "I don't understand what you mean by that. Would you please explain it to me?") *These techniques reveal to the client how he or she is being perceived by others, and the responsibility for not understanding is accepted by the nurse.*

2. Maintain consistency of staff assignment over time, *to facilitate trust and the ability to understand client's actions and communication.*

3. In a nonthreatening manner, explain to client how his or her behavior and verbalizations are viewed by and may alienate others.

4. If client is unable or unwilling to speak (mutism), use of the technique of *verbalizing the implied* is therapeutic. (*Example:* "That must have been very difficult for you when....") *This may help to convey empathy, develop trust, and eventually encourage client to discuss painful issues.*

5. Anticipate and fulfill client's needs until satisfactory communication patterns return. *Client comfort and safety are nursing priorities.*

Outcome Criteria

1. Client is able to communicate in a manner that is understood by others.

2. Client's nonverbal messages are congruent with verbalizations.

3. Client is able to recognize that disorganized thinking and impaired verbal communication occur at times of increased anxiety and intervene to interrupt the process.

• SELF-CARE DEFICIT (Identify Specific Area)

Definition: Impaired ability to perform or complete [activities of daily living (ADLs)].

Possible Etiologies ("related to")
[Withdrawal into the self]
[Regression to an earlier level of development]
[Panic level of anxiety]
Perceptual or cognitive impairment
[Inability to trust]

Defining Characteristics ("evidenced by")
[Difficulty in bringing or] inability to bring food from receptacle to mouth
Inability [or refusal] to wash body or body parts
[Impaired ability or lack of interest in selecting appropriate clothing to wear, dressing, grooming, or maintaining appearance at a satisfactory level]
[Inability or unwillingness to carry out toileting procedures without assistance]

Goals/Objectives
Short-term Goal
Client will verbalize a desire to perform ADLs by end of 1 week.
Long-term Goal
By time of discharge from treatment, client will be able to perform ADLs in an independent manner and demonstrate a willingness to do so.

Interventions with *Selected Rationales*
1. Encourage client to perform normal ADLs to his or her level of ability. *Successful performance of independent activities enhances self-esteem.*
2. Encourage independence, but intervene when client is unable to perform. *Client comfort and safety are nursing priorities.*
3. Offer recognition and positive reinforcement for independent accomplishments. (*Example:* "Mrs. J., I see you have put on a clean dress and combed your hair.") *Positive reinforcement enhances self-esteem and encourages repetition of desirable behaviors.*
4. Show client, on concrete level, how to perform activities with which he or she is having difficulty. (*Example:* If client is not

eating, place spoon in his or her hand, scoop some food into it, and say, "Now, eat a bite of mashed potatoes (or other food)." *Because concrete thinking prevails, explanations must be provided at the client's concrete level of comprehension.*

5. Keep strict records of food and fluid intake. *This information is necessary to acquire an accurate nutritional assessment.*

6. Offer nutritious snacks and fluids between meals. *Client may be unable to tolerate large amounts of food at mealtimes and may therefore require additional nourishment at other times during the day to receive adequate nutrition.*

7. If client is not eating because of suspiciousness and fears of being poisoned, provide canned foods and allow client to open them; or, if possible, suggest that food be served family-style *so that client may see everyone eating from the same servings.*

8. If client is soiling self, establish routine schedule for toileting needs. Assist client to bathroom on hourly or bi-hourly schedule, as need is determined, until he or she is able to fulfill this need without assistance.

Outcome Criteria

1. Client feeds self without assistance.
2. Client selects appropriate clothing, dresses, and grooms self daily without assistance.
3. Client maintains optimal level of personal hygiene by bathing daily and carrying out essential toileting procedures without assistance.

● INSOMNIA

Definition: A disruption in amount and quality of sleep that impairs functioning.

Possible Etiologies ("related to")

[Panic level of anxiety]
[Repressed fears]
[Hallucinations]
[Delusional thinking]

Defining Characteristics ("evidenced by")

[Difficulty falling asleep]
[Awakening very early in the morning]
[Pacing; other signs of increasing irritability caused by lack of sleep]
[Frequent yawning, nodding off to sleep]

Goals/Objectives

Short-term Goal

Within first week of treatment, client will fall asleep within 30 minutes of retiring and sleep 5 hours without awakening, with use of sedative if needed.

Long-term Goal

By time of discharge from treatment, client will be able to fall asleep within 30 minutes of retiring and sleep 6 to 8 hours without a sleeping aid.

Interventions with *Selected Rationales*

1. Keep strict records of sleeping patterns. *Accurate baseline data are important in planning care to assist client with this problem.*
2. Discourage sleep during the day *to promote more restful sleep at night.*
3. Administer antipsychotic medication at bedtime *so client does not become drowsy during the day.*
4. Assist with measures that promote sleep, such as warm, non-stimulating drinks; light snacks; warm baths; and back rubs.
5. Performing relaxation exercises to soft music may be helpful prior to sleep.
6. Limit intake of caffeinated drinks such as tea, coffee, and colas. *Caffeine is a CNS stimulant and may interfere with the client's achievement of rest and sleep.*

Outcome Criteria

1. Client is able to fall asleep within 30 minutes after retiring.
2. Client sleeps at least 6 consecutive hours without waking.
3. Client does not require a sedative to fall asleep.

@ INTERNET REFERENCES

- Additional information about schizophrenia may be located at the following websites:
  a. http://www.schizophrenia.com
  b. http://www.nimh.nih.gov
  c. http://www.nami.org/schizophrenia
  d. http://mentalhealth.com
  e. http://www.narsad.org
- Additional information about medications to treat schizophrenia may be located at the following websites:
  a. http://www.medicinenet.com/medications/article.htm
  b. http://www.fadavis.com/townsend
  c. http://www.nlm.nih.gov/medlineplus

Movie Connections

I Never Promised You a Rose Garden (schizophrenia) • *A Beautiful Mind (schizophrenia)* • *The Fisher King (schizophrenia)* • *Benny & Joon (schizophrenia)* • *Out of Darkness (schizophrenia)* • *Conspiracy Theory (paranoia)* • *The Fan (delusional disorder)*

Mood Disorders: Depression

● **BACKGROUND ASSESSMENT DATA**

"Mood" is defined as an individual's sustained emotional tone, which significantly influences behavior, personality, and perception. A disturbance in mood is the predominant feature of the mood disorders (American Psychiatric Association [APA], 2000). Mood disorders are classified as depressive or bipolar.

Major Depressive Disorder

Major depressive disorder is described as a disturbance of mood involving depression or loss of interest or pleasure in the usual activities and pastimes. There is evidence of interference in social and occupational functioning for at least 2 weeks. There is no history of manic behavior and the symptoms cannot be attributed to use of substances or a general medical condition. The following specifiers may be used to further describe the depressive episode:

1. **Single Episode or Recurrent:** This specifier identifies whether the individual has experienced prior episodes of depression.
2. **Mild, Moderate, or Severe:** These categories are identified by the number and severity of symptoms.
3. **With Psychotic Features:** Impairment of reality testing is evident. The individual experiences hallucinations and/or delusions.
4. **With Catatonic Features:** This category identifies the presence of psychomotor disturbances, such as severe psychomotor retardation, with or without the presence of waxy flexibility or stupor or excessive motor activity. The client also may manifest symptoms of negativism, mutism, echolalia, or echopraxia.
5. **With Melancholic Features:** This is a typically severe form of major depressive episode. Symptoms are exaggerated. There is a loss of interest in all activities. Depression is

regularly worse in the morning. There is a history of major depressive episodes that have responded well to somatic antidepressant therapy.
6. **Chronic:** This classification applies when the current episode of depressed mood has been evident continuously for at least the past 2 years.
7. **With Seasonal Pattern:** This diagnosis indicates the presence of depressive symptoms during the fall or winter months. This diagnosis is made when the number of seasonal depressive episodes substantially outnumbers the non–seasonal depressive episodes that have occurred over the individual's lifetime (APA, 2000). This disorder has previously been identified in the literature as seasonal affective disorder (SAD).
8. **With Postpartum Onset:** This specifier is used when symptoms of major depression occur within 4 weeks postpartum.

Dysthymic Disorder
Dysthymic disorder is a mood disturbance with characteristics similar to, if somewhat milder than, those ascribed to major depressive disorder. There is no evidence of psychotic symptoms.

Depressive Disorder Due to General Medical Condition
This disorder is characterized by a prominent and persistent depressed mood that is judged to be the direct result of the physiological effects of a general medical condition (APA, 2000).

Substance-Induced Depressed Mood Disorder
The depressed mood associated with this disorder is considered to be the direct result of the physiological effects of a substance (e.g., use or abuse of a drug or a medication, or toxin exposure).

● PREDISPOSING FACTORS TO DEPRESSION
1. **Physiological**
   a. *Genetic:* Numerous studies have been conducted that support the involvement of heredity in depressive illness. The disorder is 1.5 to 3 times more common among first-degree relatives of individuals with the disorder than among the general population (APA, 2000).
   b. *Biochemical:* A biochemical theory implicates the biogenic amines norepinephrine, dopamine, and serotonin. The levels of these chemicals have been found to be deficient in individuals with depressive illness.
   c. *Neuroendocrine Disturbances:* Elevated levels of serum cortisol and decreased levels of thyroid-stimulating

hormone have been associated with depressed mood in some individuals.

d. **Medication Side Effects:** A number of drugs can produce a depressive syndrome as a side effect. Common ones include anxiolytics, antipsychotics, and sedative-hypnotics. Antihypertensive medications such as propranolol and reserpine have been known to produce depressive symptoms.

e. **Other Physiological Conditions:** Depressive symptoms may occur in the presence of electrolyte disturbances, hormonal disturbances, nutritional deficiencies, and with certain physical disorders, such as cardiovascular accident, systemic lupus erythematosus, hepatitis, and diabetes mellitus.

2. **Psychosocial**

a. **Psychoanalytical:** Freud observed that melancholia occurs after the loss of a loved object, either actually by death or emotionally by rejection, or the loss of some other abstraction of value to the individual. Freud indicated that in clients with melancholia, the depressed person's rage is internally directed because of identification with the lost object (Sadock & Sadock, 2007).

b. **Cognitive:** Beck and colleagues (1979) proposed that depressive illness occurs as a result of impaired cognition. Disturbed thought processes foster a negative evaluation of self by the individual. The perceptions are of inadequacy and worthlessness. Outlook for the future is one of pessimism and hopelessness.

c. **Learning Theory:** Learning theory (Seligman, 1973) proposes that depressive illness is predisposed by the individual's belief that there is a lack of control over his or her life situation. It is thought that this belief arises out of experiences that result in failure (either perceived or real). Following numerous failures, the individual feels helpless to succeed at any endeavor and therefore gives up trying. This "learned helplessness" is viewed as a predisposition to depressive illness.

d. **Object Loss Theory:** The theory of object loss suggests that depressive illness occurs as a result of having been abandoned by, or otherwise separated from, a significant other during the first 6 months of life. Because during this period the mother represents the child's main source of security, she is the "object." The response occurs not only with a physical loss. This absence of attachment, which may be either physical or emotional, leads to feelings of helplessness and despair that contribute to lifelong patterns of depression in response to loss.

● SYMPTOMATOLOGY (SUBJECTIVE AND OBJECTIVE DATA)

1. The affect of a depressed person is one of sadness, dejection, helplessness, and hopelessness. The outlook is gloomy and pessimistic. A feeling of worthlessness prevails.
2. Thoughts are slowed and concentration is difficult. Obsessive ideas and rumination of negative thoughts are common. In severe depression (major depressive disorder or bipolar depression), psychotic features such as hallucinations and delusions may be evident, reflecting misinterpretations of the environment.
3. Physically, there is evidence of weakness and fatigue—very little energy to carry on activities of daily living (ADLs). The individual may express an exaggerated concern over bodily functioning, seemingly experiencing heightened sensitivity to somatic sensations.
4. Some individuals may be inclined toward excessive eating and drinking, whereas others may experience anorexia and weight loss. In response to a general slowdown of the body, digestion is often sluggish, constipation is common, and urinary retention is possible.
5. Sleep disturbances are common, either insomnia or hypersomnia.
6. At the less severe level (dysthymic disorder), individuals tend to feel their best early in the morning, then continually feel worse as the day progresses. The opposite is true of persons experiencing severe depression. The exact cause of this phenomenon is unknown, but it is thought to be related to the circadian rhythm of the hormones and their effects on the body.
7. A general slowdown of motor activity commonly accompanies depression (called *psychomotor retardation*). Energy level is depleted, movements are lethargic, and performance of daily activities is extremely difficult. Regression is common, evidenced by withdrawal into the self and retreat to the fetal position. Severely depressed persons may manifest psychomotor activity through symptoms of agitation. These are constant, rapid, purposeless movements, out of touch with the environment.
8. Verbalizations are limited. When depressed persons do speak, the content may be either ruminations regarding their own life regrets or, in psychotic clients, a reflection of their delusional thinking.
9. Social participation is diminished. The depressed client has an inclination toward egocentrism and narcissism—an intense focus on the self. This discourages others from

pursuing a relationship with the individual, which increases his or her feelings of worthlessness and penchant for isolation.

Common Nursing Diagnoses and Interventions for Depression

(Interventions are applicable to various health-care settings, such as inpatient and partial hospitalization, community outpatient clinic, home health, and private practice.)

● RISK FOR SUICIDE

Definition: At risk for self-inflicted, life-threatening injury.

Related/Risk Factors ("related to")
[Depressed mood]
Grief; hopelessness; social isolation
History of prior suicide attempt
[Has a suicide plan and means to carry it out]
Widowed or divorced
Chronic or terminal illness
Psychiatric illness or substance abuse
States desire to die
Threats of killing self

Goals/Objectives
Short-term Goals
1. Client will seek out staff when feeling urge to harm self.
2. Client will make short-term verbal (or written) contract with nurse not to harm self.
3. Client will not harm self.

Long-term Goal
Client will not harm self.

Interventions with *Selected Rationales*
1. Ask client directly: "Have you thought about harming yourself in any way? If so, what do you plan to do? Do you have the means to carry out this plan?" *The risk of suicide is greatly increased if the client has developed a plan and particularly if means exist for the client to execute the plan.*
2. Create a safe environment for the client. Remove all potentially harmful objects from client's access (sharp objects, straps, belts, ties, glass items). Supervise closely during meals and medication administration. Perform room searches as deemed necessary. *Client safety is a nursing priority.*

3. Formulate a short-term verbal or written contract with the client that he or she will not harm self during specific time period. When that contract expires, make another, and so forth. *Discussion of suicidal feelings with a trusted individual provides some relief to the client. A contract gets the subject out in the open and places some of the responsibility for the client's safety with the client. An attitude of acceptance of the client as a worthwhile individual is conveyed.*

4. Secure promise from client that he or she will seek out a staff member or support person if thoughts of suicide emerge. *Suicidal clients are often very ambivalent about their feelings. Discussion of feelings with a trusted individual may provide assistance before the client experiences a crisis situation.*

5. Maintain close observation of client. Depending on level of suicide precaution, provide one-to-one contact, constant visual observation, or every-15-minute checks. Place client in room close to nurse's station; do not assign to private room. Accompany client to off-unit activities if attendance is indicated. May need to accompany client to bathroom. *Close observation is necessary to ensure that client does not harm self in any way. Being alert for suicidal and escape attempts facilitates being able to prevent or interrupt harmful behavior.*

6. Maintain special care in administration of medications. *Prevents saving up to overdose or discarding and not taking.*

7. Make rounds at frequent, *irregular* intervals (especially at night, toward early morning, at change of shift, or other predictably busy times for staff). *Prevents staff surveillance from becoming predictable. To be aware of client's location is important, especially when staff is busy, unavailable, or less observable.*

8. Encourage verbalizations of honest feelings. Through exploration and discussion, help client to identify symbols of hope in his or her life.

9. Encourage client to express angry feelings within appropriate limits. Provide safe method of hostility release. Help client to identify true source of anger and to work on adaptive coping skills for use outside the treatment setting. *Depression and suicidal behaviors may be viewed as anger turned inward on the self. If this anger can be verbalized in a nonthreatening environment, the client may be able to eventually resolve these feelings.*

10. Identify community resources that client may use as support system and from whom he or she may request help

if feeling suicidal. *Having a concrete plan for seeking assistance during a crisis may discourage or prevent self-destructive behaviors.*

11. Orient client to reality, as required. Point out sensory misperceptions or misinterpretations of the environment. Take care not to belittle client's fears or indicate disapproval of verbal expressions.

12. Most important, spend time with client. *This provides a feeling of safety and security, while also conveying the message, "I want to spend time with you because I think you are a worthwhile person."*

Outcome Criteria

1. Client verbalizes no thoughts of suicide.
2. Client commits no acts of self-harm.
3. Client is able to verbalize names of resources outside the hospital from whom he or she may request help if feeling suicidal.

● COMPLICATED GRIEVING

Definition: A disorder that occurs after the death of a significant other [or any other loss of significance to the individual], in which the experience of distress accompanying bereavement fails to follow normative expectations and manifests in functional impairment.

Possible Etiologies ("related to")

[Real or perceived loss of any concept of value to the individual]
[Bereavement overload (cumulative grief from multiple unresolved losses)]
[Thwarted grieving response to a loss]
[Absence of anticipatory grieving]
[Feelings of guilt generated by ambivalent relationship with lost entity]

Defining Characteristics ("evidenced by")

[Idealization of lost entity]
[Denial of loss]
[Excessive anger, expressed inappropriately]
[Obsessions with past experiences]
[Ruminations of guilt feelings, excessive and exaggerated out of proportion to the situation]
[Developmental regression]
[Difficulty in expressing loss]
[Prolonged difficulty coping following a loss]

[Reliving of past experiences with little or no reduction of intensity of the grief]

[Prolonged interference with life functioning, with onset or exacerbation of somatic or psychosomatic responses]

[Labile affect]

[Alterations in eating habits, sleep patterns, dream patterns, activity level, libido]

Goals/Objectives

Short-term Goal

Client will express anger toward lost entity.

Long-term Goals

1. Client will be able to verbalize behaviors associated with the normal stages of grief.
2. Client will be able to recognize own position in grief process as he or she progresses at own pace toward resolution.

Interventions with Selected Rationales

1. Determine stage of grief in which client is fixed. Identify behaviors associated with this stage. *Accurate baseline assessment data are necessary to effectively plan care for the grieving client.*
2. Develop trusting relationship with client. Show empathy and caring. Be honest and keep all promises. *Trust is the basis for a therapeutic relationship.*
3. Convey an accepting attitude, and enable the client to express feelings openly. *An accepting attitude conveys to the client that you believe he or she is a worthwhile person. Trust is enhanced.*
4. Encourage client to express anger. Do not become defensive if initial expression of anger is displaced on nurse or therapist. Assist client to explore angry feelings so that they may be directed toward the intended object or person. *Verbalization of feelings in a nonthreatening environment may help client come to terms with unresolved issues.*
5. Assist client to discharge pent-up anger through participation in large motor activities (e.g., brisk walks, jogging, physical exercises, volleyball, punching bag, exercise bike). *Physical exercise provides a safe and effective method for discharging pent-up tension.*
6. Teach the normal stages of grief and behaviors associated with each stage. Help client to understand that feelings such as guilt and anger toward the lost entity are appropriate and acceptable during the grief process. *Knowledge of acceptability of the feelings associated with normal grieving may help to relieve some of the guilt that these responses generate.*

7. Encourage client to review relationship with the lost entity. With support and sensitivity, point out reality of the situation in areas where misrepresentations are expressed. *Client must give up an idealized perception and be able to accept both positive and negative aspects about the lost entity before the grief process is complete.*

8. Communicate to client that crying is acceptable. Use of touch is therapeutic and appropriate with most clients. Knowledge of cultural influences specific to the client is important before using this technique.

9. Assist client in problem solving as he or she attempts to determine methods for more adaptive coping with the experienced loss. Provide positive feedback for strategies identified and decisions made. *Positive feedback increases self-esteem and encourages repetition of desirable behaviors.*

10. Encourage client to reach out for spiritual support during this time in whatever form is desirable to him or her. Assess spiritual needs of client and assist as necessary in the fulfillment of those needs.

Outcome Criteria

1. Client is able to verbalize normal stages of the grief process and behaviors associated with each stage.

2. Client is able to identify own position within the grief process and express honest feelings related to the lost entity.

3. Client is no longer manifesting exaggerated emotions and behaviors related to complicated grieving and is able to carry out ADLs independently.

● LOW SELF-ESTEEM

Definition: Negative self-evaluation/feelings about self or self-capabilities.

Possible Etiologies ("related to")

[Lack of positive feedback]
[Feelings of abandonment by significant other]
[Numerous failures (learned helplessness)]
[Underdeveloped ego and punitive superego]
[Impaired cognition fostering negative view of self]

Defining Characteristics ("evidenced by")

[Difficulty accepting positive reinforcement]
[Withdrawal into social isolation]
[Being highly critical and judgmental of self and others]

[Expressions of worthlessness]
[Fear of failure]
[Inability to recognize own accomplishments]
[Setting self up for failure by establishing unrealistic goals]
[Unsatisfactory interpersonal relationships]
[Negative, pessimistic outlook]
[Hypersensitive to slight or criticism]
[Grandiosity]

Goals/Objectives

Short-term Goals

1. Within reasonable time period, client will discuss fear of failure with nurse.
2. Within reasonable time period, client will verbalize things he or she likes about self.

Long-term Goals

1. By time of discharge from treatment, client will exhibit increased feelings of self-worth as evidenced by verbal expression of positive aspects of self, past accomplishments, and future prospects.
2. By time of discharge from treatment, client will exhibit increased feelings of self-worth by setting realistic goals and trying to reach them, thereby demonstrating a decrease in fear of failure.

Interventions with *Selected Rationales*

1. Be accepting of client and his or her negativism. *An attitude of acceptance enhances feelings of self-worth.*
2. Spend time with client *to convey acceptance and contribute toward feelings of self-worth.*
3. Help client to recognize and focus on strengths and accomplishments. Minimize attention given to past (real or perceived) failures. *Lack of attention may help to eliminate negative ruminations.*
4. Encourage participation in group activities *from which client may receive positive feedback and support from peers.*
5. Help client identify areas he or she would like to change about self, and assist with problem solving toward this effort. *Low self-worth may interfere with client's perception of own problem-solving ability. Assistance may be required.*
6. Ensure that client is not becoming increasingly dependent and that he or she is accepting responsibility for own behaviors. *Client must be able to function independently if he or she is to be successful within the less-structured community environment.*

7. Ensure that therapy groups offer client simple methods of achievement. Offer recognition and positive feedback for actual accomplishments. *Successes and recognition increase self-esteem.*

8. Teach assertiveness techniques: the ability to recognize the differences among passive, assertive, and aggressive behaviors, and the importance of respecting the human rights of others while protecting one's own basic human rights. *Self-esteem is enhanced by the ability to interact with others in an assertive manner.*

9. Teach effective communication techniques, such as the use of "I" messages. "I-statements" can be used to take ownership for one's feelings rather than saying they are caused by the other person. *Example*: "I feel angry when you criticize me in front of other people, and I would prefer that you stop doing that." "You-statements" put the other individual on the defensive. *Example*: "You are a jerk for criticizing me in front of other people!"

10. Assist client in performing aspects of self-care when required. Offer positive feedback for tasks performed independently. *Positive feedback enhances self-esteem and encourages repetition of desirable behaviors.*

Outcome Criteria

1. Client is able to verbalize positive aspects of self.
2. Client is able to communicate assertively with others.
3. Client expresses some optimism and hope for the future.
4. Client sets realistic goals for self and demonstrates willing attempt to reach them.

• SOCIAL ISOLATION/IMPAIRED SOCIAL INTERACTION

Definition: Social isolation is the condition of aloneness experienced by the individual and perceived as imposed by others and as a negative or threatened state; impaired social interaction is an insufficient or excessive quantity or ineffective quality of social exchange.

Possible Etiologies ("related to")

[Developmental regression]

[Egocentric behaviors (which offend others and discourage relationships)]

Disturbed thought processes [delusional thinking]

[Fear of rejection or failure of the interaction]

[Impaired cognition fostering negative view of self]

[Unresolved grief]
Absence of significant others

Defining Characteristics ("evidenced by")

Sad, dull affect
Being uncommunicative, withdrawn; lacking eye contact
Preoccupation with own thoughts; performance of repetitive, meaningless actions
Seeking to be alone
[Assuming fetal position]
Expression of feelings of aloneness or rejection
Discomfort in social situations
Dysfunctional interaction with others

Goals/Objectives

Short-term Goal

Client will develop trusting relationship with nurse or counselor within time period to be individually determined.

Long-term Goals

1. Client will voluntarily spend time with other clients and nurse or therapist in group activities by time of discharge from treatment.
2. Client will refrain from using egocentric behaviors that offend others and discourage relationships by time of discharge from treatment.

Interventions with *Selected Rationales*

1. Spend time with client. This may mean just sitting in silence for a while. *Your presence may help improve client's perception of self as a worthwhile person.*
2. Develop a therapeutic nurse-client relationship through frequent, brief contacts and an accepting attitude. Show unconditional positive regard. *Your presence, acceptance, and conveyance of positive regard enhance the client's feelings of self-worth.*
3. After client feels comfortable in a one-to-one relationship, encourage attendance in group activities. May need to attend with client the first few times to offer support. Accept client's decision to remove self from group situation if anxiety becomes too great. *The presence of a trusted individual provides emotional security for the client.*
4. Verbally acknowledge client's absence from any group activities. *Knowledge that his or her absence was noticed may reinforce the client's feelings of self-worth.*
5. Teach assertiveness techniques. Interactions with others may be discouraged by client's use of passive or aggressive

behaviors. *Knowledge of the use of assertive techniques could improve client's relationships with others.*

6. Provide direct feedback about client's interactions with others. Do this in a nonjudgmental manner. Help client learn how to respond more appropriately in interactions with others. Teach client skills that may be used to approach others in a more socially acceptable manner. Practice these skills through role-play. *Client may not realize how he or she is being perceived by others. Direct feedback from a trusted individual may help to alter these behaviors in a positive manner. Having practiced these skills in role-play facilitates their use in real situations.*

7. The depressed client must have lots of structure in his or her life because of the impairment in decision-making and problem-solving ability. Devise a plan of therapeutic activities and provide client with a written time schedule. *Remember:* The client who is moderately depressed feels best early in the day, whereas later in the day is a better time for the severely depressed individual to participate in activities. *It is important to plan activities at a time when the client has more energy and is more likely to gain from the experience.*

8. Provide positive reinforcement for client's voluntary interactions with others. *Positive reinforcement enhances self-esteem and encourages repetition of desirable behaviors.*

Outcome Criteria

1. Client demonstrates willingness and desire to socialize with others.
2. Client voluntarily attends group activities.
3. Client approaches others in appropriate manner for one-to-one interaction.

● POWERLESSNESS

Definition: Perception that one's own action will not significantly affect an outcome; a perceived lack of control over a current situation or immediate happening.

Possible Etiologies ("related to")

Lifestyle of helplessness
Healthcare environment
[Complicated grieving process]
[Lack of positive feedback]
[Consistent negative feedback]

Defining Characteristics ("evidenced by")

Verbal expressions of having no control (e.g., over self-care, situation, outcome)

Nonparticipation in care or decision making when opportunities are provided

Expression of doubt regarding role performance

Reluctance to express true feelings

Apathy

Dependence on others that may result in irritability, resentment, anger, and guilt

Passivity

Goals/Objectives

Short-term Goal

Client will participate in decision making regarding own care within 5 days.

Long-term Goal

Client will be able to effectively problem solve ways to take control of his or her life situation by time of discharge from treatment, thereby decreasing feelings of powerlessness.

Interventions with *Selected Rationales*

1. Encourage client to take as much responsibility as possible for own self-care practices. ***Providing client with choices will increase his or her feelings of control.***
   Examples:
   a. Include client in setting the goals of care he or she wishes to achieve.
   b. Allow client to establish own schedule for self-care activities.
   c. Provide client with privacy as need is determined.
   d. Provide positive feedback for decisions made. Respect client's right to make those decisions independently, and refrain from attempting to influence him or her toward those that may seem more logical.
2. Help client set realistic goals. ***Unrealistic goals set the client up for failure and reinforce feelings of powerlessness.***
3. Help client identify areas of life situation that he or she can control. ***Client's emotional condition interferes with his or her ability to solve problems. Assistance is required to perceive the benefits and consequences of available alternatives accurately.***
4. Help client identify areas of life situation that are not within his or her ability to control. Encourage verbalization of feelings related to this inability *in an effort to deal with unresolved issues and accept what cannot be changed.*

5. Identify ways in which client can achieve. Encourage participation in these activities, and provide positive reinforcement for participation, as well as for achievement. *Positive reinforcement enhances self-esteem and encourages repetition of desirable behaviors.*

Outcome Criteria
1. Client verbalizes choices made in a plan to maintain control over his or her life situation.
2. Client verbalizes honest feelings about life situations over which he or she has no control.
3. Client is able to verbalize system for problem solving as required for adequate role performance.

• DISTURBED THOUGHT PROCESSES

Definition: Disruption in cognitive operations and activities.

Possible Etiologies ("related to")
[Withdrawal into the self]
[Underdeveloped ego; punitive superego]
[Impaired cognition fostering negative perception of self and the environment]

Defining Characteristics ("evidenced by")
Inaccurate interpretation of environment
[Delusional thinking]
Hypovigilance
[Altered attention span]—distractibility
Egocentricity
[Impaired ability to make decisions, problem solve, reason]
[Negative ruminations]

Goals/Objectives
Short-term Goal
Client will recognize and verbalize when interpretations of the environment are inaccurate within 1 week.

Long-term Goal
By time of discharge from treatment, client's verbalizations will reflect reality-based thinking with no evidence of delusional or distorted ideation.

Interventions with *Selected Rationales*
1. Convey your acceptance of client's need for the false belief, while letting him or her know that you do not share the delusion. *A positive response would convey to the client that you accept the delusion as reality.*

2. Do not argue or deny the belief. Use *reasonable doubt* as a therapeutic technique: "I understand that you believe this is true, but I personally find it hard to accept." *Arguing with the client or denying the belief serves no useful purpose, as delusional ideas are not eliminated by this approach, and the development of a trusting relationship may be impeded.*

3. Use the techniques of *consensual validation* and *seeking clarification* when communication reflects alteration in thinking. (*Examples:* "Is it that you mean . . . ?" or "I don't understand what you mean by that. Would you please explain?") *These techniques reveal to the client how he or she is being perceived by others, while the responsibility for not understanding is accepted by the nurse.*

4. Reinforce and focus on reality. Talk about real events and real people. Use real situations and events to divert client away from long, purposeless, repetitive verbalizations of false ideas.

5. Give positive reinforcement as client is able to differentiate between reality-based and non–reality-based thinking. *Positive reinforcement enhances self-esteem and encourages repetition of desirable behaviors.*

6. Teach client to intervene, using thought-stopping techniques, when irrational or negative thoughts prevail. *Thought stopping* involves using the command "stop!" or a loud noise (such as hand clapping) to interrupt unwanted thoughts. *This noise or command distracts the individual from the undesirable thinking that often precedes undesirable emotions or behaviors.*

7. Use touch cautiously, particularly if thoughts reveal ideas of persecution. *Clients who are suspicious may perceive touch as threatening and may respond with aggression.*

Outcome Criteria

1. Client's thinking processes reflect accurate interpretation of the environment.
2. Client is able to recognize negative or irrational thoughts and intervene to "stop" their progression.

● IMBALANCED NUTRITION, LESS THAN BODY REQUIREMENTS

Definition: Intake of nutrients insufficient to meet metabolic needs.

Possible Etiologies ("related to")

Inability to ingest food because of:
    [Depressed mood]
    [Loss of appetite]

[Energy level too low to meet own nutritional needs]
[Regression to lower level of development]
[Ideas of self-destruction]

Defining Characteristics ("evidenced by")

Loss of weight
Lack of interest in food
Pale mucous membranes
Poor muscle tone
[Amenorrhea]
[Poor skin turgor]
[Edema of extremities]
[Electrolyte imbalances]
[Weakness]
[Constipation]
[Anemias]

Goals/Objectives

Short-term Goal

Client will gain 2 lb per week for the next 3 weeks.

Long-term Goal

Client will exhibit no signs or symptoms of malnutrition by time of discharge from treatment (e.g., electrolytes and blood counts will be within normal limits; a steady weight gain will be demonstrated; constipation will be corrected; client will exhibit increased energy in participation in activities).

Interventions with *Selected Rationales*

1. In collaboration with dietitian, determine number of calories required to provide adequate nutrition and realistic (according to body structure and height) weight gain.
2. To prevent constipation, ensure that diet includes foods high in fiber content. Encourage client to increase fluid consumption and physical exercise to promote normal bowel functioning. *Depressed clients are particularly vulnerable to constipation because of psychomotor retardation. Constipation is also a common side effect of many antidepressant medications.*
3. Keep strict documentation of intake, output, and calorie count. *This information is necessary to make an accurate nutritional assessment and maintain client safety.*
4. Weigh client daily. *Weight loss or gain is important assessment information.*
5. Determine client's likes and dislikes, and collaborate with dietitian to provide favorite foods. *Client is more likely to eat foods that he or she particularly enjoys.*

6. Ensure that client receives small, frequent feedings, including a bedtime snack, rather than three larger meals. *Large amounts of food may be objectionable, or even intolerable, to the client.*
7. Administer vitamin and mineral supplements and stool softeners or bulk extenders, as ordered by physician.
8. If appropriate, ask family members or significant others to bring in special foods that client particularly enjoys.
9. Stay with client during meals *to assist as needed and to offer support and encouragement.*
10. Monitor laboratory values, and report significant changes to physician. *Laboratory values provide objective data regarding nutritional status.*
11. Explain the importance of adequate nutrition and fluid intake. *Client may have inadequate or inaccurate knowledge regarding the contribution of good nutrition to overall wellness.*

Outcome Criteria

1. Client has shown a slow, progressive weight gain during hospitalization.
2. Vital signs, blood pressure, and laboratory serum studies are within normal limits.
3. Client is able to verbalize importance of adequate nutrition and fluid intake.

● DISTURBED SLEEP PATTERN

Definition: Time-limited interruptions of sleep amount and quality due to [internal] or external factors.

Possible Etiologies ("related to")

[Depression]
[Repressed fears]
[Feelings of hopelessness]
[Anxiety]
[Hallucinations]
[Delusional thinking]

Defining Characteristics ("evidenced by")

[Verbal complaints of difficulty falling asleep]
[Awakening earlier or later than desired]
[Interrupted sleep]
Verbal complaints of not feeling well rested
[Awakening very early in the morning and being unable to go back to sleep]

[Excessive yawning and desire to nap during the day]
[Hypersomnia; using sleep as an escape]

Goals/Objectives

Short-term Goal

Client will be able to sleep 4 to 6 hours with the aid of a sleeping medication within 5 days.

Long-term Goal

Client will be able to fall asleep within 30 minutes of retiring and obtain 6 to 8 hours of uninterrupted sleep each night without medication by time of discharge from treatment.

Interventions with *Selected Rationales*

1. Keep strict records of sleeping patterns. *Accurate baseline data are important in planning care to assist client with this problem.*
2. Discourage sleep during the day *to promote more restful sleep at night.*
3. Administer antidepressant medication at bedtime *so client does not become drowsy during the day.*
4. Assist with measures that may promote sleep, such as warm, nonstimulating drinks, light snacks, warm baths, back rubs.
5. Performing relaxation exercises to soft music may be helpful prior to sleep.
6. Limit intake of caffeinated drinks, such as tea, coffee, and colas. *Caffeine is a central nervous system (CNS) stimulant that may interfere with the client's achievement of rest and sleep.*
7. Administer sedative medications, as ordered, *to assist client to achieve sleep until normal sleep pattern is restored.*
8. Some depressed clients may use excessive sleep as an escape. For the client experiencing hypersomnia, set limits on time spent in room. Plan stimulating diversionary activities on a structured, daily schedule. Explore fears and feelings that sleep is helping to suppress.

Outcome Criteria

1. Client is sleeping 6 to 8 hours per night without medication.
2. Client is able to fall asleep within 30 minutes of retiring.
3. Client is dealing with fears and feelings rather than escaping from them through excessive sleep.

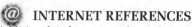

INTERNET REFERENCES

Additional information about depressive disorders, including psychosocial and pharmacological treatment of these disorders, may be located at the following websites:

a. http://depression.about.com/
b. http://www.dbsalliance.org/
c. http://www.fadavis.com/townsend
d. http://www.mentalhealth.com/
e. http://www.mental-health-matters.com/disorders/
f. http://www.mentalhelp.net
g. http://www.nlm.nih.gov/medlineplus
h. http://www.cmellc.com/topics/depress.html

Movie Connections

Prozac Nation (depression) • *The Butcher Boy (depression)*
• *'night, Mother (depression)* • *The Prince of Tides (depression/suicide)*

Mood Disorders: Bipolar Disorders

● **BACKGROUND ASSESSMENT DATA**

Mood is defined as an individual's sustained emotional tone, which significantly influences behavior, personality, and perception. A disturbance in mood is the predominant feature of the mood disorders American Psychiatric Association (APA, 2000). Mood disorders are classified as depressive or bipolar.

Bipolar Disorders

Bipolar disorders are characterized by mood swings from profound depression to extreme euphoria (mania), with intervening periods of normalcy.

During an episode of *mania*, the mood is elevated, expansive, or irritable. Motor activity is excessive and frenzied. Psychotic features may be present. A somewhat milder form is called *hypomania*. It is usually not severe enough to require hospitalization, and it does not include psychotic features.

The diagnostic picture for *bipolar depression* is identical to that described for major depressive disorder, with one exception—the client must have a history of one or more manic episodes.

When the symptom presentation includes rapidly alternating moods (sadness, irritability, euphoria) accompanied by symptoms associated with both depression and mania, the individual is given a diagnosis of *bipolar disorder, mixed*.

Bipolar I Disorder

Bipolar I disorder is the diagnosis given to an individual who is experiencing, or has experienced, a full syndrome of manic or mixed symptoms. The client may also have experienced episodes of depression.

Bipolar II Disorder

Bipolar II disorder is characterized by recurrent bouts of major depression with the episodic occurrence of hypomania. This individual has never experienced a full syndrome of manic or mixed symptoms.

145

Cyclothymic Disorder

The essential feature is a chronic mood disturbance of at least 2 years' duration, involving numerous periods of depression and hypomania, but not of sufficient severity and duration to meet the criteria for either bipolar I or II disorder. There is an absence of psychotic features.

Bipolar Disorder due to General Medical Condition

This disorder is characterized by a prominent and persistent disturbance in mood (bipolar symptomatology) that is judged to be the direct result of the physiological effects of a general medical condition (APA, 2000).

Substance-Induced Bipolar Disorder

The bipolar symptoms associated with this disorder are considered to be the direct result of the physiological effects of a substance (e.g., use or abuse of a drug or a medication, or toxin exposure).

● PREDISPOSING FACTORS TO BIPOLAR DISORDER

1. **Biological**
   a. *Genetics.* Twin studies have indicated a concordance rate for bipolar disorder among monozygotic twins at 60% to 80% compared to 10% to 20% in dizygotic twins. Family studies have shown that if one parent has bipolar disorder, the risk that a child will have the disorder is around 28% (Dubovsky, Davies, & Dubovsky, 2003). If both parents have the disorder, the risk is two to three times as great. Bipolar disorder appears to be equally common in men and women (APA, 2000). Increasing evidence continues to support the role of genetics in the predisposition to bipolar disorder.
   b. *Biochemical.* Just as there is an indication of lowered levels of norepinephrine and dopamine during an episode of depression, the opposite appears to be true of an individual experiencing a manic episode. Thus, the behavioral responses of elation and euphoria may be caused by an excess of these biogenic amines in the brain. It has also been suggested that manic individuals have increased intracellular sodium and calcium. These electrolyte imbalances may be related to abnormalities in cellular membrane function in bipolar disorder.
2. **Physiological**
   a. *Neuroanatomical factors.* Right-sided lesions in the limbic system, temporobasal areas, basal ganglia, and thalamus have been shown to induce secondary

mania. Magnetic resonance imaging studies have revealed enlarged third ventricles and subcortical white matter and periventricular hyperintensities in clients with bipolar disorder (Dubovsky, Davies, & Dubovsky, 2003).

3. **Medication Side Effects**. Certain medications used to treat somatic illnesses have been known to trigger a manic response. The most common of these are the steroids frequently used to treat chronic illnesses such as multiple sclerosis and systemic lupus erythematosus. Some clients whose first episode of mania occurred during steroid therapy have reported spontaneous recurrence of manic symptoms years later. Amphetamines, antidepressants, and high doses of anticonvulsants and narcotics also have the potential for initiating a manic episode (Dubovsky, Davies, & Dubovsky, 2003).

● SYMPTOMATOLOGY (SUBJECTIVE AND OBJECTIVE DATA)

(Note: The symptoms and treatment of bipolar depression are comparable to those of major depression, which are addressed in Chapter 6. This chapter will focus on the symptoms and treatment of bipolar mania.)

1. The affect of a manic individual is one of elation and euphoria—a continuous "high." However, the affect is very labile and may change quickly to hostility (particularly in response to attempts at limit setting), or to sadness, ruminating about past failures.

2. Alterations in thought processes and communication patterns are manifested by the following:
   a. **Flight of Ideas**. There is a continuous, rapid shift from one topic to another.
   b. **Loquaciousness**. The pressure of the speech is so forceful and strong that it is difficult to interrupt maladaptive thought processes.
   c. **Delusions of Grandeur**. The individual believes he or she is all important, all powerful, with feelings of greatness and magnificence.
   d. **Delusions of Persecution**. The individual believes someone or something desires to harm or violate him or her in some way.

3. Motor activity is constant. The individual is literally moving at all times.

4. Dress is often inappropriate: bright colors that do not match, clothing inappropriate for age or stature, excessive makeup and jewelry.

5. The individual has a meager appetite, despite excessive activity level. He or she is unable or unwilling to stop moving in order to eat.

6. Sleep patterns are disturbed. Client becomes oblivious to feelings of fatigue, and rest and sleep are abandoned for days or weeks.
7. Spending sprees are common. Individual spends large amounts of money, which is not available, on numerous items, which are not needed.
8. Usual inhibitions are discarded in favor of sexual and behavioral indiscretions.
9. Manipulative behavior and limit testing are common in the attempt to fulfill personal desires. Verbal or physical hostility may follow failure in these attempts.
10. Projection is a major defense mechanism. The individual refuses to accept responsibility for the negative consequences of personal behavior.
11. There is an inability to concentrate because of a limited attention span. The individual is easily distracted by even the slightest stimulus in the environment.
12. Alterations in sensory perception may occur, and the individual may experience hallucinations.
13. As agitation increases, symptoms intensify. Unless the client is placed in a protective environment, death can occur from exhaustion or injury.

● **COMMON NURSING DIAGNOSES
   AND INTERVENTIONS FOR MANIA**

(Interventions are applicable to various health-care settings, such as inpatient and partial hospitalization, community outpatient clinic, home health, and private practice.)

● **RISK FOR INJURY**

Definition: At risk of injury as a result of environmental conditions interacting with the individual's adaptive and defensive resources

Related/Risk Factors ("related to")
Biochemical dysfunction
Psychological (affective orientation)
[Extreme hyperactivity]
[Destructive behaviors]
[Anger directed at the environment]
[Hitting head (hand, arm, foot, etc.) against wall when angry]
[Temper tantrums—becomes destructive of inanimate objects]
[Increased agitation and lack of control over purposeless, and potentially injurious, movements]

Goals/Objectives

Short-term Goal

Client will no longer exhibit potentially injurious movements after 24 hours with administration of tranquilizing medication.

Long-term Goal

Client will experience no physical injury.

Interventions with *Selected Rationales*

1. Reduce environmental stimuli. Assign a private room, if possible, with soft lighting, low noise level, and simple room decor. *In the hyperactive state, the client is extremely distractible, and responses to even the slightest stimuli are exaggerated.*
2. Assign to a quiet unit, if possible. *Milieu unit may be too distracting.*
3. Limit group activities. Help client try to establish one or two close relationships. *Client's ability to interact with others is impaired. He or she feels more secure in a one-to-one relationship that is consistent over time.*
4. Remove hazardous objects and substances from client's environment (including smoking materials). *Client's rationality is impaired, and he or she may harm self inadvertently. Client safety is a nursing priority.*
5. Stay with the client *to offer support and provide a feeling of security* as agitation grows and hyperactivity increases.
6. Provide structured schedule of activities that includes established rest periods throughout the day. *A structured schedule provides a feeling of security for the client.*
7. Provide physical activities as a substitution for purposeless hyperactivity (examples: brisk walks, housekeeping chores, dance therapy, aerobics). *Physical exercise provides a safe and effective means of relieving pent-up tension.*
8. Administer tranquilizing medication, as ordered by physician. Antipsychotic drugs are commonly prescribed for rapid relief of agitation and hyperactivity. Atypical forms commonly used include olanzapine, ziprasidone, and aripiprazole. Examples of the typical forms include haloperidol and chlorpromazine. Observe for effectiveness and evidence of adverse side effects (see Chapter 28).

Outcome Criteria

1. Client is no longer exhibiting signs of physical agitation.
2. Client exhibits no evidence of physical injury obtained while experiencing hyperactive behavior.

● RISK FOR SELF-DIRECTED OR OTHER-DIRECTED VIOLENCE

Definition: At risk for behaviors in which an individual demonstrates that he or she can be physically, emotionally, and/or sexually harmful [either to self or to others]

Related/Risk Factors ("related to")

[Manic excitement]
[Biochemical alterations]
[Threat to self-concept]
[Suspicion of others]
[Paranoid ideation]
[Delusions]
[Hallucinations]
[Rage reactions]
Body language (e.g., rigid posture, clenching of fists and jaw, hyperactivity, pacing, breathlessness, threatening stances)
[History or threats of violence toward self or others or of destruction to the property of others]
Impulsivity
Suicidal ideation, plan, available means
[Repetition of verbalizations (continuous complaints, requests, and demands)]

Goals/Objectives

Short-term Goal

Client's agitation will be maintained at manageable level with the administration of tranquilizing medication during first week of treatment (decreasing risk of violence to self or others).

Long-term Goal

Client will not harm self or others.

Interventions with *Selected Rationales*

1. Maintain low level of stimuli in client's environment (low lighting, few people, simple decor, low noise level). *Anxiety and agitation rise in a stimulating environment. Individuals may be perceived as threatening by a suspicious, agitated client.*
2. Observe client's behavior frequently (every 15 minutes). *Close observation is required so that intervention can occur if required to ensure client's (and others') safety.*
3. Remove all dangerous objects from client's environment (sharp objects, glass or mirrored items, belts, ties, smoking

materials) *so that in his or her agitated, hyperactive state, client may not use them to harm self or others.*

4. Try to redirect the violent behavior with physical outlets for the client's hostility (e.g., punching bag). *Physical exercise is a safe and effective way of relieving pent-up tension.*

5. Intervene at the first sign of increased anxiety, agitation, or verbal or behavioral aggression. Offer empathetic response to client's feelings: "You seem anxious (or frustrated, or angry) about this situation. How can I help?" *Validation of the client's feelings conveys a caring attitude and offering assistance reinforces trust.*

6. Staff should maintain and convey a calm attitude to the client. Respond matter-of-factly to verbal hostility. *Anxiety is contagious and can be transmitted from staff to client.*

7. Have sufficient staff available to indicate a show of strength to client if necessary. *This conveys to the client evidence of control over the situation and provides some physical security for staff.*

8. Administer tranquilizing medications as ordered by physician. Monitor medication for effectiveness and for adverse side effects.

9. If the client is not calmed by "talking down" or by medication, use of mechanical restraints may be necessary. The avenue of the "least restrictive alternative" must be selected when planning interventions for a violent client. Restraints should be used only as a last resort, after all other interventions have been unsuccessful, and the client is clearly at risk of harm to self or others.

10. If restraint is deemed necessary, ensure that sufficient staff is available to assist. Follow protocol established by the institution. The Joint Commission formerly, the Joint Commission on Accreditation of Healthcare Organizations [JCAHO]) requires that an in-person evaluation (by a physician, clinical psychologist, or other licensed independent practitioner responsible for the care of the patient) be conducted within 1 hour of initiating restraint or seclusion (The Joint Commission, 2010). The physician must reissue a new order for restraints every 4 hours for adults and every 1 to 2 hours for children and adolescents.

11. The Joint Commision requires that the client in restraints be observed every 15 minutes to ensure that circulation to extremities is not compromised (check temperature, color, pulses); to assist client with needs related to nutrition, hydration, and elimination; and to position client so that comfort is facilitated and aspiration can be prevented. Some

institutions may require continuous one-to-one monitoring of restrained clients, particularly those who are highly agitated, and for whom there is a high risk of self- or accidental injury. ***Client safety is a nursing priority.***

12. As agitation decreases, assess client's readiness for restraint removal or reduction. Remove one restraint at a time, while assessing client's response. ***This procedure minimizes the risk of injury to client and staff.***

Outcome Criteria
1. Client is able to verbalize anger in an appropriate manner.
2. There is no evidence of violent behavior to self or others.
3. Client is no longer exhibiting hyperactive behaviors.

● IMBALANCED NUTRITION, LESS THAN BODY REQUIREMENTS

Definition: Intake of nutrients insufficient to meet metabolic needs

Possible Etiologies ("related to")
[Refusal or inability to sit still long enough to eat meals]
[Lack of appetite]
[Excessive physical agitation]
[Physical exertion in excess of energy produced through caloric intake]
[Lack of interest in food]

Defining Characteristics ("evidenced by")
Loss of weight
Pale mucous membranes
Poor muscle tone
[Amenorrhea]
[Poor skin turgor]
[Anemias]
[Electrolyte imbalances]

Goals/Objectives
Short-term Goal
Client will consume sufficient finger foods and between-meal snacks to meet recommended daily allowances of nutrients.

Long-term Goal
Client will exhibit no signs or symptoms of malnutrition.

Interventions with *Selected Rationales*

1. In collaboration with dietitian, determine the number of calories required to provide adequate nutrition for maintenance or realistic (according to body structure and height) weight gain.
2. Provide client with high-protein, high-calorie, nutritious finger foods and drinks that can be consumed "on the run." *Because of hyperactive state, client has difficulty sitting still long enough to eat a meal. The likelihood is greater that he or she will consume food and drinks that can be carried around and eaten with little effort.*
3. Have juice and snacks available on the unit at all times. *Nutritious intake is required on a regular basis to compensate for increased caloric requirements due to hyperactivity.*
4. Maintain accurate record of intake, output, and calorie count. *This information is necessary to make an accurate nutritional assessment and maintain client's safety.*
5. Weigh client daily. *Weight loss or gain is important nutritional assessment information.*
6. Determine client's likes and dislikes, and collaborate with dietitian to provide favorite foods. *Client is more likely to eat foods that he or she particularly enjoys.*
7. Administer vitamin and mineral supplements, as ordered by physician, *to improve nutritional state.*
8. Pace or walk with client as finger foods are taken. As agitation subsides, sit with client during meals. Offer support and encouragement. Assess and record amount consumed. *Presence of a trusted individual may provide feeling of security and decrease agitation. Encouragement and positive reinforcement increase self-esteem and foster repetition of desired behaviors.*
9. Monitor laboratory values, and report significant changes to physician. *Laboratory values provide objective nutritional assessment data.*
10. Explain the importance of adequate nutrition and fluid intake. *Client may have inadequate or inaccurate knowledge regarding the contribution of good nutrition to overall wellness.*

Outcome Criteria

1. Client has gained (maintained) weight during hospitalization.
2. Vital signs, blood pressure, and laboratory serum studies are within normal limits.
3. Client is able to verbalize importance of adequate nutrition and fluid intake.

• DISTURBED THOUGHT PROCESSES

Definition: Disruption in cognitive operations and activities

Possible Etiologies ("related to")

[Biochemical alterations]
[Electrolyte imbalance]
[Psychotic process]
[Sleep deprivation]

Defining Characteristics ("evidenced by")

Inaccurate interpretation of environment
Hypervigilance
[Altered attention span]—distractibility
Egocentricity
[Decreased ability to grasp ideas]
[Impaired ability to make decisions, problem-solve, reason]
[Delusions of grandeur]
[Delusions of persecution]
[Suspiciousness]

Goals/Objectives

Short-term Goal

Within 1 week, client will be able to recognize and verbalize when thinking is non–reality-based.

Long-term Goal

By time of discharge from treatment, client's verbalizations will reflect reality-based thinking with no evidence of delusional ideation.

Interventions with *Selected Rationales*

1. Convey your acceptance of client's need for the false belief, while letting him or her know that you do not share the delusion. *A positive response would convey to the client that you accept the delusion as reality.*

2. Do not argue or deny the belief. Use *reasonable doubt* as a therapeutic technique: "I understand that you believe this is true, but I personally find it hard to accept." *Arguing with the client or denying the belief serves no useful purpose, because delusional ideas are not eliminated by this approach and the development of a trusting relationship may be impeded.*

3. Use the techniques of *consensual validation* and *seeking clarification* when communication reflects alteration in thinking. (*Examples:* "Is it that you mean...?" or "I don't understand what you mean by that. Would you please explain?")

These techniques reveal to the client how he or she is being perceived by others, and the responsibility for not understanding is accepted by the nurse.

4. Reinforce and focus on reality. Talk about real events and real people. Use real situations and events to divert client from long, tedious, repetitive verbalizations of false ideas.

5. Give positive reinforcement as client is able to differentiate between reality-based and non–reality-based thinking. *Positive reinforcement enhances self-esteem and encourages repetition of desirable behaviors.*

6. Teach client to intervene, using thought-stopping techniques, when irrational thoughts prevail. Thought stopping involves using the command "Stop!" or a loud noise (such as hand clapping) to interrupt unwanted thoughts. *This noise or command distracts the individual from the undesirable thinking, which often precedes undesirable emotions or behaviors.*

7. Use touch cautiously, particularly if thoughts reveal ideas of persecution. *Clients who are suspicious may perceive touch as threatening and may respond with aggression.*

Outcome Criteria

1. Thought processes reflect an accurate interpretation of the environment.
2. Client is able to recognize thoughts that are not based in reality and intervene to stop their progression.

● DISTURBED SENSORY PERCEPTION

Definition: Change in the amount or patterning of incoming stimuli [either internally or externally initiated] accompanied by a diminished, exaggerated, distorted, or impaired response to such stimuli

Possible Etiologies ("related to")

Biochemical imbalance
Electrolyte imbalance
[Sleep deprivation]
[Psychotic process]

Defining Characteristics ("evidenced by")

Change in usual response to stimuli
Hallucinations
Disorientation

[Inappropriate responses]
[Rapid mood swings]
[Exaggerated emotional responses]
[Visual and auditory distortions]
[Talking and laughing to self]
[Listening pose (tilting head to one side as if listening)]
[Stops talking in middle of sentence to listen]

Goals/Objectives
Short-term Goal
Client will be able to recognize and verbalize when he or she is interpreting the environment inaccurately.

Long-term Goal
Client will be able to define and test reality, eliminating the occurrence of sensory misperceptions.

Interventions with *Selected Rationales*

1. Observe client for signs of hallucinations (listening pose, laughing or talking to self, stopping in midsentence). *Early intervention may prevent aggressive responses to command hallucinations.*
2. Avoid touching the client before warning him or her that you are about to do so. *Client may perceive touch as threatening and respond in an aggressive manner.*
3. An attitude of acceptance will encourage the client to share the content of the hallucination with you. *This is important in order to prevent possible injury to the client or others from command hallucinations.*
4. Do not reinforce the hallucination. Use words such as "the voices" instead of "they" when referring to the hallucination. *Words like "they" validate that the voices are real.*

> **CLINICAL PEARL** Let the client who is "hearing voices" know that you do not share the perception.
> Say, "Even though I realize that the voices are real to you, I do not hear any voices speaking." The nurse must be honest with the client so that he or she may realize that the hallucinations are not real.

5. Try to connect the times of the misperceptions to times of increased anxiety. Help client to understand this connection. *If client can learn to interrupt the escalating anxiety, reality orientation may be maintained.*
6. Try to distract the client away from the misperception. *Involvement in interpersonal activities and explanation of the actual situation may bring the client back to reality.*

Outcome Criteria

1. Client is able to differentiate between reality and unrealistic events or situations.
2. Client is able to refrain from responding to false sensory perceptions.

● IMPAIRED SOCIAL INTERACTION

Definition: Insufficient or excessive quantity or ineffective quality of social exchange

Possible Etiologies ("related to")

Disturbed thought processes
[Delusions of grandeur]
[Delusions of persecution]
Self-concept disturbance

Defining Characteristics ("evidenced by")

Discomfort in social situations
Inability to receive or communicate a satisfying sense of social engagement (e.g., belonging, caring, interest, or shared history)
Use of unsuccessful social interaction behaviors
Dysfunctional interaction with others
[Excessive use of projection—does not accept responsibility for own behavior]
[Verbal manipulation]
[Inability to delay gratification]

Goals/Objectives

Short-term Goal

Client will verbalize which of his or her interaction behaviors are appropriate and which are inappropriate within 1 week.

Long-term Goal

Client will demonstrate use of appropriate interaction skills as evidenced by lack of, or marked decrease in, manipulation of others to fulfill own desires.

Interventions with *Selected Rationales*

1. Recognize the purpose these behaviors serve for the client: to reduce feelings of insecurity by increasing feelings of power and control. *Understanding the motivation behind the manipulation may facilitate acceptance of the individual and his or her behavior.*

2. Set limits on manipulative behaviors. Explain to client what you expect and what the consequences are if the limits are violated. Limits must be agreed upon by all staff who will be working with the client. *Client is unable to establish own limits, so this must be done for him or her. Unless administration of consequences for violation of limits is consistent, manipulative behavior will not be eliminated.*
3. Do not argue, bargain, or try to reason with the client. Merely state the limits and expectations. Be sure to follow through with consequences if limits are violated. *Consistency is essential for success of this intervention.* Do not let this "charmer" talk you out of it. *Ignoring these attempts may work to decrease manipulative behaviors.*
4. Provide positive reinforcement for nonmanipulative behaviors. Explore feelings, and help the client seek more appropriate ways of dealing with them. *Positive reinforcement enhances self-esteem and promotes repetition of desirable behaviors.*
5. Help client recognize consequences of own behaviors and refrain from attributing them to others. *Client must accept responsibility for own behaviors before adaptive change can occur.*
6. Help client identify positive aspects about self, recognize accomplishments, and feel good about them. *As self-esteem is increased, client will feel less need to manipulate others for own gratification.*

Outcome Criteria
1. Client is able to verbalize positive aspects of self.
2. Client accepts responsibility for own behaviors.
3. Client does not manipulate others for gratification of own needs.

● INSOMNIA

Definition: A disruption in amount and quality of sleep that impairs functioning

Possible Etiologies ("related to")
[Excessive hyperactivity]
[Agitation]
[Biochemical alterations]

Defining Characteristics ("evidenced by")
Difficulty falling asleep
[Pacing in hall during sleeping hours]

[Sleeping only short periods at a time]
[Numerous periods of wakefulness during the night]
[Awakening and rising extremely early in the morning; exhibiting signs of restlessness]

Goals/Objectives

Short-term Goal

Within 3 days, with the aid of a sleeping medication, client will sleep 4 to 6 hours without awakening.

Long-term Goal

By time of discharge from treatment, client will be able to acquire 6 to 8 hours of uninterrupted sleep without sleeping medication.

Interventions with *Selected Rationales*

1. Provide a quiet environment, with a low level of stimulation. *Hyperactivity increases and ability to achieve sleep and rest are hindered in a stimulating environment.*
2. Monitor sleep patterns. Provide structured schedule of activities that includes established times for naps or rest. *Accurate baseline data are important in planning care to help client with this problem. A structured schedule, including time for naps, will help the hyperactive client achieve much-needed rest.*
3. Assess client's activity level. Client may ignore or be unaware of feelings of fatigue. Observe for signs such as increasing restlessness, fine tremors, slurred speech, and puffy, dark circles under eyes. *Client can collapse from exhaustion if hyperactivity is uninterrupted and rest is not achieved.*
4. Before bedtime, provide nursing measures that promote sleep, such as back rub; warm bath; warm, nonstimulating drinks; soft music; and relaxation exercises.
5. Prohibit intake of caffeinated drinks, such as tea, coffee, and colas. *Caffeine is a CNS stimulant and may interfere with the client's achievement of rest and sleep.*
6. Administer sedative medications, as ordered, to assist client achieve sleep until normal sleep pattern is restored.

Outcome Criteria

1. Client is sleeping 6 to 8 hours per night without sleeping medication.
2. Client is able to fall asleep within 30 minutes of retiring.
3. Client is dealing openly with fears and feelings rather than manifesting denial of them through hyperactivity.

INTERNET REFERENCES

Additional information about bipolar disorders, including psychosocial and pharmacological treatment of these disorders, may be located at the following websites:

a. http://www.dbsalliance.org/
b. http://www.fadavis.com/townsend
c. http://www.mentalhealth.com/
d. http://www.cmellc.com/topics/bipolar.html
e. http://www.mental-health-matters.com/disorders/
f. http://www.mentalhelp.net
g. http://www.nlm.nih.gov/medlineplus

 Movie Connections

Lust for Life (bipolar disorder) ● *Call Me Anna (bipolar disorder)*
● *Blue Sky (bipolar disorder)* ● *A Woman Under the Influence (bipolar disorder)*

Anxiety Disorders

● **BACKGROUND ASSESSMENT DATA**

The characteristic features of this group of disorders are symptoms of anxiety and avoidance behavior. Anxiety disorders are categorized in the following manner:

Panic Disorder (with or without Agoraphobia)

Panic disorder is characterized by recurrent panic attacks, the onset of which are unpredictable, and manifested by intense apprehension, fear, or terror, often associated with feelings of impending doom, and accompanied by intense physical discomfort. The attacks usually last minutes or, more rarely, hours. If accompanied by agoraphobia, there is a fear of being in places or situations from which escape might be difficult or in which help might not be available in the event of a panic attack (American Psychiatric Association [APA], 2000). Common agoraphobic situations include being outside the home alone; being in a crowd or standing in a line; being on a bridge; and traveling in a bus, train, or car.

Agoraphobia without History of Panic Disorder

The APA (2000) *Diagnostic and Statistical Manual of Mental Disorders, Fourth Edition, Text Revision (DSM-IV-TR)* identifies the essential feature of this disorder as fear of being in places or situations from which escape might be difficult or in which help might not be available in the event of suddenly developing a symptom(s) that could be incapacitating or extremely embarrassing. Travel is restricted or the individual needs a companion when away from home or else endures agoraphobic situations despite intense anxiety.

Social Phobia

Social phobia is characterized by a persistent fear of behaving or performing in the presence of others in a way that will be humiliating or embarrassing to the individual. The individual has extreme concerns about being exposed to possible scrutiny by others and fears social or performance situations in which embarrassment may occur (APA, 2000). Exposure to the phobic situation is avoided, or it is endured with intense anxiety. Common social phobias include speaking or writing in front of a group of people, eating in the presence of others, and using public restrooms.

Specific Phobia

Formerly called *simple phobia*, this disorder is characterized by persistent fears of specific objects or situations. These phobias are fairly widespread among the general population, the most common being fear of animals (zoophobia), fear of closed places (claustrophobia), and fear of heights (acrophobia). Exposure to the phobic stimulus is avoided or endured with intense anxiety.

Obsessive-Compulsive Disorder

This disorder is characterized by involuntary recurring thoughts or images that the individual is unable to ignore and by recurring impulse to perform a seemingly purposeless activity. These obsessions and compulsions serve to prevent extreme anxiety on the part of the individual.

Posttraumatic Stress Disorder

Posttraumatic stress disorder (PTSD) is characterized by the development of physiological and behavioral symptoms following a psychologically traumatic event that is generally outside the range of usual human experience. The stressor, which would be considered markedly distressing to almost anyone, has usually been experienced with intense fear, terror, and helplessness. If duration of the symptoms is 3 months or longer, the diagnosis is specified as "chronic." If there is a delay of 6 months or longer in the onset of symptoms, the diagnosis is specified as "delayed onset."

Acute Stress Disorder

Acute stress disorder is characterized by the development of physiological and behavioral symptoms similar to those of PTSD. The major difference in the diagnoses lies in the length of time the symptoms exist. With acute stress disorder, the symptoms must subside within 4 weeks of occurrence of the stressor. If they last longer than 4 weeks, the individual is given the diagnosis of PTSD.

Generalized Anxiety Disorder

This disorder is characterized by chronic, unrealistic, and excessive anxiety and worry. The symptoms must have occurred more days than not for at least 6 months and must cause clinically significant distress or impairment in social, occupational, or other important areas of functioning (APA, 2000). Symptoms include restlessness, feeling "on edge," becoming easily fatigued, difficulty concentrating, and irritability.

Anxiety Disorder Due to a General Medical Condition

The symptoms of this disorder are judged to be the direct physiological consequence of a general medical condition. Symptoms may include prominent generalized anxiety symptoms, panic attacks, or obsessions or compulsions (APA, 2000). Medical conditions that have been known to cause anxiety disorders include endocrine, cardiovascular, respiratory, metabolic, and neurological disorders.

Substance-Induced Anxiety Disorder

The *DSM-IV-TR* (APA, 2000) describes the essential features of this disorder as prominent anxiety symptoms that are judged to be caused by the direct physiological effects of a substance (i.e., a drug of abuse, a medication, or toxin exposure). The symptoms may occur during substance intoxication or withdrawal and may involve intense anxiety, panic attacks, phobias, or obsessions or compulsions.

● PREDISPOSING FACTORS TO ANXIETY DISORDERS

1. **Physiological**
   a. *Biochemical:* Increased levels of norepinephrine have been noted in panic and generalized anxiety disorders. Abnormal elevations of blood lactate have also been noted in clients with panic disorder. Decreased levels of serotonin have been implicated in the etiology of obsessive-compulsive disorder.
   b. *Genetic:* Studies suggest that anxiety disorders are prevalent within the general population. It has been shown that they are more common among first-degree biological relatives of people with the disorders than among the general population (APA, 2000).
   c. *Medical or Substance-Induced:* Anxiety disorders may be caused by a variety of medical conditions or the ingestion of various substances. (Refer to previous section on categories of anxiety disorders.)
2. **Psychosocial**
   a. *Psychodynamic Theory:* The psychodynamic view focuses on the inability of the ego to intervene when conflict occurs between the id and the superego, producing anxiety. For

various reasons (unsatisfactory parent-child relationship; conditional love or provisional gratification), ego development is delayed. When developmental defects in ego functions compromise the capacity to modulate anxiety, the individual resorts to unconscious mechanisms to resolve the conflict. Overuse or ineffective use of ego defense mechanisms results in maladaptive responses to anxiety.

b. ***Cognitive Theory:*** The main thesis of the cognitive view is that faulty, distorted, or counterproductive thinking patterns accompany or precede maladaptive behaviors and emotional disorders (Sadock & Sadock, 2007). When there is a disturbance in this central mechanism of cognition, there is a consequent disturbance in feeling and behavior. Because of distorted thinking, anxiety is maintained by erroneous or dysfunctional appraisal of a situation. There is a loss of ability to reason regarding the problem, whether it is physical or interpersonal. The individual feels vulnerable in a given situation, and the distorted thinking results in an irrational appraisal, fostering a negative outcome.

● SYMPTOMATOLOGY (SUBJECTIVE AND OBJECTIVE DATA)

An individual may experience a panic attack under any of the following conditions:

- As the predominant disturbance, with no apparent precipitant
- When exposed to a phobic stimulus
- When attempts are made to curtail ritualistic behavior
- Following a psychologically traumatic event

Symptoms include the following (APA, 2000):

- Pounding, rapid heart rate
- Feeling of choking or smothering
- Difficulty breathing
- Pain in the chest
- Feeling dizzy or faint
- Increased perspiration
- Feeling of numbness or tingling in the extremities
- Trembling
- Fear that one is dying or going crazy
- Sense of impending doom
- Feelings of unreality (derealization and/or depersonalization)

Other symptoms of anxiety disorders include the following:

1. Restlessness, feeling "on edge," excessive worry, being easily fatigued, difficulty concentrating, irritability, and sleep disturbances (generalized anxiety disorder).

2. Recurrent and intrusive recollections or dreams about the traumatic event, feeling of reliving the trauma (flashback episodes), difficulty feeling emotion (a "numbing" affect), insomnia, and irritability or outbursts of anger (PTSD).
3. Repetitive, obsessive thoughts, common ones being related to violence, contamination, and doubt; repetitive, compulsive performance of purposeless activity, such as handwashing, counting, checking, and touching (obsessive-compulsive disorder).
4. Marked and persistent fears of specific objects or situations (specific phobia), social or performance situations (social phobia), or being in a situation from which one has difficulty escaping (agoraphobia).

Common Nursing Diagnoses and Interventions

(Interventions are applicable to various health-care settings, such as inpatient and partial hospitalization, community outpatient clinic, home health, and private practice.)

● ANXIETY (PANIC)

Definition: Vague uneasy feeling of discomfort or dread accompanied by an autonomic response (the source often nonspecific or unknown to the individual); a feeling of apprehension caused by anticipation of danger. It is an alerting signal that warns of impending danger and enables the individual to take measures to deal with threat.

Possible Etiologies ("related to")

Unconscious conflict about essential values and goals of life
Situational and maturational crises
[Real or perceived] threat to self-concept
[Real or perceived] threat of death
Unmet needs
[Being exposed to a phobic stimulus]
[Attempts at interference with ritualistic behaviors]
[Traumatic experience]

Defining Characteristics ("evidenced by")

Increased respiration
Increased pulse
Decreased or increased blood pressure
Nausea
Confusion

Increased perspiration
Faintness
Trembling or shaking
Restlessness
Insomnia
[Nightmares or visual perceptions of traumatic event]
[Fear of dying, going crazy, or doing something uncontrolled during an attack]

Goals/Objectives
Short-term Goal
Client will verbalize ways to intervene in escalating anxiety within 1 week.

Long-term Goal
Client will be able to recognize symptoms of onset of anxiety and intervene before reaching panic stage by time of discharge from treatment.

Interventions with *Selected Rationales*

1. Maintain a calm, nonthreatening manner while working with client. *Anxiety is contagious and may be transferred from staff to client or vice versa. Client develops feeling of security in presence of calm staff person.*
2. Reassure client of his or her safety and security. This can be conveyed by physical presence of nurse. Do not leave client alone at this time. *Client may fear for his or her life. Presence of a trusted individual provides client with feeling of security and assurance of personal safety.*
3. Use simple words and brief messages, spoken calmly and clearly, to explain hospital experiences to client. *In an intensely anxious situation, client is unable to comprehend anything but the most elementary communication.*
4. Keep immediate surroundings low in stimuli (dim lighting, few people, simple decor). *A stimulating environment may increase level of anxiety.*
5. Administer tranquilizing medication, as ordered by physician. Assess medication for effectiveness and for adverse side effects.
6. When level of anxiety has been reduced, explore with client possible reasons for occurrence. *Recognition of precipitating factor(s) is the first step in teaching client to interrupt escalation of the anxiety.*
7. Encourage client to talk about traumatic experience under nonthreatening conditions. Help client work through feelings of guilt related to the traumatic event. Help client understand that this was an event to which most people

would have responded in like manner. Support client during flashbacks of the experience. *Verbalization of feelings in a nonthreatening environment may help client come to terms with unresolved issues.*

8. Teach signs and symptoms of escalating anxiety, and ways to interrupt its progression (e.g., relaxation techniques, deep-breathing exercises, physical exercises, brisk walks, jogging, meditation).

Outcome Criteria

1. Client is able to maintain anxiety at level in which problem solving can be accomplished.
2. Client is able to verbalize signs and symptoms of escalating anxiety.
3. Client is able to demonstrate techniques for interrupting the progression of anxiety to the panic level.

● FEAR

Definition: Response to perceived threat that is consciously recognized as a danger.

Possible Etiologies ("related to")

Phobic stimulus
[Being in place or situation from which escape might be difficult]
[Causing embarrassment to self in front of others]

Defining Characteristics ("evidenced by")

[Refuses to leave own home alone]
[Refuses to eat in public]
[Refuses to speak or perform in public]
[Refuses to expose self to (specify phobic object or situation)]
Identifies object of fear
[Symptoms of apprehension or sympathetic stimulation in presence of phobic object or situation]

Goals/Objectives

Short-term Goal

Client will discuss phobic object or situation with nurse or therapist within 5 days.

Long-term Goal

Client will be able to function in presence of phobic object or situation without experiencing panic anxiety by time of discharge from treatment.

Interventions with *Selected Rationales*

1. Reassure client of his or her safety and security. *At panic level of anxiety, client may fear for own life.*
2. Explore client's perception of threat to physical integrity or threat to self-concept. *It is important to understand the client's perception of the phobic object or situation in order to assist with the desensitization process.*
3. Discuss reality of the situation with client in order to recognize aspects that can be changed and those that cannot. *Client must accept the reality of the situation (aspects that cannot change) before the work of reducing the fear can progress.*
4. Include client in making decisions related to selection of alternative coping strategies. (*Example:* Client may choose either to avoid the phobic stimulus or attempt to eliminate the fear associated with it.) *Allowing the client choices provides a measure of control and serves to increase feelings of self-worth.*
5. If the client elects to work on elimination of the fear, techniques of desensitization may be employed. This is a systematic plan of behavior modification, designed to expose the individual gradually to the situation or object (either in reality or through fantasizing) until the fear is no longer experienced. This is also sometimes accomplished through implosion therapy, in which the individual is "flooded" with stimuli related to the phobic situation or object (rather than in gradual steps) until anxiety is no longer experienced in relation to the object or situation. *Fear is decreased as the physical and psychological sensations diminish in response to repeated exposure to the phobic stimulus under nonthreatening conditions.*
6. Encourage client to explore underlying feelings that may be contributing to irrational fears. Help client to understand how facing these feelings, rather than suppressing them, can result in more adaptive coping abilities. *Verbalization of feelings in a nonthreatening environment may help client come to terms with unresolved issues.*

Outcome Criteria

1. Client does not experience disabling fear when exposed to phobic object or situation, *or*
2. Client verbalizes ways in which he or she will be able to avoid the phobic object or situation with minimal change in lifestyle.
3. Client is able to demonstrate adaptive coping techniques that may be used to maintain anxiety at a tolerable level.

● INEFFECTIVE COPING

Definition: Inability to form a valid appraisal of the stressors, inadequate choices of practiced responses, and/or inability to use available resources.

Possible Etiologies ("related to")
[Underdeveloped ego; punitive superego]
[Fear of failure]
Situational crises
Maturational crises
[Personal vulnerability]
[Inadequate support systems]
[Unmet dependency needs]

Defining Characteristics ("evidenced by")
[Ritualistic behavior]
[Obsessive thoughts]
Inability to meet basic needs
Inability to meet role expectations
Inadequate problem solving
[Alteration in societal participation]

Goals/Objectives
Short-term Goal
Within 1 week, client will decrease participation in ritualistic behavior by half.

Long-term Goal
By time of discharge from treatment, client will demonstrate ability to cope effectively without resorting to obsessive-compulsive behaviors or increased dependency.

Interventions with *Selected Rationales*
1. Assess client's level of anxiety. Try to determine the types of situations that increase anxiety and result in ritualistic behaviors. *Recognition of precipitating factors is the first step in teaching the client to interrupt the escalating anxiety.*
2. Initially meet client's dependency needs as required. Encourage independence and give positive reinforcement for independent behaviors. *Sudden and complete elimination of all avenues for dependency would create intense anxiety on the part of the client. Positive reinforcement enhances self-esteem and encourages repetition of desired behaviors.*
3. In the beginning of treatment allow plenty of time for rituals. Do not be judgmental or verbalize disapproval of the

behavior. *To deny client this activity may precipitate panic level of anxiety.*

4. Support client's efforts to explore the meaning and purpose of the behavior. *Client may be unaware of the relationship between emotional problems and compulsive behaviors. Recognition is important before change can occur.*
5. Provide structured schedule of activities for the client, including adequate time for completion of rituals. *Structure provides a feeling of security for the anxious client.*
6. Gradually begin to limit the amount of time allotted for ritualistic behavior as client becomes more involved in unit activities. *Anxiety is minimized when client is able to replace ritualistic behaviors with more adaptive ones.*
7. Give positive reinforcement for nonritualistic behaviors. *Positive reinforcement enhances self-esteem and encourages repetition of desired behaviors.*
8. Encourage recognition of situations that provoke obsessive thoughts or ritualistic behaviors. Explain ways of interrupting these thoughts and patterns of behavior (e.g., thought-stopping techniques, relaxation techniques, physical exercise, or other constructive activity with which client feels comfortable).

Outcome Criteria

1. Client is able to verbalize signs and symptoms of increasing anxiety and intervene to maintain anxiety at manageable level.
2. Client demonstrates ability to interrupt obsessive thoughts and refrain from ritualistic behaviors in response to stressful situations.

● POWERLESSNESS

Definition: The perception that one's own action will not significantly affect an outcome; a perceived lack of control over a current situation or immediate happening.

Possible Etiologies ("related to")

Lifestyle of helplessness
[Fear of disapproval from others]
[Unmet dependency needs]
[Lack of positive feedback]
[Consistent negative feedback]

Defining Characteristics ("evidenced by")

Verbal expressions of having no control (e.g., over self-care, situation, outcome)

Nonparticipation in care or decision making when opportunities are provided

Expression of doubt regarding role performance

Reluctance to express true feelings

Apathy

Dependence on others that may result in irritability, resentment, anger, and guilt

Passivity

Goals/Objectives

Short-term Goal

Client will participate in decision making regarding own care within 5 days.

Long-term Goal

Client will be able to effectively problem-solve ways to take control of his or her life situation by discharge, thereby decreasing feelings of powerlessness.

Interventions with *Selected Rationales*

1. Allow client to take as much responsibility as possible for own self-care practices. *Providing client with choices will increase his or her feelings of control.*

   Examples are as follows:
   a. Include client in setting the goals of care he or she wishes to achieve.
   b. Allow client to establish own schedule for self-care activities.
   c. Provide client with privacy as need is determined.
   d. Provide positive feedback for decisions made. Respect client's right to make those decisions independently, and refrain from attempting to influence him or her toward those that may seem more logical.

2. Help client set realistic goals. *Unrealistic goals set the client up for failure and reinforce feelings of powerlessness.*

3. Help identify areas of life situation that client can control. *Client's emotional condition interferes with his or her ability to solve problems. Assistance is required to perceive the benefits and consequences of available alternatives accurately.*

4. Help client identify areas of life situation that are not within his or her ability to control. Encourage verbalization of feelings related to this inability *in an effort to deal with unresolved issues and accept what cannot be changed.*

5. Identify ways in which client can achieve. Encourage participation in these activities, and provide positive reinforcement for participation, as well as for achievement. *Positive*

reinforcement enhances self-esteem and encourages repetition of desirable behaviors.

Outcome Criteria

1. Client verbalizes choices made in a plan to maintain control over his or her life situation.
2. Client verbalizes honest feelings about life situations over which he or she has no control.
3. Client is able to verbalize system for problem-solving as required for adequate role performance.

• SOCIAL ISOLATION

Definition: Aloneness experienced by the individual and perceived as imposed by others and as a negative or threatening state.

Possible Etiologies ("related to")

[Panic level of anxiety]
[Past experiences of difficulty in interactions with others]
[Need to engage in ritualistic behavior in order to keep anxiety under control]
[Repressed fears]

Defining Characteristics ("evidenced by")

[Stays alone in room]
Uncommunicative
Withdrawn
No eye contact
Developmentally [or culturally] inappropriate behaviors
Preoccupation with own thoughts; repetitive, meaningless actions
Expression of feelings of rejection or of aloneness imposed by others
Experiences feelings of differences from others
Insecurity in public

Goals/Objectives

Short-term Goal

Client will willingly attend therapy activities accompanied by trusted support person within 1 week.

Long-term Goal

Client will voluntarily spend time with other clients and staff members in group activities by time of discharge from treatment.

Interventions with *Selected Rationales*

1. Convey an accepting attitude by making brief, frequent contacts. *An accepting attitude increases feelings of self-worth and facilitates trust.*
2. Show unconditional positive regard. *This conveys your belief in the client as a worthwhile human being.*
3. Be with the client to offer support during group activities that may be frightening or difficult for him or her. *The presence of a trusted individual provides emotional security for the client.*
4. Be honest and keep all promises. *Honesty and dependability promote a trusting relationship.*
5. Be cautious with touch. Allow client extra space and an avenue for exit if he or she becomes too anxious. *A person in panic anxiety may perceive touch as a threatening gesture.*
6. Administer tranquilizing medications as ordered by physician. Monitor for effectiveness and for adverse side effects. *Short-term use of antianxiety medications, such as diazepam, chlordiazepoxide, or alprazolam, helps to reduce level of anxiety in most individuals, thereby facilitating interactions with others.*
7. Discuss with client the signs of increasing anxiety and techniques for interrupting the response (e.g., relaxation exercises, thought stopping). *Maladaptive behaviors, such as withdrawal and suspiciousness, are manifested during times of increased anxiety.*
8. Give recognition and positive reinforcement for client's voluntary interactions with others. *Positive reinforcement enhances self-esteem and encourages repetition of acceptable behaviors.*

Outcome Criteria

1. Client demonstrates willingness or desire to socialize with others.
2. Client voluntarily attends group activities.
3. Client approaches others in appropriate manner for one-to-one interaction.

• SELF-CARE DEFICIT (IDENTIFY SPECIFIC AREA)

Definition: Impaired ability to perform or complete [activities of daily living (ADL) independently].

Possible Etiologies ("related to")

[Withdrawal; isolation from others]
[Unmet dependency needs]

[Excessive ritualistic behavior]
[Disabling anxiety]
[Irrational fears]

Defining Characteristics ("evidenced by")

[Unwillingness to bathe regularly]
[Uncombed hair; dirty clothes; offensive body and breath odor; disheveled appearance]
[Eating only a few bites of food off meal tray]
[Lack of interest in selecting appropriate clothing to wear, dressing, grooming, or maintaining appearance at a satisfactory level]
[Incontinence]

Goals/Objectives
Short-term Goal
Client will verbalize desire to take control of self-care activities within 5 days.
Long-term Goal
Client will be able to take care of own ADLs and demonstrate a willingness to do so by time of discharge from treatment.

Interventions with *Selected Rationales*

1. Urge client to perform normal ADLs to his or her level of ability. *Successful performance of independent activities enhances self-esteem.*
2. Encourage independence, but intervene when client is unable to perform. *Client comfort and safety are nursing priorities.*
3. Offer recognition and positive reinforcement for independent accomplishments. (*Example:* "Mrs. J., I see you have put on a clean dress and combed your hair.") *Positive reinforcement enhances self-esteem and encourages repetition of desired behaviors.*
4. Show client how to perform activities with which he or she is having difficulty. *When anxiety is high, client may require simple, concrete demonstrations of activities that would be performed without difficulty under normal conditions.*
5. Keep strict records of food and fluid intake. *This information is necessary to formulate an accurate nutritional assessment.*
6. Offer nutritious snacks and fluids between meals. *Client may be unable to tolerate large amounts of food at mealtimes and may therefore require additional nourishment at other times during the day to receive adequate nutrition.*
7. If client is incontinent, establish routine schedule for toileting needs. Assist client to bathroom on hourly or bihourly schedule, as need is determined, until he or she is able to fulfill this need without assistance.

Outcome Criteria

1. Client feeds self, leaving no more than a few bites of food on food tray.
2. Client selects appropriate clothing and dresses and grooms self daily.
3. Client maintains optimal level of personal hygiene by bathing daily and carrying out essential toileting procedures without assistance.

@ INTERNET REFERENCES

• Additional information about anxiety disorders and medications to treat these disorders may be located at the following websites:
   a. http://www.adaa.org
   b. http://www.mentalhealth.com
   c. http://www.nimh.nih.gov
   d. http://www.anxietynetwork.com/pdhome.html
   e. http://www.fadavis.com/townsend
   f. http://www.drugs.com/condition/anxiety.html

Movie Connections

As Good as It Gets (OCD) • *The Aviator (OCD)* • *What About Bob? (phobias)* • *Copycat (agoraphobia)* • *Analyze This (panic disorder)* • *Vertigo (specific phobia)* • *Born on the Fourth of July (PTSD)* • *The Deer Hunter (PTSD)*

Somatoform Disorders

● BACKGROUND ASSESSMENT DATA

Somatoform disorders are characterized by physical symptoms suggesting medical disease but without demonstrable organic pathology or a known pathophysiological mechanism to account for them. They are classified as mental disorders because pathophysiological processes are not demonstrable or understandable by existing laboratory procedures, and there is either evidence or strong presumption that psychological factors are the major cause of the symptoms. It is now well documented that a large proportion of clients in general medical outpatient clinics and private medical offices do not have organic disease requiring medical treatment. It is likely that many of these clients have somatoform disorders, but they do not perceive themselves as having a psychiatric problem and thus do not seek treatment from psychiatrists. The American Psychiatric Association (APA, 2000) *Diagnostic and Statistical Manual of Mental Disorders, Fourth Edition, Text Revision (DSM-IV-TR)* identifies the following categories of somatoform disorders:

● SOMATOFORM DISORDERS
Somatization Disorder

Somatization disorder is a chronic syndrome of multiple somatic symptoms that cannot be explained medically and are associated with psychosocial distress and long-term seeking of assistance from health-care professionals. Symptoms can represent virtually any organ system but commonly are expressed as neurological, gastrointestinal, psychosexual, or cardiopulmonary disorders. Onset of the disorder is usually in adolescence or early adulthood and is more common in women than in men. The disorder usually runs a fluctuating course, with periods of remission and exacerbation.

Pain Disorder

The essential feature of pain disorder is severe and prolonged pain that causes clinically significant distress or impairment in social, occupational, or other important areas of functioning (APA, 2000). This diagnosis is made when psychological factors have been judged to have a major role in the onset, severity, exacerbation, or maintenance of the pain, even when the physical examination reveals pathology that is associated with the pain.

Hypochondriasis

Hypochondriasis is an unrealistic preoccupation with the fear of having a serious illness. The *DSM-IV-TR* suggests that this fear arises out of an unrealistic interpretation of physical signs and symptoms. Occasionally medical disease may be present, but in the hypochondriacal individual, the symptoms are grossly disproportionate to the degree of pathology. Individuals with hypochondriasis often have a long history of "doctor shopping" and are convinced that they are not receiving the proper care.

Conversion Disorder

Conversion disorder is a loss of or change in body function resulting from a psychological conflict, the physical symptoms of which cannot be explained by any known medical disorder or pathophysiological mechanism. The most common conversion symptoms are those that suggest neurological disease such as paralysis, aphonia, seizures, coordination disturbance, akinesia, dyskinesia, blindness, tunnel vision, anosmia, anesthesia, and paresthesia.

Body Dysmorphic Disorder

This disorder, formerly called dysmorphophobia, is characterized by the exaggerated belief that the body is deformed or defective in some specific way. The most common complaints involve imagined or slight flaws of the face or head, such as thinning hair, acne, wrinkles, scars, vascular markings, facial swelling or asymmetry, or excessive facial hair (APA, 2000).

● PREDISPOSING FACTORS TO SOMATOFORM DISORDERS

1. **Physiological**
   a. *Genetic*. Studies have shown an increased incidence of somatization disorder, conversion disorder, and hypochondriasis in first-degree relatives, implying a possible inheritable predisposition (Sadock & Sadock, 2007; Soares & Grossman, 2007; Yutzy, 2003).
   b. ***Biochemical***. Decreased levels of serotonin and endorphins may play a role in the etiology of pain disorder.

2. **Psychosocial**
    a. ***Psychodynamic.*** Some psychodynamicists view hypochon-
       driasis as an ego defense mechanism. They hypothesize
       that physical complaints are the expression of low self-
       esteem and feelings of worthlessness and that the individual
       believes it is easier to feel something is wrong with the body
       than to feel something is wrong with the self.

       The psychodynamic theory of conversion disorder pro-
       poses that emotions associated with a traumatic event that
       the individual cannot express because of moral or ethical
       unacceptability are "converted" into physical symptoms.
       The unacceptable emotions are repressed and converted
       to a somatic hysterical symptom that is symbolic in some
       way of the original emotional trauma.
    b. ***Family Dynamics.*** Some families have difficulty expressing
       emotions openly and resolving conflicts verbally. When this
       occurs, the child may become ill, and a shift in focus is made
       from the open conflict to the child's illness, leaving unre-
       solved the underlying issues that the family cannot confront
       openly. Thus, somatization by the child brings some stabil-
       ity to the family, as harmony replaces discord and the child's
       welfare becomes the common concern. The child in turn
       receives positive reinforcement for the illness.
    c. ***Sociocultural/Familial Factors.*** Somatic complaints are
       often reinforced when the sick role relieves the individual
       from the need to deal with a stressful situation, whether it
       be within society or within the family. When the sick per-
       son is allowed to avoid stressful obligations and postpone
       unwelcome challenges, is excused from troublesome du-
       ties, or becomes the prominent focus of attention because
       of the illness, positive reinforcement virtually guarantees
       repetition of the response.
    d. ***Past Experience with Physical Illness.*** Personal experi-
       ence, or the experience of close family members, with seri-
       ous or life-threatening illness can predispose an individual
       to hypochondriasis. Once an individual has experienced a
       threat to biological integrity, he or she may develop a fear
       of recurrence. The fear of recurring illness generates an
       exaggerated response to minor physical changes, leading
       to hypochondriacal behaviors.
    e. ***Cultural and Environmental Factors.*** Some cultures and
       religions carry implicit sanctions against verbalizing or
       directly expressing emotional states, thereby indirectly
       encouraging "more acceptable" somatic behaviors. Cross-
       cultural studies have shown that the somatization symp-
       toms associated with depression are relatively similar,
       but the "cognitive" or emotional symptoms such as guilt

are predominantly seen in Western societies. In Middle Eastern and Asian cultures, depression is almost exclusively manifested by somatic or vegetative symptoms.

Environmental influences may be significant in the predisposition to somatization disorder. Some studies have suggested that a tendency toward somatization appears to be more common in individuals who have low socioeconomic, occupational, and educational status.

● SYMPTOMATOLOGY (SUBJECTIVE AND OBJECTIVE DATA)

1. Any physical symptom for which there is no organic basis but for which evidence exists for the implication of psychological factors.
2. Depressed mood is common.
3. Loss or alteration in physical functioning, with no organic basis. Examples include the following:
   a. Blindness or tunnel vision
   b. Paralysis
   c. Anosmia (inability to smell)
   d. Aphonia (inability to speak)
   e. Seizures
   f. Coordination disturbances
   g. Pseudocyesis (false pregnancy)
   h. Akinesia or dyskinesia
   i. Anesthesia or paresthesia
4. "La belle indifference"—a relative lack of concern regarding the severity of the symptoms just described (e.g., a person is suddenly blind but shows little anxiety over the situation).
5. "Doctor shopping"
6. Excessive use of analgesics
7. Requests for surgery
8. Assumption of an invalid role
9. Impairment in social or occupational functioning because of preoccupation with physical complaints
10. Psychosexual dysfunction (impotence, dyspareunia [painful coitus], sexual indifference)
11. Excessive dysmenorrhea
12. Excessive preoccupation with physical defect that is out of proportion to the actual condition

Common Nursing Diagnoses and Interventions

(Interventions are applicable to various health-care settings, such as inpatient and partial hospitalization, community outpatient clinic, home health, and private practice.)

• CHRONIC PAIN

Definition: Unpleasant sensory and emotional experience arising from actual or potential tissue damage or described in terms of such damage (International Association for the Study of Pain); sudden or slow onset of any intensity from mild to severe, constant or recurring without an anticipated or predictable end and a duration of greater than 6 months.

Possible Etiologies ("related to")

[Severe level of anxiety, repressed]
[Low self-esteem]
[Unmet dependency needs]
[Secondary gains from the sick role]

Defining Characteristics ("evidenced by")

Verbal report of pain [in the absence of pathophysiological evidence]
Reduced interaction with people
Facial mask [of pain]
Guarding behavior
[Demanding behaviors]
[Refuses to attend therapeutic activities because of pain]
[History of seeking assistance from numerous health-care professionals]
[Excessive use of analgesics, without relief of pain]
Self-focusing

Goals/Objectives

Short-term Goal

Within 2 weeks, client will verbalize understanding of correlation between pain and psychological problems.

Long-term Goal

By time of discharge from treatment, client will verbalize a noticeable, if not complete, relief from pain.

Interventions with *Selected Rationales*

1. Monitor physician's ongoing assessments and laboratory reports *to ascertain that organic pathology is clearly ruled out.*
2. Recognize and accept that the pain is real to the individual, even though no organic cause can be identified. *Denying the client's feelings is nontherapeutic and hinders the development of a trusting relationship.*
3. Observe and record the duration and intensity of the pain. Note factors that precipitate the onset of pain. *Identification of the precipitating stressor is important*

for assessment purposes. This information will be used to develop a plan for assisting the client to cope more adaptively.

4. Provide pain medication as prescribed by physician. *Client comfort and safety are nursing priorities.*

5. Assist with comfort measures, such as back rub, warm bath, and heating pad. Be careful, however, not to respond in a way that reinforces the behavior. *Secondary gains from physical symptoms may prolong maladaptive behaviors.*

6. Offer your attention at times when client is not focusing on pain. *Positive reinforcement encourages repetition of adaptive behaviors.*

7. Identify activities that serve to distract client from focus on self and pain. *These distractors serve in a therapeutic manner as a transition from focus on self or physical manifestations to focus on unresolved psychological issues.*

8. Encourage verbalization of feelings. Explore meaning that pain holds for client. Help client connect symptoms of pain to times of increased anxiety and to identify specific situations that cause anxiety to rise. *Verbalization of feelings in a nonthreatening environment facilitates expression and resolution of disturbing emotional issues.*

9. Encourage client to identify alternative methods of coping with stress. *These may avert the physical pain as a maladaptive response to stress.*

10. Explore ways to intervene as symptoms begin to intensify, so that pain does not become disabling (e.g., visual or auditory distractions, mental imagery, deep-breathing exercises, application of hot or cold compresses, relaxation exercises).

11. Provide positive reinforcement for adaptive behaviors. *Positive reinforcement enhances self-esteem and encourages repetition of desired behaviors.*

Outcome Criteria

1. Client verbalizes that pain does not interfere with completion of daily activities.

2. Client verbalizes an understanding of the relationship between pain and emotional problems.

3. Client demonstrates ability to intervene as anxiety rises, to prevent the onset or increase in severity of pain.

● INEFFECTIVE COPING

Definition: Inability to form a valid appraisal of the stressors, inadequate choices of practiced responses, and/or inability to use available resources.

Possible Etiologies ("related to")

[Severe level of anxiety, repressed]
[Low self-esteem]
[Unmet dependency needs]
[History of self or loved one having experienced a serious illness or disease]
[Regression to, or fixation in, an earlier level of development]
[Retarded ego development]
[Inadequate coping skills]

Defining Characteristics ("evidenced by")

[Numerous physical complaints verbalized, in the absence of any pathophysiological evidence]
[Total focus on the self and physical symptoms]
[History of doctor shopping]
[Demanding behaviors]
[Refuses to attend therapeutic activities]
[Does not correlate physical symptoms with psychological problems]
Inability to meet basic needs
Inability to meet role expectations
Inadequate problem-solving
Sleep disturbance

Goals/Objectives

Short-term Goal

Within 2 weeks, client will verbalize understanding of correlation between physical symptoms and psychological problems.

Long-term Goal

By time of discharge from treatment, client will demonstrate ability to cope with stress by means other than preoccupation with physical symptoms.

Interventions with *Selected Rationales*

1. Monitor physician's ongoing assessments, laboratory reports, and other data to maintain assurance that possibility of organic pathology is clearly ruled out. *Knowledge of these data is vital for the provision of adequate and appropriate client care.*
2. Recognize and accept that the physical complaint is indeed real to the individual, even though no organic cause can be identified. *Denial of the client's feelings is nontherapeutic and interferes with establishment of a trusting relationship.*
3. Identify gains that the physical symptom is providing for the client: increased dependency, attention, distraction from other problems. *These are important assessment data to be used in assisting the client with problem resolution.*

4. Initially, fulfill client's most urgent dependency needs. *Failure to do this may cause client to become extremely anxious, with an increase in maladaptive behaviors.*
5. Gradually withdraw attention to physical symptoms. Minimize time given in response to physical complaints. *Lack of positive response will discourage repetition of undesirable behaviors.*
6. Explain to client that any new physical complaints will be referred to the physician, and give no further attention to them. Be sure to note physician's assessment of the complaint. *The possibility of organic pathology must always be taken into consideration. Failure to do so could jeopardize client's safety.*
7. Encourage client to verbalize fears and anxieties. Explain that attention will be withdrawn if rumination about physical complaints begins. Follow through. *Without consistency of limit setting, change will not occur.*
8. Help client observe that physical symptoms occur because of, or are exacerbated by, specific stressors. Discuss alternative coping responses to these stressors.
9. Give positive reinforcement for adaptive coping strategies. *Positive reinforcement encourages repetition of desired behaviors.*
10. Help client identify ways to achieve recognition from others without resorting to physical symptoms. *Positive recognition from others enhances self-esteem and minimizes the need for attention through maladaptive behaviors.*
11. Discuss how interpersonal relationships are affected by client's narcissistic behavior. Explain how this behavior alienates others. *Client may not realize how he or she is perceived by others.*
12. Provide instruction in relaxation techniques and assertiveness skills. *These approaches decrease anxiety and increase self-esteem, which facilitate adaptive responses to stressful situations.*

Outcome Criteria

1. Client is able to demonstrate techniques that may be used in response to stress to prevent the occurrence or exacerbation of physical symptoms.
2. Client verbalizes an understanding of the relationship between emotional problems and physical symptoms.

• DISTURBED BODY IMAGE

Definition: Confusion in mental picture of one's physical self.

Possible Etiologies ("related to")
[Severe level of anxiety, repressed]
[Low self-esteem]
[Unmet dependency needs]

Defining Characteristics ("evidenced by")
[Preoccupation with real or imagined change in bodily structure or function]
[Verbalizations about physical appearance that are out of proportion to any actual physical abnormality that may exist]
Fear of reaction by others
Negative feelings about body
Change in social involvement

Goals/Objectives
Short-term Goal
Client will verbalize understanding that changes in bodily structure or function are exaggerated out of proportion to the change that actually exists. (Time frame for this goal must be determined according to individual client's situation.)

Long-term Goal
Client will verbalize perception of own body that is realistic to actual structure or function by time of discharge from treatment.

Interventions with *Selected Rationales*
1. Establish trusting relationship with client. ***Trust enhances therapeutic interactions between nurse and client.***
2. If there is actual change in structure or function, encourage client to progress through stages of grieving. Assess level of knowledge and provide information regarding normal grieving process and associated feelings. ***Knowledge of acceptable feelings facilitates progression through the grieving process.***
3. Identify misperceptions or distortions client has regarding body image. Correct inaccurate perceptions in a matter-of-fact, nonthreatening manner. Withdraw attention when preoccupation with distorted image persists. ***Lack of attention may encourage elimination of undesirable behaviors.***
4. Help client recognize personal body boundaries. ***Use of touch may help him or her recognize acceptance of the individual by others and reduce fear of rejection because of changes in bodily structure or function.***
5. Encourage independent self-care activities, providing assistance as required. ***Self-care activities accomplished independently enhance self-esteem and also create the necessity for client to confront reality of his or her bodily condition.***

6. Provide positive reinforcement for client's expressions of realistic bodily perceptions. *Positive reinforcement enhances self-esteem and encourages repetition of desired behaviors.*

Outcome Criteria

1. Client verbalizes realistic perception of bodily condition.
2. Client demonstrates acceptance of changes in bodily structure or function, as evidenced by expression of positive feelings about body, ability or willingness to perform self-care activities independently, and a focus on personal achievements rather than preoccupation with distorted body image.

● DISTURBED SENSORY PERCEPTION

Definition: Change in the amount or patterning of incoming stimuli [either internally or externally initiated] accompanied by a diminished, exaggerated, distorted, or impaired response to such stimuli.

Possible Etiologies ("related to")

[Severe level of anxiety, repressed]
[Low self-esteem]
[Unmet dependency needs]
[Regression to, or fixation in, an earlier level of development]
[Retarded ego development]
[Inadequate coping skills]
Psychological stress [narrowed perceptual fields caused by anxiety]

Defining Characteristics ("evidenced by")

[Loss or alteration in physical functioning suggesting a physical disorder (often neurological in nature) but for which organic pathology is not evident. Common alterations include paralysis, anosmia, aphonia, deafness, blindness]
[La belle indifference]

Goals/Objectives

Short-term Goal

Client will verbalize understanding of emotional problems as a contributing factor to alteration in physical functioning within 10 days.

Long-term Goal

Client will demonstrate recovery of lost function.

Interventions with *Selected Rationales*

1. Monitor physician's ongoing assessments, laboratory reports, and other data to maintain assurance that possibility of organic pathology is clearly ruled out. *Failure to do so may jeopardize client's safety.*

2. Identify gains that the physical symptom is providing for the client: increased dependency, attention, distraction from other problems. *These are important assessment data to be used in assisting the client with problem resolution.*

3. Fulfill client's needs related to activities of daily living (ADLs) with which the physical symptom is interfering. *Client comfort and safety are nursing priorities.*

4. Do not focus on the disability, and allow client to be as independent as possible. Intervene only when client requires assistance. *Positive reinforcement would encourage continual use of the maladaptive response for secondary gains, such as dependency.*

5. Encourage client to participate in therapeutic activities to the best of his or her ability. Do not allow client to use the disability as a manipulative tool. Withdraw attention if client continues to focus on physical limitation. Reinforce reality as required, but ensure maintenance of a nonthreatening environment.

6. Encourage client to verbalize fears and anxieties. Help client to recognize that the physical symptom appears at a time of extreme stress and is a mechanism used for coping. *Client may be unaware of the relationship between physical symptom and emotional stress.*

7. Help client identify coping mechanisms that he or she could use when faced with stressful situations rather than retreating from reality with a physical disability.

8. Explain assertiveness techniques and practice use of same through role-playing. *Use of assertiveness techniques enhances self-esteem and minimizes anxiety in interpersonal relationships.*

9. Help client identify a satisfactory support system within the community from which he or she may seek assistance as needed to cope with overwhelming stress.

Outcome Criteria

1. Client is no longer experiencing symptoms of altered physical functioning.

2. Client verbalizes an understanding of the relationship between extreme psychological stress and loss of physical functioning.

3. Client is able to verbalize adaptive ways of coping with stress and identify community support systems to which he or she may go for help.

● SELF-CARE DEFICIT (IDENTIFY SPECIFIC AREA)

Definition: Impaired ability to perform or complete [activities of daily living ADLs independently]

Possible Etiologies ("related to")

[Paralysis of body part]
[Inability to see]
[Inability to hear]
[Inability to speak]
Pain, discomfort

Defining Characteristics ("evidenced by")

Inability to bring food from a receptacle to the mouth
Inability to wash body or body parts; obtain or get to water sources; regulate temperature or flow
Impaired ability to put on or take off necessary items of clothing; obtain or replace articles of clothing; fasten clothing; maintain appearance at a satisfactory level
Inability to get to toilet or commode [impaired mobility]
Inability to manipulate clothing for toileting
Inability to flush toilet or commode
Inability to sit on or rise from toilet or commode
Inability to carry out proper toilet hygiene

Goals/Objectives

Short-term Goal

Client will perform self-care needs independently, to the extent that physical ability will allow, within 5 days.

Long-term Goal

By discharge from treatment, client will be able to perform ADLs independently and demonstrate a willingness to do so.

Interventions with *Selected Rationales*

1. Assess client's level of disability; note areas of strength and impairment. *This knowledge is required to develop adequate plan of care for client.*
2. Encourage client to perform normal ADLs to his or her level of ability. *Successful performance of independent activities enhances self-esteem.*
3. Encourage independence, but intervene when client is unable to perform. *Client comfort and safety are nursing priorities.*
4. Ensure that nonjudgmental attitude is conveyed as nursing assistance with self-care activities is provided. Remember

that the physical symptom is real to the client. It is not within the client's conscious control. *A judgmental attitude interferes with the nurse's ability to provide therapeutic care for this client.*

5. Feed client, if necessary, and provide assistance with containers, positioning, and other matters, as required. *Client comfort and safety are nursing priorities.*

6. Bathe client, or assist with bath, depending on his or her level of ability. *Client comfort and safety are nursing priorities.*

7. Assist client with dressing, oral hygiene, combing hair, and applying makeup, as required. *Client comfort and safety are nursing priorities.*

8. Provide bedpan, commode, or assistance to bathroom as determined by client's level of ability. *Client comfort and safety are nursing priorities.*

9. Provide positive reinforcement for ADLs performed independently. *Positive reinforcement enhances self-esteem and encourages repetition of desired behaviors.*

10. Take precautions against fostering dependency by intervening when client is capable of performing independently. Allow ample time for client to complete these activities to the best of his or her ability without assistance. *Allowing the client to maintain dependency may provide secondary gains and delay recovery from the disability.*

11. Encourage client to discuss feelings regarding the disability and the need for dependency it creates. Help client to see the purpose this disability is serving for him or her. *Self-disclosure and exploration of feelings with a trusted individual may help client fulfill unmet needs and confront unresolved issues.*

Outcome Criteria

1. Client feeds self without assistance.
2. Client selects appropriate clothing and dresses and grooms self daily.
3. Client maintains optimal level of personal hygiene by bathing daily and carrying out essential toileting procedures without assistance.

● DEFICIENT KNOWLEDGE (PSYCHOLOGICAL CAUSES FOR PHYSICAL SYMPTOMS)

Definition: Absence or deficiency of cognitive information related to a specific topic.

Possible Etiologies ("related to")
Lack of interest in learning
[Severe level of anxiety]

Defining Characteristics ("evidenced by")
[Denial of emotional problems]
[Statements such as, "I don't know why the doctor put me on the psychiatric unit. I have a physical problem."]
[History of "shopping" for a doctor who will substantiate symptoms as pathophysiological]
[Noncompliance with psychiatric treatment plan]

Goals/Objectives
Short-term Goal
Client will verbalize an understanding that no pathophysiological condition exists to substantiate physical symptoms.

Long-term Goal
By time of discharge from treatment, client will be able to verbalize psychological cause(s) for physical symptoms.

Interventions with *Selected Rationales*
1. Assess client's level of knowledge regarding effects of psychological problems on the body. *An adequate database is necessary for the development of an effective teaching plan.*
2. Assess client's level of anxiety and readiness to learn. *Learning does not occur beyond the moderate level of anxiety.*
3. Discuss physical examinations and laboratory tests that have been conducted. Explain purpose and results of each.
4. Explore feelings and fears held by client. Go slowly. These feelings may have been suppressed or repressed for a very long time and their disclosure will undoubtedly be a painful experience. Be supportive. *Verbalization of feelings in a nonthreatening environment may help client come to terms with long-unresolved issues.*
5. Have client keep a diary of appearance, duration, and intensity of physical symptoms. A separate record of situations that the client finds especially stressful should also be kept. *Comparison of these records may provide objective data from which to observe the relationship between physical symptoms and stress.*
6. Help client identify needs that are being met through the sick role. Together, formulate a more adaptive means for fulfilling these needs. Practice by role-playing. *Change cannot occur until the client realizes that physical symptoms are used to fulfill unmet needs. Anxiety is relieved by*

role-playing, since the client is able to anticipate responses to stressful situations.

7. Explain assertiveness techniques to the client. Discuss the importance of recognizing the differences among passive, assertive, and aggressive behaviors, and of respecting the human rights of others while protecting one's own basic human rights. *Use of these techniques enhances self-esteem and facilitates client's interpersonal relationships.*

8. Discuss adaptive methods of stress management: relaxation techniques, physical exercise, meditation, breathing exercises, or mental imagery. *These techniques may be employed in an attempt to relieve anxiety and discourage the use of physical symptoms as a maladaptive response.*

Outcome Criteria

1. Client verbalizes an understanding of the relationship between psychological stress and physical symptoms.
2. Client demonstrates the ability to use therapeutic techniques in the management of stress.

@ INTERNET REFERENCES

- Additional information about somatoform disorders may be located at the following websites:
  a. http://psyweb.com/Mdisord/jsp/somatd.jsp
  b. http://www.uib.no/med/avd/med_a/gastro/wilhelms/hypochon.html
  c. http://emedicine.medscape.com/article/805361-overview
  d. http://psychological.com/somatofom_disorders.htm
  e. http://emedicine.medscape.com/article/917864-overview
  f. http://findarticles.com/p/articles/mi_g2601/is_0012/ai_2601001276

Movie Connections

Bandits (hypochondriasis) • *Hannah and Her Sisters (hypochondriasis)* • *Send Me No Flowers (hypochondriasis)*

Dissociative Disorders

● BACKGROUND ASSESSMENT DATA

The essential feature of the dissociative disorders is a disruption in the usually integrated functions of consciousness, memory, identity, or perception (APA, 2000). During periods of intolerable stress, the individual blocks off part of his or her life from consciousness. The stressful emotion becomes a separate entity, as the individual "splits" from it and mentally drifts into a fantasy state. The following categories are defined in the *Diagnostic and Statistical Manual of Mental Disorders, Fourth Edition, Text Revision (DSM-IV-TR)* (APA, 2000):

1. **Dissociative Amnesia:** An inability to recall important personal information, usually of a traumatic or stressful nature. The extent of the disturbance is too great to be explained by ordinary forgetfulness. Types of impairment in recall include the following:
   a. *Localized Amnesia:* Inability to recall all incidents associated with a traumatic event for a specific time period following the event (usually a few hours to a few days).
   b. *Selective Amnesia:* Inability to recall only certain incidents associated with a traumatic event for a specific period following the event.
   c. *Continuous Amnesia:* Inability to recall events subsequent to a specific time up to and including the present. (The memory does not return after a short period, as in localized amnesia. The individual is unable to form new memories.)
   d. *Systematized Amnesia:* With this type of amnesia, the individual cannot remember events that relate to a specific category of information, such as one's family, or to one particular person or event.
   e. *Generalized Amnesia:* Failure of recall encompassing one's entire life.
2. **Dissociative Fugue.** A sudden, unexpected travel away from home or customary work locale with assumption of a new identity and an inability to recall one's previous identity. Following recovery, there is no recollection of events that

191

took place during the fugue. Course is typically brief—hours to days, and rarely, months. Recurrences are rare.

3. **Dissociative Identity Disorder (DID).** The existence within the individual of two or more distinct personalities, each of which is dominant at a particular time. The original personality usually is not aware (at least initially) of the existence of subpersonalities. When there are more than two subpersonalities, however, they are usually aware of each other. Transition from one personality to another is usually sudden and often associated with psychosocial stress. The course tends to be more chronic than in the other dissociative disorders.

4. **Depersonalization Disorder.** Characterized by a temporary change in the quality of self-awareness, which often takes the form of feelings of unreality, changes in body image, feelings of detachment from the environment, or a sense of observing oneself from outside the body.

● **PREDISPOSING FACTORS TO DISSOCIATIVE DISORDER**

1. **Physiological**
   a. *Genetics.* The *DSM-IV-TR* suggests that DID is more common in first-degree relatives of people with the disorder than in the general population. The disorder is often seen in more than one generation of a family.
   b. *Neurobiological.* Some clinicians have suggested a possible correlation between neurological alterations and dissociative disorders. Although available information is inadequate, it is possible that dissociative amnesia and dissociative fugue may be related to alterations in certain areas of the brain that have to do with memory. These include the hippocampus, mammillary bodies, amygdala, fornix, thalamus, and frontal cortex. Some studies have suggested a possible link between DID and certain neurological conditions, such as temporal lobe epilepsy and severe migraine headaches. Electroencephalographic abnormalities have been observed in some clients with DID.

2. **Psychosocial**
   a. *Psychodynamic Theory.* Freud (1962) believed that dissociative behaviors occurred when individuals repressed distressing mental contents from conscious awareness. He believed that the unconscious was a dynamic entity in which repressed mental contents were stored and unavailable to conscious recall. Current psychodynamic explanations of dissociation are based on Freud's concepts.
   b. *Psychological Trauma.* A growing body of evidence points to the etiology of DID as a set of traumatic experiences that overwhelms the individual's capacity to cope

by any means other than dissociation. These experiences usually take the form of severe physical, sexual, and/or psychological abuse by a parent or significant other in the child's life. DID is thought to serve as a survival strategy for the child in this traumatic environment, whereby he or she creates a new being who is able to experience the overwhelming pain of the cruel reality, while the primary self can then escape awareness of the pain. It has been suggested that the number of an individual's alternate personalities may be related to the number of different types of abuse he or she suffered as a child. Individuals with many personalities have usually been severely abused well into adolescence.

● SYMPTOMATOLOGY (SUBJECTIVE AND OBJECTIVE DATA)

1. Impairment in recall.
   a. Inability to remember specific incidents.
   b. Inability to recall any of one's past life, including one's identity.
2. Sudden travel away from familiar surroundings; assumption of new identity, with inability to recall past.
3. Assumption of additional identities within the personality; behavior involves transition from one identity to another as a method of dealing with stressful situations.
4. Feeling of unreality; detachment from a stressful situation— may be accompanied by dizziness, depression, obsessive rumination, somatic concerns, anxiety, fear of going insane, and a disturbance in the subjective sense of time (APA, 2000).

Common Nursing Diagnoses and Interventions

(Interventions are applicable to various health-care settings, such as inpatient and partial hospitalization, community outpatient clinic, home health, and private practice.)

● INEFFECTIVE COPING

Definition: Inability to form a valid appraisal of the stressors, inadequate choices of practiced responses, and/or inability to use available resources

Possible Etiologies ("related to")

[Severe level of anxiety, repressed]
[Childhood trauma]
[Childhood abuse]

[Low self-esteem]
[Unmet dependency needs]
[Regression to, or fixation in, an earlier level of development]
[Inadequate coping skills]

Defining Characteristics ("evidenced by")

[Dissociating self from painful situation by experiencing:
   Memory loss (partial or complete)
   Sudden travel away from home with inability to recall
      previous identity
   The presence of more than one personality within the
      individual
   Detachment from reality]
Inadequate problem-solving
Inability to meet role expectations
[Inappropriate use of defense mechanisms]

Goals/Objectives

Short-term Goal

1. Client will verbalize understanding that he or she is employing dissociative behaviors in times of psychosocial stress.
2. Client will verbalize more adaptive ways of coping in stressful situations than resorting to dissociation.

Long-term Goal

Client will demonstrate ability to cope with stress (employing means other than dissociation).

Interventions with *Selected Rationales*

1. Reassure client of safety and security by your presence. Dissociative behaviors may be frightening to the client. *Presence of a trusted individual provides feeling of security and assurance of freedom from harm.*
2. Identify stressor that precipitated severe anxiety. *This information is necessary to the development of an effective plan of client care and problem resolution.*
3. Explore feelings that client experienced in response to the stressor. Help client understand that the disequilibrium felt is acceptable—indeed, even expected—in times of severe stress. *Client's self-esteem is preserved by the knowledge that others may experience these behaviors in similar circumstances.*
4. As anxiety level decreases (and memory returns), use exploration and an accepting, nonthreatening environment to encourage client to identify repressed traumatic experiences that contribute to chronic anxiety.
5. Have client identify methods of coping with stress in the past and determine whether the response was adaptive or

maladaptive. *In times of extreme anxiety, client is unable to evaluate appropriateness of response. This information is necessary for client to develop a plan of action for the future.*

6. Help client define more adaptive coping strategies. Make suggestions of alternatives that might be tried. Examine benefits and consequences of each alternative. Assist client in the selection of those that are most appropriate for him or her. *Depending on current level of anxiety, client may require assistance with problem-solving and decision-making.*

7. Provide positive reinforcement for client's attempts to change. *Positive reinforcement enhances self-esteem and encourages repetition of desired behaviors.*

8. Identify community resources to which the individual may go for support if past maladaptive coping patterns return.

Outcome Criteria

1. Client is able to demonstrate techniques that may be used in response to stress to prevent dissociation.
2. Client verbalizes an understanding of the relationship between severe anxiety and the dissociative response.

• DISTURBED THOUGHT PROCESSES

Definition: Disruption in cognitive operations and activities

Possible Etiologies ("related to")

[Severe level of anxiety, repressed]
[Childhood trauma]
[Childhood abuse]
[Threat to physical integrity]
[Threat to self-concept]

Defining Characteristics ("evidenced by")

[Memory loss—inability to recall selected events related to a stressful situation]
[Memory loss—inability to recall events associated with entire life]
[Memory loss—inability to recall own identity]

Goals/Objectives

Short-term Goal

Client will verbalize understanding that loss of memory is related to stressful situation and begin discussing stressful situation with nurse or therapist.

Long-term Goal

Client will recover deficits in memory and develop more adaptive coping mechanisms to deal with stressful situations.

Interventions with *Selected Rationales*

1. Obtain as much information as possible about client from family and significant others (likes, dislikes, important people, activities, music, pets). *A baseline assessment is important for the development of an effective plan of care.*
2. Do not flood client with data regarding his or her past life. *Individuals who are exposed to painful information from which the amnesia is providing protection may decompensate even further into a psychotic state.*
3. Instead, expose client to stimuli that represent pleasant experiences from the past, such as smells associated with enjoyable activities, beloved pets, and music known to have been pleasurable to client.
4. As memory begins to return, engage client in activities that may provide additional stimulation. *Recall may occur during activities that simulate life experiences.*
5. Encourage client to discuss situations that have been especially stressful and to explore the feelings associated with those times. *Verbalization of feelings in a nonthreatening environment may help client come to terms with unresolved issues that may be contributing to the dissociative process.*
6. Identify specific conflicts that remain unresolved, and assist client to identify possible solutions. *Unless these underlying conflicts are resolved, any improvement in coping behaviors must be viewed as only temporary.*
7. Provide instruction regarding more adaptive ways to respond to anxiety *so that dissociative behaviors are no longer needed.*

Outcome Criteria

1. Client is able to recall all events of past life.
2. Client is able to demonstrate adaptive coping strategies that may be used in response to severe anxiety to avert amnestic behaviors.

● DISTURBED PERSONAL IDENTITY

Definition: Inability to maintain an integrated and complete perception of self

Possible Etiologies ("related to")
[Severe level of anxiety, repressed]
[Childhood trauma]
[Childhood abuse]
[Threat to physical integrity]
[Threat to self-concept]

Defining Characteristics ("evidenced by")
[Presence of more than one personality within the individual]

Goals/Objectives
Short-term Goal
Client will verbalize understanding of the existence of multiple personalities within the self and be able to recognize stressful situations that precipitate transition from one to another.

Long-term Goal
Client will verbalize understanding of the need for, enter into, and cooperate with long-term therapy for this disorder, with the ultimate goal being integration into one personality.

Interventions with *Selected Rationales*
1. The nurse must develop a trusting relationship with the original personality and with each of the subpersonalities. *Trust is the basis of a therapeutic relationship. Each of the personalities views itself as a separate entity and must initially be treated as such.*
2. Help the client understand the existence of the subpersonalities. *Client may be unaware of this dissociative response to stressful situations.*
3. Help client identify the need each subpersonality serves in the personal identity of the individual. *Knowledge of these unfulfilled needs is the first step toward integration of the personalities and the client's ability to face unresolved issues without dissociation.*
4. Help the client identify stressful situations that precipitate the transition from one personality to another. Carefully observe and record these transitions. *This knowledge is required to assist the client in responding more adaptively and to eliminate the need for transition to another personality.*
5. Use nursing interventions necessary to deal with maladaptive behaviors associated with individual subpersonalities. For example, if one personality is suicidal, precautions must be taken to guard against client's self-harm. If another personality has a

tendency toward physical hostility, precautions must be taken for the protection of others. *Safety of the client and others is a nursing priority.*

CLINICAL PEARL It may be possible to seek assistance from one of the personalities. For example, a strong-willed personality may help to control the behaviors of a "suicidal" personality.

6. Help subpersonalities to understand that their "being" will not be destroyed, but integrated into a unified identity within the individual. *Because subpersonalities function as separate entities, the idea of total elimination generates fear and defensiveness.*
7. Provide support during disclosure of painful experiences and reassurance when the client becomes discouraged with lengthy treatment.

Outcome Criteria
1. Client recognizes the existence of more than one personality.
2. Client is able to verbalize the purpose these personalities serve.
3. Client verbalizes the intention of seeking long-term outpatient psychotherapy.

● DISTURBED SENSORY PERCEPTION (KINESTHETIC)

Definition: Change in the amount or patterning of incoming stimuli [either internally or externally initiated] accompanied by a diminished, exaggerated, distorted, or impaired response to such stimuli.

Possible Etiologies ("related to")
[Severe level of anxiety, repressed]
[Childhood trauma]
[Childhood abuse]
[Threat to physical integrity]
[Threat to self-concept]

Defining Characteristics ("evidenced by")
[Alteration in the perception or experience of the self]
[Loss of one's own sense of reality]
[Loss of the sense of reality of the external world]

Goals/Objectives

Short-term Goal
Client will verbalize adaptive ways of coping with stress.

Long-term Goal
By time of discharge from treatment, client will demonstrate the ability to perceive stimuli correctly and maintain a sense of reality during stressful situations.

Interventions with *Selected Rationales*

1. Provide support and encouragement during times of depersonalization. The client manifesting these symptoms may express fear and anxiety at experiencing such behaviors. They do not understand the response and may express a fear of "going insane." *Support and encouragement from a trusted individual provide a feeling of security when fears and anxieties are manifested.*

2. Explain the depersonalization behaviors and the purpose they usually serve for the client. *This knowledge may help to minimize fears and anxieties associated with their occurrence.*

3. Explain the relationship between severe anxiety and depersonalization behaviors. *The client may be unaware that the occurrence of depersonalization behaviors is related to severe anxiety.*

4. Help client relate these behaviors to times of severe psychological stress that he or she has experienced personally. *Knowledge of this relationship is the first step in the process of behavioral change.*

5. Explore past experiences and possibly repressed painful situations such as trauma or abuse. *It is thought that traumatic experiences predispose individuals to dissociative disorders.*

6. Discuss these painful experiences with the client and encourage him or her to deal with the feelings associated with these situations. Work to resolve the conflicts these repressed feelings have nurtured. *These interventions serve to decrease the need for the dissociative response to anxiety.*

7. Discuss ways the client may more adaptively respond to stress and role-play with him or her to practice using these new methods. *Having practiced through role-play helps to prepare client to face stressful situations by using these new behaviors when they occur in real life.*

Outcome Criteria

1. Client perceives stressful situations correctly and is able to maintain a sense of reality.
2. Client demonstrates use of adaptive strategies for coping with stress.

@ INTERNET REFERENCES

- Additional information about Dissociative Disorders may be located at the following websites:
    a. http://www.human-nature.com/odmh/dissociative.html
    b. http://www.nami.org/Content/ContentGroups/Helpline1/Dissociative_Disorders.htm
    c. http://www.mental-health-matters.com/disorders
    d. http://www.issd.org/
    e. http://www.sidran.org/didbr.html
    f. http://emedicine.medscape.com/article/294508-overview
    g. http://findarticles.com/p/articles/mi_g2601/is_0004/ai_2601000438

Movie Connections

Dead Again (amnesia) • *Mirage (amnesia)* • *Suddenly Last Summer (amnesia)* • *The Three Lives of Karen (fugue)* • *Sybil (DID)* • *The Three Faces of Eve (DID)* • *Identity (DID)*

Sexual and Gender Identity Disorders

● BACKGROUND ASSESSMENT DATA

The American Psychiatric Association (APA, 2000) *Diagnostic and Statistical Manual of Mental Disorders, Fourth Edition, Text Revision (DSM-IV-TR)* identifies two categories of sexual disorders: paraphilias and sexual dysfunctions. *Paraphilias* are characterized by recurrent, intense sexual urges, fantasies, or behaviors that involve unusual objects, activities, or situations (APA, 2000). *Sexual dysfunction disorders* can be described as an impairment or disturbance in any of the phases of the sexual response cycle. These include disorders of desire, arousal, and orgasm and disorders that relate to the experience of genital pain during intercourse. Gender identity disorders are characterized by strong and persistent cross-gender identification accompanied by persistent discomfort with one's assigned sex (APA, 2000).

Paraphilias

The term "paraphilia" is used to identify repetitive or preferred sexual fantasies or behaviors that involve any of the following:

1. The preference for use of a nonhuman object.
2. Repetitive sexual activity with humans involving real or simulated suffering or humiliation.
3. Repetitive sexual activity with nonconsenting partners.

Types of paraphilias include the following:

1. **Exhibitionism**. The major symptoms include recurrent, intense sexual urges, behaviors, or sexually arousing fantasies, of at least 6 months' duration, involving the exposure of one's genitals to an unsuspecting stranger (APA, 2000). Masturbation may occur during the exhibitionism. Most individuals with paraphilias are men, and the behavior is generally established in adolescence (Andreasen & Black, 2006).
2. **Fetishism**. Fetishism involves recurrent, intense sexual urges or behaviors, or sexually arousing fantasies, of at least

6 months' duration, involving the use of nonliving objects (APA, 2000). Common fetish objects include bras, women's underpants, stockings, shoes, boots, or other wearing apparel. The fetish object is generally used during masturbation or incorporated into sexual activity with another person to produce sexual excitation. When the fetish involves cross-dressing, the disorder is called **transvestic fetishism.**

3. **Frotteurism**. This disorder is defined as the recurrent preoccupation with intense sexual urges or fantasies, of at least 6 months' duration, involving touching or rubbing against a nonconsenting person (APA, 2000). Sexual excitement is derived from the actual touching or rubbing, not from the coercive nature of the act.

4. **Pedophilia**. The *DSM-IV-TR* describes the essential feature of pedophilia as recurrent sexual urges, behaviors, or sexually arousing fantasies, of at least 6 months' duration, involving sexual activity with a prepubescent child. The age of the molester is 16 or older and is at least 5 years older than the child. This category of paraphilia is the most common of sexual assaults.

5. **Sexual Masochism**. The identifying feature of this disorder is recurrent, intense sexual urges, behaviors, or sexually arousing fantasies, of at least 6 months' duration, involving the act of being humiliated, beaten, bound, or otherwise made to suffer (APA, 2000). These masochistic activities may be fantasized, solitary, or with a partner. Examples include becoming sexually aroused by self-inflicted pain or by being restrained, raped, or beaten by a sexual partner.

6. **Sexual Sadism**. The essential feature of sexual sadism is identified as recurrent, intense, sexual urges, behaviors, or sexually arousing fantasies, of at least 6 months' duration, involving acts in which the psychological or physical suffering (including humiliation) of the victim is sexually exciting (APA, 2000). The sadistic activities may be fantasized or acted on with a consenting or nonconsenting partner. In all instances, sexual excitation occurs in response to the suffering of the victim. Examples include rape, beating, torture, or even killing.

7. **Voyeurism**. This disorder is identified by recurrent, intense sexual urges, behaviors, or sexually arousing fantasies, of at least 6 months' duration, involving the act of observing an unsuspecting person who is naked, in the process of disrobing, or engaging in sexual activity (APA, 2000). Sexual excitement is achieved through the act of looking, and no contact with the person is attempted. Masturbation usually accompanies the "window peeping" but may

occur later as the individual fantasizes about the voyeuristic act.

Predisposing Factors to Paraphilias

1. **Physiological**
   a. ***Biological Factors:*** Various studies have implicated several organic factors in the etiology of paraphilias. Destruction of parts of the limbic system in animals has been shown to cause hypersexual behavior (Becker & Johnson, 2008). Temporal lobe diseases, such as psychomotor seizures or temporal lobe tumors, have been implicated in some individuals with paraphilias. Abnormal levels of androgens also may contribute to inappropriate sexual arousal. The majority of studies involved violent sex offenders, and the results cannot accurately be generalized.

2. **Psychosocial**
   a. ***Psychoanalytical Theory:*** The psychoanalytic approach defines a paraphiliac as one who has failed the normal developmental process toward heterosexual adjustment (Sadock & Sadock, 2007). This occurs when the individual fails to resolve the Oedipal crisis and identifies with the parent of the opposite gender. This creates intense anxiety, which leads the individual to seek sexual gratification in ways that provide a "safe substitution" for the parent (Becker & Johnson, 2008).

Symptomatology (Subjective and Objective Data)

1. Exposure of one's genitals to a stranger.
2. Sexual arousal in the presence of nonliving objects.
3. Touching and rubbing one's genitals against an unconsenting person.
4. Sexual attraction to, or activity with, a prepubescent child.
5. Sexual arousal from being humiliated, beaten, bound, or otherwise made to suffer (through fantasy, self-infliction, or by a sexual partner).
6. Sexual arousal by inflicting psychological or physical suffering on another individual (either consenting or nonconsenting).
7. Sexual arousal from dressing in the clothes of the opposite gender.
8. Sexual arousal from observing unsuspecting people either naked or engaged in sexual activity.
9. Masturbation often accompanies the activities described when they are performed solitarily.
10. The individual is markedly distressed by these activities.

Sexual Dysfunctions

Sexual dysfunctions may occur in any phase of the sexual response cycle. Types of sexual dysfunctions include the following:

1. **Sexual Desire Disorders**
   a. *Hypoactive Sexual Desire Disorder:* This disorder is defined by the *DSM-IV-TR* (APA, 2000) as a persistent or recurrent deficiency or absence of sexual fantasies and desire for sexual activity. The complaint appears to be more common among women than men.
   b. *Sexual Aversion Disorder:* This disorder is characterized by a persistent or recurrent extreme aversion to, and avoidance of, all (or almost all) genital sexual contact with a sexual partner (APA, 2000).
2. **Sexual Arousal Disorders**
   a. *Female Sexual Arousal Disorder:* This disorder is identified in the *DSM-IV-TR* (APA, 2000) as a persistent or recurrent inability to attain, or to maintain until completion of the sexual activity, an adequate lubrication or swelling response of sexual excitement.
   b. *Male Erectile Disorder:* This disorder is characterized by a persistent or recurrent inability to attain, or to maintain until completion of the sexual activity, an adequate erection (APA, 2000).
3. **Orgasmic Disorders**
   a. *Female Orgasmic Disorder (Anorgasmia):* This disorder is defined by the *DSM-IV-TR* as a persistent or recurrent delay in, or absence of, orgasm following a normal sexual excitement phase.
   b. *Male Orgasmic Disorder (Retarded Ejaculation):* With this disorder, the man is unable to ejaculate, even though he has a firm erection and has had more than adequate stimulation. The severity of the problem may range from only occasional problems ejaculating to a history of never having experienced an orgasm.
   c. *Premature Ejaculation: The DSM-IV-TR* describes this disorder as persistent or recurrent ejaculation with minimal sexual stimulation before, on, or shortly after penetration and before the person wishes it.
4. **Sexual Pain Disorders**
   a. *Dyspareunia:* Dyspareunia is defined as recurrent or persistent genital pain associated with sexual intercourse, in either a man or a woman, that is not caused by vaginismus, lack of lubrication, another general medical condition, or the physiological effects of substance use (APA, 2000).
   b. *Vaginismus:* Vaginismus is characterized by an involuntary constriction of the outer third of the vagina, which prevents penile insertion and intercourse.

Predisposing Factors to Sexual Dysfunctions

1. **Physiological Factors**
   a. *Sexual Desire Disorders:* In men, these disorders have been linked to low levels of serum testosterone and to elevated levels of serum prolactin. Evidence also exists that suggests a relationship between serum testosterone and increased female libido. Various medications, such as antihypertensives, antipsychotics, antidepressants, anxiolytics, and anticonvulsants, as well as chronic use of drugs such as alcohol and cocaine, have also been implicated in sexual desire disorders.
   b. *Sexual Arousal Disorders:* These may occur in response to decreased estrogen levels in postmenopausal women. Medications such as antihistamines and cholinergic blockers may produce similar results. Erectile dysfunctions in men may be attributed to arteriosclerosis, diabetes, temporal lobe epilepsy, multiple sclerosis, some medications (antihypertensives, antidepressants, tranquilizers), spinal cord injury, pelvic surgery, and chronic use of alcohol.
   c. *Orgasmic Disorders:* In women these may be attributed to some medical conditions (hypothyroidism, diabetes, and depression) and certain medications (antihypertensives, antidepressants). Medical conditions that may interfere with male orgasm include genitourinary surgery (e.g., prostatectomy), Parkinson's disease, and diabetes. Various medications have also been implicated, including antihypertensives, antidepressants, and antipsychotics. Transient cases of the disorder may occur with excessive alcohol intake.
   d. *Sexual Pain Disorders:* In women these can be caused by disorders of the vaginal entrance, irritation or damage to the clitoris, vaginal or pelvic infections, endometriosis, tumors, or cysts. Painful intercourse in men may be attributed to penile infections, phimosis, urinary tract infections, or prostate problems.

2. **Psychosocial Factors**
   a. *Sexual Desire Disorders:* Phillips (2000) has identified a number of individual and relationship factors that may contribute to hypoactive sexual desire disorder. Individual causes include religious orthodoxy; sexual identity conflicts; past sexual abuse; financial, family, or job problems; depression; and aging-related concerns (e.g., changes in physical appearance). Among the relationship causes are interpersonal conflicts; current physical, verbal, or sexual abuse; extramarital affairs; and desire or practices different from partner.

b. *Sexual Arousal Disorders:* In the female these may be attributed to doubts, fears, guilt, anxiety, shame, conflict, embarrassment, tension, disgust, resentment, grief, anger toward the partner, and puritanical or moralistic upbringing. A history of sexual abuse may also be an important etiologic factor (Leiblum, 1999). The etiology of male erectile disorder may be related to chronic stress, anxiety, or depression. Early developmental factors that promote feelings of inadequacy and a sense of being unloving or unlovable may also result in impotence. Difficulties in the relationship may also be a contributing factor.

c. *Orgasmic Disorders:* A number of factors have been implicated in the etiology of female orgasm disorders. They include fear of becoming pregnant, hostility toward men, negative cultural conditioning, childhood exposure to rigid religious orthodoxy, and traumatic sexual experiences during childhood or adolescence. Orgasm disorders in men may be related to a rigid, puritanical background where sex was perceived as sinful and the genitals as dirty; or interpersonal difficulties, such as ambivalence about commitment, fear of pregnancy, or unexpressed hostility, may be implicated.

d. *Sexual Pain Disorders:* Vaginismus may occur after having experienced painful intercourse for any organic reason, after which involuntary constriction of the vagina occurs in anticipation and fear of recurring pain. Other psychosocial factors that have been implicated in the etiology of vaginismus include negative childhood conditioning of sex as dirty, sinful, and shameful; early childhood sexual trauma; homosexual orientation; traumatic experience with an early pelvic examination; pregnancy phobia; sexually transmitted disease phobia; or cancer phobia (Phillips, 2000; King, 2005; Leiblum, 1999; Sadock & Sadock, 2007).

Symptomatology (Subjective and Objective Data)

1. Absence of sexual fantasies and desire for sexual activity.
2. Discrepancy between partners' levels of desire for sexual activity.
3. Feelings of disgust, anxiety, or panic responses to genital contact.
4. Inability to produce adequate lubrication for sexual activity.
5. Absence of a subjective sense of sexual excitement during sexual activity.

6. Failure to attain or maintain penile erection until completion of sexual activity.

7. Inability to achieve orgasm (in men, to ejaculate) following a period of sexual excitement judged adequate in intensity and duration to produce such a response.

8. Ejaculation occurs with minimal sexual stimulation or before, on, or shortly after penetration and before the individual wishes it.

9. Genital pain occurring before, during, or after sexual intercourse.

10. Constriction of the outer third of the vagina prevents penile penetration.

Common Nursing Diagnoses and Interventions for Paraphilias and Sexual Dysfunctions

(Interventions are applicable to various health-care settings, such as inpatient and partial hospitalization, community outpatient clinic, home health, and private practice.)

● SEXUAL DYSFUNCTION

Definition: The state in which an individual experiences a change in sexual function during the sexual response phases of desire, excitation, and/or orgasm, which is viewed as unsatisfying, unrewarding, or inadequate.

Possible Etiologies ("related to")

Ineffectual or absent role models

Physical [or sexual] abuse

Psychosocial abuse

Values conflict

Lack of privacy

Lack of significant other

Altered body structure or function (pregnancy, recent childbirth, drugs, surgery, anomalies, disease process, trauma, radiation)

Misinformation or deficient knowledge

[Depression]

[Pregnancy phobia]

[Sexually transmitted disease phobia]

[Cancer phobia]

[Previous painful experience]

[Severe anxiety]

[Relationship difficulties]

Defining Characteristics ("evidenced by")

Verbalization of problem:
- [Absence of desire for sexual activity
- Feelings of disgust, anxiety, or panic responses to genital contact
- Absence of lubrication or subjective sense of sexual excitement during sexual activity
- Failure to attain or maintain penile erection during sexual activity
- Inability to achieve orgasm or ejaculation
- Premature ejaculation
- Genital pain during intercourse
- Constriction of the vagina that prevents penile penetration]

Inability to achieve desired satisfaction

Goals/Objectives

Short-term Goals

1. Client will identify stressors that may contribute to loss of sexual function within 1 week *or*
2. Client will discuss pathophysiology of disease process that contributes to sexual dysfunction within 1 week.

For client with permanent dysfunction due to disease process:

3. Client will verbalize willingness to seek professional assistance from a sex therapist in order to learn alternative ways of achieving sexual satisfaction with partner by (time is individually determined).

Long-term Goal

Client will resume sexual activity at level satisfactory to self and partner by (time is individually determined).

Interventions with *Selected Rationales*

1. Assess client's sexual history and previous level of satisfaction in sexual relationship. *This establishes a database from which to work and provides a foundation for goal setting.*
2. Assess client's perception of the problem. *Client's idea of what constitutes a problem may differ from the nurse's. It is the client's perception on which the goals of care must be established.*
3. Help client determine time dimension associated with the onset of the problem and discuss what was happening in his or her life situation at that time. *Stress in any areas of life can affect sexual functioning. Client may be unaware of correlation between stress and sexual dysfunction.*
4. Assess client's mood and level of energy. *Depression and fatigue decrease desire and enthusiasm for participation in sexual activity.*

5. Review medication regimen; observe for side effects. *Many medications can affect sexual functioning. Evaluation of drug and individual response is important to ascertain whether drug may be contributing to the problem.*

6. Encourage client to discuss disease process that may be contributing to sexual dysfunction. Ensure that client is aware that alternative methods of achieving sexual satisfaction exist and can be learned through sex counseling if he or she and partner desire to do so. *Client may be unaware that satisfactory changes can be made in his or her sex life. He or she may also be unaware of the availability of sex counseling.*

7. Encourage client to ask questions regarding sexuality and sexual functioning that may be troubling him or her. *Increasing knowledge and correcting misconceptions can decrease feelings of powerlessness and anxiety and facilitate problem resolution.*

8. Make referral to sex therapist, if necessary. Client may even request that an initial appointment be made for him or her. *Complex problems are likely to require assistance from an individual who is specially trained to treat problems related to sexuality. Client and partner may be somewhat embarrassed to seek this kind of assistance. Support from a trusted nurse can provide the impetus for them to pursue the help they need.*

Outcome Criteria
1. Client is able to correlate physical or psychosocial factors that interfere with sexual functioning.
2. Client is able to communicate with partner about their sexual relationship without discomfort.
3. Client and partner verbalize willingness and desire to seek assistance from professional sex therapist *or*
4. Client verbalizes resumption of sexual activity at level satisfactory to self and partner.

• INEFFECTIVE SEXUALITY PATTERN

Definition: Expressions of concern regarding own sexuality.

Possible Etiologies ("related to")
Lack of significant other
Ineffective or absent role models
[Illness-related alterations in usual sexuality patterns]
Conflicts with sexual orientation or variant preferences
[Unresolved Oedipal conflict]
[Delayed sexual adjustment]

Defining Characteristics ("evidenced by")

Reported difficulties, limitations, or changes in sexual behaviors or activities

[Expressed dissatisfaction with sexual behaviors]

[Reports that sexual arousal can only be achieved through variant practices, such as pedophilia, fetishism, masochism, sadism, frotteurism, exhibitionism, voyeurism]

[Desires to experience satisfying sexual relationship with another individual without need for arousal through variant practices]

Goals/Objectives

(Time elements to be determined by individual situation.)

Short-term Goals

1. Client will verbalize aspects about sexuality that he or she would like to change.
2. Client and partner will communicate with each other ways in which each believes their sexual relationship could be improved.

Long-term Goals

1. Client will express satisfaction with own sexuality pattern.
2. Client and partner will express satisfaction with sexual relationship.

Interventions with *Selected Rationales*

1. Take sexual history, noting client's expression of areas of dissatisfaction with sexual pattern. *Knowledge of what client perceives as the problem is essential for providing the type of assistance he or she may need.*
2. Assess areas of stress in client's life and examine relationship with sexual partner. *Variant sexual behaviors are often associated with added stress in the client's life. Relationship with partner may deteriorate as individual eventually gains sexual satisfaction only from variant practices.*
3. Note cultural, social, ethnic, racial, and religious factors that may contribute to conflicts regarding variant sexual practices. *Client may be unaware of the influence these factors exert in creating feelings of discomfort, shame, and guilt regarding sexual attitudes and behavior.*
4. Be accepting and nonjudgmental. *Sexuality is a very personal and sensitive subject. The client is more likely to share this information if he or she does not fear being judged by the nurse.*
5. Assist therapist in plan of behavior modification to help client who desires to decrease variant sexual behaviors. *Individuals with paraphilias are treated by specialists who have*

experience in modifying variant sexual behaviors. Nurses can intervene by providing assistance with implementation of the plan for behavior modification.

6. If altered sexuality patterns are related to illness or medical treatment, provide information to client and partner regarding the correlation between the illness and the sexual alteration. Explain possible modifications in usual sexual patterns that client and partner may try in an effort to achieve a satisfying sexual experience in spite of the limitation. *Client and partner may be unaware of alternate possibilities for achieving sexual satisfaction, or anxiety associated with the limitation may interfere with rational problem solving.*

7. Explain to client that sexuality is a normal human response and does not relate exclusively to the sex organs or sexual behavior. Sexuality involves complex interrelationships among one's self-concept, body image, personal history, and family and cultural influences; and all interactions with others. *If client feels "abnormal" or very unlike everyone else, the self-concept is likely to be very low—he or she may even feel worthless. To increase the client's feelings of self-worth and desire to change behavior, help him or her to see that even though the behavior is variant, feelings and motivations are common.*

Outcome Criteria

1. Client is able to verbalize fears about abnormality and inappropriateness of sexual behaviors.
2. Client expresses desire to change variant sexual behavior and cooperates with plan of behavior modification.
3. Client and partner verbalize modifications in sexual activities in response to limitations imposed by illness or medical treatment.
4. Client expresses satisfaction with own sexuality pattern or a satisfying sexual relationship with another.

Gender Identity Disorders

Gender identity is the sense of knowing to which gender one belongs—that is, the awareness of one's masculinity or femininity. Gender identity disorders occur when there is incongruity between anatomic sex and gender identity. An individual with gender identity disorder has an intense desire to be, or insists that he or she is of, the other gender. The *DSM-IV-TR* (APA, 2000) identifies two categories of the disorder: gender identity disorder in children and gender identity disorder in adolescents and adults.

Intervention with adolescents and adults with gender identity disorder is difficult. Adolescents commonly act out and rarely have the motivation required to alter their cross-gender roles.

Adults generally seek therapy to learn how to cope with their altered sexual identity, not to correct it.

Treatment of children with the disorder is aimed at helping them to become more comfortable with their assigned gender and to avoid the possible development of gender dissatisfaction in adulthood.

Predisposing Factors to Gender Identity Disorder

1. **Physiological**
   a. Studies of genetics and physiological alterations have been conducted in an attempt to determine whether or not a biological predisposition to gender identity disorder exists. To date, no clear evidence has been demonstrated.
2. **Psychosocial**
   a. ***Family Dynamics:*** It appears that family dynamics plays the most influential role in the etiology of gender disorders. Sadock and Sadock (2007) state, "Children develop a gender identity consonant with their sex of rearing (also known as assigned sex)." Gender roles are culturally determined, and parents encourage masculine or feminine behaviors in their children. Although "temperament" may play a role with certain behavioral characteristics being present at birth, mothers usually foster a child's pride in their gender. Sadock and Sadock (2007) state:

      > The father's role is also important in the early years, and his presence normally helps the separation-individuation process. Without a father, mother and child may remain overly close. For a girl, the father is normally the prototype of future love objects; for a boy, the father is a model for male identification" (p. 719).

   b. ***Psychoanalytical Theory.*** This theory suggests that gender identity problems begin during the struggle of the Oedipal/Electra conflict. Problems may reflect both real family events and those created in the child's imagination. These conflicts, whether real or imagined, interfere with the child's loving of the opposite-gender parent and identifying with the same-gender parent, and ultimately with normal gender identity.

Symptomatology (Subjective and Objective Data)

In children or adolescents:
1. Repeatedly stating intense desire to be of the opposite gender.
2. Insistence that one is of the opposite gender.
3. Preference in males for cross-dressing or simulating female attire.
4. Insistence by females on wearing only stereotypical masculine clothing.

5. Fantasies of being of the opposite gender.
6. Strong desire to participate only in the stereotypical games and pastimes of the opposite gender.
7. Strong preference for playmates (peers) of the opposite gender.

In adults:

1. A stated desire to be of the opposite gender.
2. Frequently passing as the opposite gender.
3. Desire to live or be treated as the opposite gender.
4. Stated conviction that one has the typical feelings and reactions of the opposite gender.
5. Persistent discomfort with or sense of inappropriateness in the assigned gender role.
6. Request for opposite gender hormones or surgery to alter sexual characteristics.

Common Nursing Diagnoses and Interventions for Gender Identity Disorder

(Interventions are applicable to various health-care settings, such as inpatient and partial hospitalization, community outpatient clinic, home health, and private practice.)

NOTE: Because adults and adolescents rarely have the desire or motivation to modify their gender identity, nursing interventions in this section are focused on working with gender-disordered children. Becker and Johnson (2008) state, "It is important to note that not all children with gender identity disorder become adults with gender identity disorder." (p. 733).

● DISTURBED PERSONAL IDENTITY

Definition: Inability to maintain an integrated and complete perception of self.

Possible Etiologies ("related to")

[Parenting patterns that encourage culturally unacceptable behaviors for assigned gender]
[Unresolved Oedipal/Electra conflict]

Defining Characteristics ("evidenced by")

[Statements of desire to be opposite gender]
[Statements that one is the opposite gender]
[Cross-dressing, or passing as the opposite gender]
[Strong preference for playmates (peers) of the opposite gender]
[Stated desire to be treated as the opposite gender]
[Statements of having feelings and reactions of the opposite gender]

Goals/Objectives

Short-term Goals

1. Client will verbalize knowledge of behaviors that are appropriate and culturally acceptable for assigned gender.
2. Client will verbalize desire for congruence between personal feelings and behavior and assigned gender.

Long-term Goals

1. Client will demonstrate behaviors that are appropriate and culturally acceptable for assigned gender.
2. Client will express personal satisfaction and feelings of being comfortable in assigned gender.

Interventions with *Selected Rationales*

1. Spend time with client and show positive regard. *Trust and unconditional acceptance are essential to the establishment of a therapeutic nurse-client relationship.*
2. Be aware of own feelings and attitudes toward this client and his or her behavior. *Attitudes influence behavior. The nurse must not allow negative attitudes to interfere with the effectiveness of interventions.*
3. Allow client to describe his or her perception of the problem. *It is important to know how the client perceives the problem before attempting to correct misperceptions.*
4. Discuss with the client the types of behaviors that are more culturally acceptable. Practice these behaviors through role-playing or with play therapy strategies (e.g., male and female dolls). Positive reinforcement or social attention may be given for use of appropriate behaviors. No response is given for stereotypical opposite-gender behaviors. *The goal is to enhance culturally appropriate same-gender behaviors, but not necessarily to extinguish all coexisting opposite-gender behaviors.*

Outcome Criteria

1. Client demonstrates behaviors that are culturally appropriate for assigned gender.
2. Client verbalizes and demonstrates self-satisfaction with assigned gender role.
3. Client demonstrates development of a close relationship with the parent of the same gender.

• IMPAIRED SOCIAL INTERACTION

Definition: Insufficient or excessive quantity or ineffective quality of social exchange.

Possible Etiologies ("related to")

[Socially and culturally unacceptable behavior]
[Negative role modeling]
[Low self-esteem]

Defining Characteristics ("evidenced by")

Discomfort in social situations
Inability to receive or communicate a satisfying sense of belonging, caring, interest, or shared history
Use of unsuccessful social interaction behaviors
Dysfunctional interaction with others

Goals/Objectives

Short-term Goal

Client will verbalize possible reasons for ineffective interactions with others.

Long-term Goal

Client will interact with others using culturally acceptable behaviors.

Interventions with *Selected Rationales*

1. Once client feels comfortable with the new behaviors in role playing or one-to-one nurse-client interactions, the new behaviors may be tried in group situations. If possible, remain with the client during initial interactions with others. *Presence of a trusted individual provides security for the client in a new situation. It also provides the potential for feedback to the client about his or her behavior.*
2. Observe client behaviors and the responses he or she elicits from others. Give social attention (e.g., smile, nod) to desired behaviors. Follow up these "practice" sessions with one-to-one processing of the interaction. Give positive reinforcement for efforts. *Positive reinforcement encourages repetition of desirable behaviors. One-to-one processing provides time for discussing the appropriateness of specific behaviors and why they should or should not be repeated.*
3. Offer support if client is feeling hurt from peer ridicule. Matter-of-factly discuss the behaviors that elicited the ridicule. Offer no personal reaction to the behavior. *Personal reaction from the nurse would be considered judgmental. Validation of client's feelings is important, yet it is also important that client understand why his or her behavior was the subject of ridicule and how to avoid it in the future.*

Outcome Criteria
1. Client interacts appropriately with others demonstrating culturally acceptable behaviors.
2. Client verbalizes and demonstrates comfort in assigned gender role in interactions with others.

● LOW SELF-ESTEEM

Definition: Negative self-evaluating/feelings about self or self-capabilities.

Possible Etiologies ("related to")

[Rejection by peers]
Lack of approval and/or affection
Repeated negative reinforcement
[Lack of personal satisfaction with assigned gender]

Defining Characteristics ("evidenced by")

[Inability to form close, personal relationships]
[Negative view of self]
[Expressions of worthlessness]
[Social isolation]
[Hypersensitivity to slight or criticism]
Expressions of shame or guilt
Self-negating verbalizations
Lack of eye contact

Goals/Objectives
Short-term Goal

Client will verbalize positive statements about self, including past accomplishments and future prospects.

Long-term Goal

Client will verbalize and demonstrate behaviors that indicate self-satisfaction with assigned gender, ability to interact with others, and a sense of self as a worthwhile person.

Interventions with *Selected Rationales*
1. *To enhance the child's self-esteem:*
   a. Encourage the child to engage in activities in which he or she is likely to achieve success.
   b. Help the child to focus on aspects of his or her life for which positive feelings exist. Discourage rumination about situations that are perceived as failures or over

which the client has no control. Give positive feedback for
these behaviors.

2. Help the client identify behaviors or aspects of life he or she
would like to change. If realistic, assist the child in problem
solving ways to bring about the change. ***Having some control
over his or her life may decrease feelings of powerlessness
and increase feelings of self-worth.***

3. Offer to be available for support to the child when he or she is
feeling rejected by peers. ***Having an available support person who does not judge the child's behavior and who provides
unconditional acceptance assists the child to progress toward
acceptance of self as a worthwhile person.***

Outcome Criteria

1. Client verbalizes positive perception of self.
2. Client verbalizes self-satisfaction about accomplishments
and demonstrates behaviors that reflect self-worth.

@ INTERNET REFERENCES

- Additional information about sexual disorders may be located
at the following websites:
  a. http://www.sexualhealth.com/
  b. http://www.cmellc.com/topics/sexual.html
  c. http://www.priory.com/sex.htm
  d. http://web4health.info/en/answers/sex-menu.htm
  e. http://allpsych.com/disorders/sexual/index.html
- Additional information about gender identity disorders may be
located at the following websites:
  a. http://www.avitale.com/
  b. http://www.leaderu.com/jhs/rekers.html
  c. http://emedicine.medscape.com/article/293890-overview
  d. http://psyweb.com/Mdisord/jsp/sexd.jsp

Movie Connections

Mystic River (pedophilia) ● *Blue Velvet (sexual masochism)*
● *Looking for Mr. Goodbar (sadism/masochism)* ● *Normal (transvestitism)*
● *Transamerica (transvestitism)*

CHAPTER 12

Eating Disorders

● BACKGROUND ASSESSMENT DATA

The American Psychiatric Association (APA, 2000) *Diagnostic and Statistical Manual of Mental Disorders, Fourth Edition, Text Revision (DSM-IV-TR)* identifies eating disorders as those characterized by severe disturbances in eating behavior. Two such disorders are described in the *DSM-IV-TR*: anorexia nervosa and bulimia nervosa. Obesity is not classified as a psychiatric disorder per se; however, because of the strong emotional factors associated with it, the *DSM-IV-TR* suggests that obesity may be considered within the category of *Psychological Factors Affecting Medical Condition*. A third category of eating disorder, binge eating disorder, is also being considered by the American Psychiatric Association.

Anorexia Nervosa

Defined

Anorexia nervosa is a clinical syndrome in which the person has a morbid fear of obesity. It is characterized by the individual's gross distortion of body image, preoccupation with food, and refusal to eat. The disorder occurs predominantly in females 12 to 30 years of age. Without intervention, death from starvation can occur.

Symptomatology (Subjective and Objective Data)

1. Morbid fear of obesity. Preoccupied with body size. Reports "feeling fat" even when in an emaciated condition.
2. Refusal to eat. Reports "not being hungry," although it is thought that the actual feelings of hunger do not cease until late in the disorder.
3. Preoccupation with food. Thinks and talks about food at great length. Prepares enormous amounts of food for friends and family members but refuses to eat any of it.
4. Amenorrhea is common, often appearing even before noticeable weight loss has occurred.
5. Delayed psychosexual development.
6. Compulsive behavior, such as excessive hand washing, may be present.

218

7. Extensive exercising is common.
8. Feelings of depression and anxiety often accompany this disorder.
9. May engage in the binge-and-purge syndrome from time to time (see following section on bulimia nervosa).

Bulimia Nervosa

Defined

Bulimia nervosa is an eating disorder (commonly called "the binge-and-purge syndrome") characterized by extreme over-eating, followed by self-induced vomiting and abuse of laxatives and diuretics. The disorder occurs predominantly in females and begins in adolescence or early adult life.

Symptomatology (Subjective and Objective Data)

1. Binges are usually solitary and secret, and the individual may consume thousands of calories in one episode.
2. After the binge has begun, there is often a feeling of loss of control or inability to stop eating.
3. Following the binge, the individual engages in inappropriate compensatory measures to avoid gaining weight (e.g., self-induced vomiting; excessive use of laxatives, diuretics, or enemas; fasting; and extreme exercising).
4. Eating binges may be viewed as pleasurable but are followed by intense self-criticism and depressed mood.
5. Individuals with bulimia are usually within normal weight range, some a few pounds underweight, some a few pounds overweight.
6. Obsession with body image and appearance is a predominant feature of this disorder. Individuals with bulimia display undue concern with sexual attractiveness and how they will appear to others.
7. Binges usually alternate with periods of normal eating and fasting.
8. Excessive vomiting may lead to problems with dehydration and electrolyte imbalance.
9. Gastric acid in the vomitus may contribute to the erosion of tooth enamel.

Predisposing Factors to Anorexia Nervosa and Bulimia Nervosa

1. **Physiological Factors**
   a. *Genetics:* A hereditary predisposition to eating disorders has been hypothesized on the basis of family histories and an apparent association with other disorders for which the likelihood of genetic influences exist. Anorexia nervosa is more common among sisters and mothers of those with

the disorder than among the general population. Several studies have reported a higher than expected frequency of mood disorders among first-degree biological relatives of people with anorexia nervosa and bulimia nervosa and of substance abuse and dependence in relatives of individuals with bulimia nervosa (APA, 2000).

b. *Neuroendocrine Abnormalities:* Some speculation has occurred regarding a primary hypothalamic dysfunction in anorexia nervosa. Studies consistent with this theory have revealed elevated cerebrospinal fluid cortisol levels and a possible impairment of dopaminergic regulation in individuals with anorexia (Halmi, 2008).

c. *Neurochemical Influences:* Neurochemical influences in bulimia may be associated with the neurotransmitters serotonin and norepinephrine. This hypothesis has been supported by the positive response these individuals have shown to therapy with the selective serotonin reuptake inhibitors (SSRIs). Some studies have found high levels of endogenous opioids in the spinal fluid of clients with anorexia, promoting the speculation that these chemicals may contribute to denial of hunger (Sadock & Sadock, 2007). Some of these individuals have been shown to gain weight when given naloxone, an opioid antagonist.

2. **Psychosocial Factors**

a. *Psychodynamic Theory*: The psychodynamic theory suggests that behaviors associated with eating disorders reflect a developmental arrest in the very early years of childhood caused by disturbances in mother-infant interactions. The tasks of trust, autonomy, and separation-individuation go unfulfilled, and the individual remains in the dependent position. Ego development is retarded. The problem is compounded when the mother responds to the child's physical and emotional needs with food. Manifestations include a disturbance in body identity and a distortion in body image. When events occur that threaten the vulnerable ego, feelings emerge of lack of control over one's body (self). Behaviors associated with food and eating provide feelings of control over one's life.

b. *Family Dynamics*: This theory proposes that the issue of control becomes the overriding factor in the family of the individual with an eating disorder. These families often consist of a passive father, a domineering mother, and an overly dependent child. A high value is placed on perfectionism in this family, and the child feels he or she must satisfy these standards. Parental criticism promotes an increase in obsessive and perfectionistic behavior on the part of the child, who continues to seek love, approval, and recognition. The child eventually begins to feel helpless and ambivalent toward the parents. In adolescence, these distorted eating patterns may represent a rebellion against the parents, viewed by the child as a means of gaining and remaining in control. The symptoms are often triggered by a stressor that the adolescent perceives as a loss of control in some aspect of his or her life.

Obesity

Defined

The following formula is used to determine the degree of obesity in an individual:

$$\text{Body mass index (BMI)} = \frac{\text{weight (kg)}}{\text{height (m)}^2}$$

The BMI range for normal weight is 20 to 24.9. Studies by the National Center for Health Statistics indicate that *overweight* is defined as a BMI of 25.0 to 29.9 (based on U.S. Dietary Guidelines for Americans). Based on criteria of the World Health Organization, *obesity* is defined as a BMI of 30.0 or greater. These guidelines, which were released by the National Heart, Lung, and Blood Institute in July 1998, markedly increased the number of Americans considered to be overweight. The average American woman has a BMI of 26, and fashion models typically have BMIs of 18 (Priesnitz, 2005).

Obesity is known to contribute to a number of health problems, including hyperlipidemia, diabetes mellitus, osteoarthritis, and increased workload on the heart and lungs.

Predisposing Factors to Obesity

1. **Physiological Factors**
   a. *Genetics:* Genetics have been implicated in the development of obesity in that 80% of offspring of two obese parents are obese (Halmi, 2008). This hypothesis has also been supported by studies of twins reared by normal and overweight parents.
   b. *Physical Factors:* Overeating and/or obesity has also been associated with lesions in the appetite and satiety centers of the hypothalamus, hypothyroidism, decreased insulin production in diabetes mellitus, and increased cortisone production in Cushing's disease.
   c. *Lifestyle Factors:* On a more basic level, obesity can be viewed as the ingestion of a greater number of calories than are expended. Weight gain occurs when caloric intake exceeds caloric output in terms of basal metabolism and physical activity. Many overweight individuals lead

sedentary lifestyles, making it very difficult to burn off calories.

2. **Psychosocial Factors**

   a. *Psychoanalytical Theory:* This theory suggests that obesity is the result of unresolved dependency needs, with the individual being fixed in the oral stage of psychosexual development. The symptoms of obesity are viewed as depressive equivalents, attempts to regain "lost" or frustrated nurturance and care.

Common Nursing Diagnoses and Interventions for Anorexia and Bulimia

(Interventions are applicable to various health-care settings, such as inpatient and partial hospitalization, community outpatient clinic, home health, and private practice.)

● IMBALANCED NUTRITION: LESS THAN BODY REQUIREMENTS

Definition: Intake of nutrients insufficient to meet metabolic needs.

Possible Etiologies ("related to")

[Refusal to eat]

[Ingestion of large amounts of food, followed by self-induced vomiting]

[Abuse of laxatives, diuretics, and/or diet pills]

[Physical exertion in excess of energy produced through caloric intake]

Defining Characteristics ("evidenced by")

[Loss of 15% of expected body weight (anorexia nervosa)]
Pale mucous membranes
Poor muscle tone
Excessive loss of hair [or increased growth of hair on body (lanugo)]
[Amenorrhea]
[Poor skin turgor]
[Electrolyte imbalances]
[Hypothermia]
[Bradycardia]
[Hypotension]
[Cardiac irregularities]
[Edema]

Goals/Objectives

Short-term Goal

Client will gain _____ lbs per week (amount to be established by client, nurse, and dietitian).

Long-term Goal

By discharge from treatment, client will exhibit no signs or symptoms of malnutrition.

Interventions with *Selected Rationales*

1. If client is unable or unwilling to maintain adequate oral intake, physician may order a liquid diet to be administered via nasogastric tube. Nursing care of the individual receiving tube feedings should be administered according to established hospital procedures. *The client's physical safety is a nursing priority, and without adequate nutrition, a life-threatening situation exists.*

For oral diet:

2. In collaboration with dietitian, determine number of calories required to provide adequate nutrition and realistic (according to body structure and height) weight gain. *Adequate calories are required to affect a weight gain of 2 to 3 lbs per week.*

3. Explain to client details of behavior modification program as outlined by physician. Explain benefits of compliance with prandial routine and consequences for noncompliance. *Behavior modification bases privileges granted or restricted directly on weight gain and loss. Focus is placed on emotional issues, rather than food and eating specifically.*

4. Sit with client during mealtimes for support and to observe amount ingested. A limit (usually 30 minutes) should be imposed on time allotted for meals. *Without a time limit, meals can become lengthy, drawn-out sessions, providing client with attention based on food and eating.*

5. Client should be observed for at least 1 hour following meals. *This time may be used by client to discard food stashed from tray or to engage in self-induced vomiting.*

6. Client may need to be accompanied to bathroom *if self-induced vomiting is suspected.*

7. Strict documentation of intake and output. *This information is required to promote client safety and plan nursing care.*

8. Weigh client daily immediately on arising and following first voiding. Always use same scale, if possible. *Client care, privileges, and restrictions will be based on accurate daily weights.*

9. Do not discuss food or eating with client, once protocol has been established. Do, however, offer support and positive reinforcement for obvious improvements in eating behaviors. ***Discussing food with client provides positive feedback for maladaptive behaviors.***

10. Client must understand that if, because of poor oral intake, nutritional status does not improve, tube feedings will be initiated ***to ensure client's safety.*** Staff must be consistent and firm with this action, using a matter-of-fact, nonpunitive approach regarding the tube insertion and subsequent feedings.

11. As nutritional status improves and eating habits are established, begin to explore with client the feelings associated with his or her extreme fear of gaining weight. ***Emotional issues must be resolved if maladaptive responses are to be eliminated.***

Outcome Criteria

1. Client has achieved and maintained at least 85% of expected body weight.
2. Vital signs, blood pressure, and laboratory serum studies are within normal limits.
3. Client verbalizes importance of adequate nutrition.

● DEFICIENT FLUID VOLUME

Definition: Decreased intravascular, interstitial, and/or intracellular fluid. This refers to dehydration, water loss alone without change in sodium.

Possible Etiologies ("related to")

[Decreased fluid intake]
[Abnormal fluid loss caused by self-induced vomiting]
[Excessive use of laxatives or enemas]
[Excessive use of diuretics]
[Electrolyte or acid-base imbalance brought about by malnourished condition or self-induced vomiting]

Defining Characteristics ("evidenced by")

Decreased urine output
[Output greater than intake]
Increased urine concentration
Elevated hematocrit
Decreased blood pressure
Increased pulse rate
Increased body temperature

Dry skin
Decreased skin turgor
Weakness
Change in mental state
Dry mucous membranes

Goals/Objectives

Short-term Goal

Client will drink 125 mL of fluid each hour during waking hours.

Long-term Goal

By discharge from treatment, client will exhibit no signs or symptoms of dehydration (as evidenced by quantity of urinary output sufficient to individual client; normal specific gravity; vital signs within normal limits; moist, pink mucous membranes; good skin turgor; and immediate capillary refill).

Interventions with *Selected Rationales*

1. Keep strict record of intake and output. Teach client importance of daily fluid intake of 2000 to 3000 mL. *This information is required to promote client safety and plan nursing care.*
2. Weigh client daily immediately on arising and following first voiding. Always use same scale, if possible. *An accurate daily weight is needed to plan nursing care for the client.*
3. Assess and document condition of skin turgor and any changes in skin integrity. *Condition of skin provides valuable data regarding client hydration.*
4. Discourage client from bathing every day if skin is very dry. *Hot water and soap are drying to the skin.*
5. Monitor laboratory serum values, and notify physician of significant alterations. *Laboratory data provide an objective measure for evaluating adequate hydration.*
6. Client should be observed for at least 1 hour following meals and may need to be accompanied to the bathroom if self-induced vomiting is suspected. *Vomiting causes active loss of body fluids and can precipitate fluid volume deficit.*
7. Assess and document moistness and color of oral mucous membranes. *Dry, pale mucous membranes may be indicative of malnutrition or dehydration.*
8. Encourage frequent oral care *to moisten mucous membranes, reducing discomfort from dry mouth, and to decrease bacterial count, minimizing risk of tissue infection.*
9. Help client identify true feelings and fears that contribute to maladaptive eating behaviors. *Emotional issues must be resolved if maladaptive behaviors are to be eliminated.*

Outcome Criteria

1. Client's vital signs, blood pressure, and laboratory serum studies are within normal limits.
2. No abnormalities of skin turgor and dryness of skin and oral mucous membranes are evident.
3. Client verbalizes knowledge regarding consequences of fluid loss due to self-induced vomiting and importance of adequate fluid intake.

● INEFFECTIVE COPING

Definition: Inability to form a valid appraisal of the stressors, inadequate choices of practiced responses, and/or inability to use available resources.

Possible Etiologies ("related to")

[Retarded ego development]
[Unfulfilled tasks of trust and autonomy]
[Dysfunctional family system]
[Unmet dependency needs]
[Feelings of helplessness and lack of control in life situation]
[Possible chemical imbalance caused by malfunction of hypothalamus]
[Unrealistic perceptions]

Defining Characteristics ("evidenced by")

[Preoccupation with extreme fear of obesity, and distortion of own body image]
[Refusal to eat]
[Obsessed with talking about food]
[Compulsive behavior (e.g., excessive hand washing)]
[Excessive overeating, followed by self-induced vomiting and/or abuse of laxatives and diuretics]
[Poor self-esteem]
[Chronic fatigue]
[Chronic anxiety]
[Chronic depression]
Inadequate problem solving
Inability to meet role expectations
Destructive behavior toward self

Goals/Objectives

Short-term Goal

Within 7 days, client will eat regular meals and attend activities without discussing food or physical appearance.

Long-term Goal
Client will be able to verbalize adaptive coping mechanisms that can be realistically incorporated into his or her lifestyle, thereby eliminating the need for maladaptive eating behaviors.

Interventions with *Selected Rationales*

1. Establish a trusting relationship with client by being honest, accepting, and available and by keeping all promises. *The therapeutic nurse-client relationship is built on trust.*
2. Acknowledge client's anger at feelings of loss of control brought about by established eating regimen (refer to INTERVENTIONS for Imbalanced Nutrition).
3. When nutritional status has improved, begin to explore with client the feelings associated with his or her extreme fear of gaining weight. *Emotional issues must be resolved if maladaptive behaviors are to be eliminated.*
4. Explore family dynamics. Help client to identify his or her role contributions and their appropriateness within the family system. Assist client to identify specific concerns within the family structure and ways to help relieve those concerns. Also, discuss importance of client's separation of self as individual within the family system, and of identifying independent emotions and accepting them as his or her own. *Client must recognize how maladaptive eating behaviors are related to emotional problems—often issues of control within the family structure.*
5. Initially, allow client to maintain dependent role. To deprive the individual of this role at this time could cause his or her anxiety to rise to an unmanageable level. As trust is developed and physical condition improves, encourage client to be as independent as possible in self-care activities. Offer positive reinforcement for independent behaviors and problem-solving and decision-making. *Client must learn to function independently. Positive reinforcement increases self-esteem and encourages the client to use behaviors that are more acceptable.*
6. Explore with client ways in which he or she may feel in control within the environment without resorting to maladaptive eating behaviors. *When client feels control over major life issues, the need to gain control through maladaptive eating behaviors will diminish.*

Outcome Criteria

1. Client is able to assess maladaptive coping behaviors accurately.
2. Client is able to verbalize adaptive coping strategies that can be used in the home environment.

● ANXIETY (Moderate to Severe)

Definition: Vague uneasy feeling of discomfort or dread accompanied by an autonomic response (the source often nonspecific or unknown to the individual); a feeling of apprehension caused by anticipation of danger. It is an alerting signal that warns of impending danger and enables the individual to take measures to deal with threat.

Possible Etiologies ("related to")

Situational and maturational crises
[Unmet dependency needs]
[Low self-esteem]
[Dysfunctional family system]
[Feelings of helplessness and lack of control in life situation]
[Unfulfilled tasks of trust and autonomy]

Defining Characteristics ("evidenced by")

Increased tension
Increased helplessness
Overexcited
Apprehensive; fearful
Restlessness
Poor eye contact
[Increased difficulty taking oral nourishment]
[Inability to learn]

Goals/Objectives

Short-term Goal

Client will demonstrate use of relaxation techniques to maintain anxiety at manageable level within 7 days.

Long-term Goal

By time of discharge from treatment, client will be able to recognize events that precipitate anxiety and intervene to prevent disabling behaviors.

Interventions with *Selected Rationales*

1. Be available to stay with client. Remain calm and provide reassurance of safety. ***Client safety and security is a nursing priority.***
2. Help client identify the situation that precipitated onset of anxiety symptoms. ***Client may be unaware that emotional issues are related to symptoms of anxiety. Recognition may be the first step in elimination of this maladaptive response.***

3. Review client's methods of coping with similar situations in the past. *In seeking to create change, it is helpful for client to identify past responses and determine whether they were successful and whether they could be employed again. Client strengths should be identified and used to his or her advantage.*
4. Provide quiet environment. Reduce stimuli: low lighting, few people. *Anxiety level may be decreased in calm atmosphere with few stimuli.*
5. Administer antianxiety medications, as ordered by physician. Monitor for effectiveness of medication as well as for adverse side effects. *Short-term use of antianxiety medications (e.g., lorazepam, chlordiazepoxide, alprazolam) provides relief from the immobilizing effects of anxiety, and facilitates client's cooperation with therapy.*
6. Teach client to recognize signs of increasing anxiety and ways to intervene for maintaining the anxiety at a manageable level (e.g., exercise, walking, jogging, relaxation techniques). *Anxiety and tension can be reduced safely and with benefit to the client through physical activities.*

Outcome Criteria

1. Client is able to verbalize events that precipitate anxiety and demonstrate techniques for its reduction.
2. Client is able to verbalize ways in which he or she may gain more control of the environment and thereby reduce feelings of helplessness.

● DISTURBED BODY IMAGE/LOW SELF-ESTEEM

Definition: Confusion in mental picture of one's physical self. Negative self-evaluating/feelings about self or self-capabilities.

Possible Etiologies ("related to")

[Lack of positive feedback]
[Perceived failures]
[Unrealistic expectations (on the part of self and others)]
[Retarded ego development]
[Unmet dependency needs]
[Threat to security caused by dysfunctional family dynamics]
[Morbid fear of obesity]
[Perceived loss of control in some aspect of life]

Defining Characteristics ("evidenced by")

[Distorted body image, views self as fat, even in the presence of normal body weight or severe emaciation]
[Denial that problem with low body weight exists]
[Difficulty accepting positive reinforcement]
[Not taking responsibility for self-care (self-neglect)]
[Nonparticipation in therapy]
[Self-destructive behavior (self-induced vomiting; abuse of laxatives or diuretics; refusal to eat)]
Lack of eye contact
[Depressed mood and self-deprecating thoughts following episode of binging and purging]
[Preoccupation with appearance and how others perceive them]

Goals/Objectives

Short-term Goal

Client will verbally acknowledge misperception of body image as "fat" within specified time (depending on severity and chronicity of condition).

Long-term Goal

Client will demonstrate an increase in self-esteem as manifested by verbalizing positive aspects of self and exhibiting less preoccupation with own appearance as a more realistic body image is developed by time of discharge from therapy.

Interventions with *Selected Rationales*

1. Help client reexamine negative perceptions of self and recognize positive attributes. *Client's own identification of strengths and positive attributes can increase sense of self-worth.*
2. Offer positive reinforcement for independently made decisions influencing client's life. *Positive reinforcement enhances self-esteem and may encourage client to continue functioning more independently.*
3. Offer positive reinforcement when honest feelings related to autonomy and dependence issues remain separated from maladaptive eating behaviors.
4. Help client develop a realistic perception of body image and relationship with food. *Client needs to recognize that his or her perception of body image is unhealthy and that maintaining control through maladaptive eating behaviors is dangerous—even life-threatening.*
5. Promote feelings of control within the environment through participation and independent decision making. Through positive feedback, help client learn to accept self as is, including weaknesses as well as strengths. *Client must come to understand that he or she is a capable, autonomous*

individual who can perform outside the family unit and who is not expected to be perfect. Control of his or her life must be achieved in other ways besides dieting and weight loss.

6. Help client realize that perfection is unrealistic, and explore this need with him or her. *As client begins to feel better about self and identifies positive self-attributes, and develops the ability to accept certain personal inadequacies, the need for unrealistic achievements should diminish.*

7. Help client claim ownership of angry feelings and recognize that expressing them is acceptable if done so in an appropriate manner. Be an effective role model. *Unexpressed anger is often turned inward on the self, resulting in depreciation of self-esteem.*

Outcome Criteria

1. Client is able to verbalize positive aspects about self.
2. Client expresses interest in welfare of others and less preoccupation with own appearance.
3. Client verbalizes that image of body as "fat" was misperception and demonstrates ability to take control of own life without resorting to maladaptive eating behaviors.

Common Nursing Diagnoses and Interventions for Obesity

(Interventions are applicable to various health-care settings, such as inpatient and partial hospitalization, community outpatient clinic, home health, and private practice.)

● IMBALANCED NUTRITION: MORE THAN BODY REQUIREMENTS

Definition: Intake of nutrients that exceeds metabolic needs.

Possible Etiologies ("related to")

[Compulsive eating]
Excessive intake in relation to metabolic needs
[Sedentary lifestyle]
[Genetics]
[Unmet dependency needs—fixation in oral developmental stage]

Defining Characteristics ("evidenced by")

Weight 20% over ideal for height and frame
[Body mass index of 30 or more]

Goals/Objectives

Short-term Goal

Client will verbalize understanding of what must be done to lose weight.

Long-term Goal

Client will demonstrate change in eating patterns resulting in a steady weight loss.

Interventions with *Selected Rationales*

1. Encourage the client to keep a diary of food intake. *A food diary provides the opportunity for the client to gain a realistic picture of the amount of food ingested and provides data on which to base the dietary program.*

2. Discuss feelings and emotions associated with eating. *This helps to identify when client is eating to satisfy an emotional need rather than a physiological one.*

3. With input from the client, formulate an eating plan that includes food from the basic food pyramid with emphasis on low-fat intake. It is helpful to keep the plan as similar to the client's usual eating pattern as possible. *Diet must eliminate calories while maintaining adequate nutrition. Client is more likely to stay on the eating plan if he or she is able to participate in its creation and it deviates as little as possible from usual types of foods.*

4. Identify realistic increment goals for weekly weight loss. *Reasonable weight loss (1 to 2 lb/wk) results in more lasting effects. Excessive, rapid weight loss may result in fatigue and irritability and may ultimately lead to failure in meeting goals for weight loss. Motivation is more easily sustained by meeting "stair-step" goals.*

5. Plan progressive exercise program tailored to individual goals and choice. *Exercise may enhance weight loss by burning calories and reducing appetite, increasing energy, toning muscles, and enhancing sense of well-being and accomplishment. Walking is an excellent choice for overweight individuals.*

6. Discuss the probability of reaching plateaus when weight remains stable for extended periods. *Client should know that this is likely to happen as changes in metabolism occur. Plateaus cause frustration, and client may need additional support during these times to remain on the weight loss program.*

7. Provide instruction about medications to assist with weight loss if ordered by the physician. *Appetite-suppressant drugs (e.g., sibutramine) and others that have weight loss as a side effect (e.g., fluoxetine; topiramate) may be helpful to*

someone who is severely overweight. Drugs should be used
for this purpose for only a short period while the individual
attempts to adjust to the new pattern of eating.

Outcome Criteria

1. Client has established a healthy pattern of eating for weight control with weight loss progressing toward a desired goal.
2. Client verbalizes plans for future maintenance of weight control.

● DISTURBED BODY IMAGE/LOW SELF-ESTEEM

Definition: Confusion in mental picture of one's physical self. Negative self-evaluating/feelings about self or self-capabilities.

Possible Etiologies ("related to")

[Dissatisfaction with appearance]
[Unmet dependency needs]
[Lack of adequate nurturing by maternal figure]

Defining Characteristics ("evidenced by")

Negative feelings about body (e.g., feelings of helplessness, hopelessness, or powerlessness)
[Verbalization of desire to lose weight]
[Failure to take responsibility for self-care (self-neglect)]
Lack of eye contact
[Expressions of low self-worth]

Goals/Objectives
Short-term Goal
Client will begin to accept self based on self-attributes rather than on appearance.

Long-term Goal
Client will pursue loss of weight as desired.

Interventions with *Selected Rationales*

1. Assess client's feelings and attitudes about being obese. *Obesity and compulsive eating behaviors may have deep-rooted psychological implications, such as compensation for lack of love and nurturing or a defense against intimacy.*
2. Ensure that the client has privacy during self-care activities. *The obese individual may be sensitive or self-conscious about his or her body.*

3. Have client recall coping patterns related to food in family of origin, and explore how these may affect current situation. *Parents are role models for their children. Maladaptive eating behaviors are learned within the family system and are supported through positive reinforcement. Food may be substituted by the parent for affection and love, and eating is associated with a feeling of satisfaction, becoming the primary defense.*

4. Determine client's motivation for weight loss and set goals. *The individual may harbor repressed feelings of hostility, which may be expressed inward on the self. Because of a poor self-concept, the person often has difficulty with relationships. When the motivation is to lose weight for someone else, successful weight loss is less likely to occur.*

5. Help client identify positive self-attributes. Focus on strengths and past accomplishments unrelated to physical appearance. *It is important that self-esteem not be tied solely to size of the body. Client needs to recognize that obesity need not interfere with positive feelings regarding self-concept and self-worth.*

6. Refer client to support or therapy group. *Support groups can provide companionship, increase motivation, decrease loneliness and social ostracism, and give practical solutions to common problems. Group therapy can be helpful in dealing with underlying psychological concerns.*

Outcome Criteria

1. Client has established a healthy pattern of eating for weight control with weight loss progressing toward a desired goal.
2. Client verbalizes plans for future maintenance of weight control.

@ INTERNET REFERENCES

- Additional information about anorexia nervosa and bulimia nervosa may be located at the following websites:
  a. http://www.aabainc.org
  b. http://healthyminds.org/multimedia/eatingdisorders.pdf
  c. http://www.mentalhealth.com/dis/p20-et01.html
  d. http://www.anred.com/
  e. http://www.mentalhealth.com/dis/p20-et02.html
  f. http://www.nimh.nih.gov/publicat/eatingdisorders.cfm
  g. http://medlineplus.nlm.nih.gov/medlineplus/eatingdisorders.html
- Additional information about obesity may be located at the following websites:
  a. http://www.shapeup.org/
  b. http://www.obesity.org/

    c. http://medlineplus.nlm.nih.gov/medlineplus/obesity
      .html
    d. http://www.asbp.org/
    e. http://win.niddk.nih.gov/publications/binge.htm

Movie Connections

The Best Little Girl in the World (anorexia nervosa) • *Kate's Secret (bulimia nnervosa)* • *For the Love of Nancy (anorexia nervosa)* • *Super Size Me (obesity)*

CHAPTER 13

Adjustment Disorder

● BACKGROUND ASSESSMENT DATA

The essential feature of adjustment disorder is a maladaptive reaction to an identifiable psychosocial stressor that occurs within 3 months after the onset of the stressor and has persisted for no longer than 6 months (American Psychiatric Association [APA], 2000). The response is considered maladaptive either because there is impairment in social or occupational functioning or because the behaviors are exaggerated beyond the usual, expected response to such a stressor. The impairment is corrected with the disappearance of, or adaptation to, the stressor. The following categories are defined:

1. **Adjustment Disorder with Depressed Mood**. This category is the most commonly diagnosed adjustment disorder. The major symptoms include depressed mood, tearfulness, and hopelessness. A differential diagnosis with the affective disorders must be considered.
2. **Adjustment Disorder with Anxiety.** The major symptom of this adjustment disorder is anxiety. Primary manifestations include nervousness, worry, and restlessness. A differential diagnosis with the anxiety disorders must be considered.
3. **Adjustment Disorder with Mixed Anxiety and Depressed Mood.** This type of adjustment disorder is identified by a combination of depression and anxiety. A differential diagnosis must be made considering the affective and anxiety disorders.
4. **Adjustment Disorder with Disturbance of Conduct.** The major response involves conduct in which there is violation of the rights of others or of major age-appropriate societal norms and rules. A differential diagnosis with conduct disorder or antisocial personality disorder must be considered.
5. **Adjustment Disorder with Mixed Disturbance of Emotions and Conduct.** The behavioral manifestations include both emotional symptoms (e.g., depression, anxiety) and disturbances in conduct.
6. **Adjustment Disorder Unspecified**. This diagnosis is used when the maladaptive reaction is not consistent with any of

the other categories of adjustment disorder. Manifestations may include physical complaints, social withdrawal, and occupational or academic inhibition, without significant depressed or anxious mood.

Predisposing Factors

1. **Physiological**
   a. ***Developmental Impairment.*** Chronic conditions, such as organic mental disorder or mental retardation, are thought to impair the ability of an individual to adapt to stress, causing increased vulnerability to adjustment disorder. Sadock and Sadock (2007) suggest that genetic factors also may influence individual risks for maladaptive response to stress.
2. **Psychosocial Theories**
   a. ***Psychoanalytical Theory.*** Some proponents of psychoanalytical theory view adjustment disorder as a maladaptive response to stress that is caused by early childhood trauma, increased dependency, and retarded ego development. Other psychoanalysts put considerable weight on the constitutional factor, or birth characteristics that contribute to the manner in which individuals respond to stress. In many instances, adjustment disorder is precipitated by a specific meaningful stressor having found a point of vulnerability in an individual of otherwise adequate ego strength.
   b. ***Developmental Model.*** Some studies relate a predisposition to adjustment disorder to factors such as developmental stage, timing of the stressor, and available support systems. When a stressor occurs, and the individual does not have the developmental maturity, available support systems, or adequate coping strategies to adapt, normal functioning is disrupted, resulting in psychological or somatic symptoms. The disorder also may be related to a dysfunctional grieving process. The individual may remain in the denial or anger stage, with inadequate defense mechanisms to complete the grieving process.
   c. ***Stress-Adaptation Model.*** This model considers the type of stressor the individual experiences, the situational context in which it occurs, and intrapersonal factors in the predisposition to adjustment disorder. It has been found that continuous stressors (those to which an individual is exposed over an extended period of time) are more commonly cited than sudden-shock stressors (those that occur without warning) as precipitants to maladaptive functioning. The situational context in which the stressor occurs may include factors such as personal and general economic

conditions; occupational and recreational opportunities; the availability of social supports, such as family, friends, and neighbors; and the availability of cultural or religious support groups. Intrapersonal factors that have been implicated in the predisposition to adjustment disorder include birth temperament, learned social skills and coping strategies, the presence of psychiatric illness, degree of flexibility, and level of intelligence.

Symptomatology (Subjective and Objective Data)

1. Depressed mood
2. Tearfulness
3. Hopelessness
4. Nervousness
5. Worry
6. Restlessness
7. Ambivalence
8. Anger, expressed inappropriately
9. Increased dependency
10. Violation of the rights of others
11. Violation of societal norms and rules, such as truancy, vandalism, reckless driving, fighting
12. Inability to function occupationally or academically
13. Manipulative behavior
14. Social isolation
15. Physical complaints, such as headache, backache, other aches and pains, fatigue

Common Nursing Diagnoses and Interventions

(Interventions are applicable to various health-care settings, such as inpatient and partial hospitalization, community outpatient clinic, home health, and private practice.)

● RISK FOR SELF-DIRECTED OR OTHER-DIRECTED VIOLENCE

Definition: At risk for behaviors in which an individual demonstrates that he or she can be physically, emotionally, and/or sexually harmful either to self or to others.

Related/Risk Factors ("related to")

[Fixation in earlier level of development]
[Negative role modeling]

[Dysfunctional family system]
[Low self-esteem]
[Unresolved grief]
[Psychic overload]
[Extended exposure to stressful situation]
[Lack of support systems]
[Biological factors, such as organic changes in the brain]
Body language (e.g., rigid posture, clenching of fists and jaw, hyperactivity, pacing, breathlessness, threatening stances)
[History or threats of violence toward self or others or of destruction to the property of others]
Impulsivity
Suicidal ideation, plan, available means
[Anger; rage]
[Increasing anxiety level]
[Depressed mood]

Goals/Objectives

Short-term Goals

1. Client will seek out staff member when hostile or suicidal feelings occur.
2. Client will verbalize adaptive coping strategies for use when hostile or suicidal feelings occur.

Long-term Goals

1. Client will demonstrate adaptive coping strategies for use when hostile or suicidal feelings occur.
2. Client will not harm self or others.

Interventions with *Selected Rationales*

1. Observe client's behavior frequently. Do this through routine activities and interactions; avoid appearing watchful and suspicious. *Close observation is required so that intervention can occur if required to ensure client's (and others') safety.*
2. Observe for suicidal behaviors: verbal statements, such as "I'm going to kill myself" and "Very soon my mother won't have to worry herself about me any longer," and nonverbal behaviors, such as giving away cherished items and mood swings. *Clients who are contemplating suicide often give clues regarding their potential behavior. The clues may be very subtle and require keen assessment skills by the nurse.*
3. Determine suicidal intent and available means. Ask direct questions, such as "Do you plan to kill yourself?" and "How do you plan to do it?" *The risk of suicide is greatly increased if the client has developed a plan and particularly if means exist for the client to execute the plan.*

4. Obtain verbal or written contract from client agreeing not to harm self and to seek out staff in the event that suicidal ideation occurs. *Discussion of suicidal feelings with a trusted individual provides some relief to the client. A contract gets the subject out in the open and places some of the responsibility for his or her safety with the client. An attitude of acceptance of the client as a worthwhile individual is conveyed.*

5. Help client recognize when anger occurs and to accept those feelings as his or her own. Have client keep an "anger notebook," in which feelings of anger experienced during a 24-hour period are recorded. Information regarding source of anger, behavioral response, and client's perception of the situation should also be noted. Discuss entries with client and suggest alternative behavioral responses for those identified as maladaptive.

6. Act as a role model for appropriate expression of angry feelings and give positive reinforcement to client for attempting to conform. *It is vital that the client express angry feelings, because suicide and other self-destructive behaviors are often viewed as the result of anger turned inward on the self.*

7. Remove all dangerous objects from client's environment (e.g., sharp items, belts, ties, straps, breakable items, smoking materials). *Client safety is a nursing priority.*

8. Try to redirect violent behavior by means of physical outlets for the client's anxiety (e.g., punching bag, jogging). *Physical exercise is a safe and effective way of relieving pent-up tension.*

9. Be available to stay with client as anxiety level and tensions begin to rise. *Presence of a trusted individual provides a feeling of security and may help to prevent rapid escalation of anxiety.*

10. Staff should maintain and convey a calm attitude to client. *Anxiety is contagious and can be transmitted from staff members to client.*

11. Have sufficient staff available to indicate a show of strength to client if necessary. *This conveys to the client evidence of control over the situation and provides some physical security for staff.*

12. Administer tranquilizing medications as ordered by physician or obtain an order if necessary. Monitor client response for effectiveness of the medication and for adverse side effects. *Short-term use of tranquilizing medications such as anxiolytics or antipsychotics can induce a calming effect on the client and may prevent aggressive behaviors.*

13. Use of mechanical restraints or isolation room may be required if less restrictive interventions are unsuccessful. Follow policy and procedure prescribed by the institution in executing this intervention. The Joint Commission

(formerly the Joint Commission on Accreditation of Health-care Organizations [JCAHO]) requires that an in-person evaluation (by a physician, clinical psychologist, or other licensed independent practitioner responsible for the care of the patient) be conducted within 1 hour of initiating restraint or seclusion (The Joint Commission, 2010). The physician must reevaluate and issue a new order for re-straints every 4 hours for adults and every 1 to 2 hours for children and adolescents.

14. Observe the client in restraints every 15 minutes (or ac-cording to institutional policy). Ensure that circulation to extremities is not compromised (check temperature, color, pulses). Assist client with needs related to nutrition, hy-dration, and elimination. Position client so that comfort is facilitated and aspiration can be prevented. *Client safety is a nursing priority.*

15. As agitation decreases, assess client's readiness for restraint removal or reduction. Remove one restraint at a time, while assessing client's response. *This minimizes risk of injury to the client and staff.*

Outcome Criteria

1. Anxiety is maintained at a level at which client feels no need for aggression.
2. Client denies any ideas of self-destruction.
3. Client demonstrates use of adaptive coping strategies when feelings of hostility or suicide occur.
4. Client verbalizes community support systems from which as-sistance may be requested when personal coping strategies are not successful.

● ANXIETY (MODERATE TO SEVERE)

Definition: Vague uneasy feeling of discomfort or dread accom-panied by an autonomic response (the source often nonspecific or unknown to the individual); a feeling of apprehension caused by antic-ipation of danger. It is an alerting signal that warns of impending dan-ger and enables the individual to take measures to deal with threat.

Possible Etiologies ("related to")

Situational and maturational crises
[Low self-esteem]
[Dysfunctional family system]
[Feelings of powerlessness and lack of control in life situation]
[Retarded ego development]
[Fixation in earlier level of development]

Defining Characteristics ("evidenced by")

Increased tension
[Increased helplessness]
Overexcited
Apprehensive; fearful
Restlessness
Poor eye contact
Feelings of inadequacy
Insomnia
Focus on the self
Increased cardiac and respiratory rates
Diminished ability to problem solve and learn

Goals/Objectives

Short-term Goal

Client will demonstrate use of relaxation techniques to maintain anxiety at manageable level within 7 days.

Long-term Goal

By time of discharge from treatment, client will be able to recognize events that precipitate anxiety and intervene to prevent disabling behaviors.

Interventions with *Selected Rationales*

1. Be available to stay with client. Remain calm and provide assurance of safety. *Client safety and security is a nursing priority.*
2. Help client identify situation that precipitated onset of anxiety symptoms. *Client may be unaware that emotional issues are related to symptoms of anxiety. Recognition may be the first step in elimination of this maladaptive response.*
3. Review client's methods of coping with similar situations in the past. Discuss ways in which client may assume control over these situations. *In seeking to create change, it would be helpful for client to identify past responses and to determine whether they were successful and if they could be employed again. A measure of control reduces feelings of powerlessness in a situation, ultimately decreasing anxiety. Client strengths should be identified and used to his or her advantage.*
4. Provide quiet environment. Reduce stimuli: low lighting, few people. *Anxiety level may be decreased in calm atmosphere with few stimuli.*
5. Administer antianxiety medications as ordered by physician, or obtain order if necessary. Monitor client's response for effectiveness of the medication as well as for adverse side effects. *Short-term use of antianxiety medications (e.g., lorazepam, chlordiazepoxide, alprazolam) provides relief*

from the immobilizing effects of anxiety and facilitates client's cooperation with therapy.

6. Discuss with client signs of increasing anxiety and ways of intervening to maintain the anxiety at a manageable level (e.g., exercise, walking, jogging, relaxation techniques). *Anxiety and tension can be reduced safely and with benefit to the client through physical activities.*

Outcome Criteria

1. Client is able to verbalize events that precipitate anxiety and to demonstrate techniques for its reduction.
2. Client is able to verbalize ways in which he or she may gain more control of the environment and thereby reduce feelings of powerlessness.

● INEFFECTIVE COPING

Definition: Inability to form a valid appraisal of the stressors, inadequate choices of practiced responses, and/or inability to use available resources.

Possible Etiologies ("related to")

Situational crises
Maturational crises
[Inadequate support systems]
[Negative role modeling]
[Retarded ego development]
[Fixation in earlier level of development]
[Dysfunctional family system]
[Low self-esteem]
[Unresolved grief]

Defining Characteristics ("evidenced by")

Inability to meet role expectations
[Alteration in societal participation]
Inadequate problem solving
[Increased dependency]
[Manipulation of others in the environment for purposes of fulfilling own desires]
[Refusal to follow rules]

Goals/Objectives
Short-term Goal

By the end of 1 week, client will comply with rules of therapy and refrain from manipulating others to fulfill own desires.

Long-term Goal

By time of discharge from treatment, client will identify, develop, and use socially acceptable coping skills.

Interventions with *Selected Rationales*

1. Discuss with client the rules of therapy and consequences of noncompliance. Carry out the consequences matter-of-factly if rules are broken. *Negative consequences may work to decrease manipulative behaviors.*

2. Do not debate, argue, rationalize, or bargain with the client regarding limit-setting on manipulative behaviors. *Ignoring these attempts may work to decrease manipulative behaviors. Consistency among all staff members is vital if this intervention is to be successful.*

3. Encourage discussion of angry feelings. Help client identify the true object of the hostility. Provide physical outlets for healthy release of the hostile feelings (e.g., punching bags, pounding boards). *Verbalization of feelings with a trusted individual may help client work through unresolved issues. Physical exercise provides a safe and effective means of releasing pent-up tension.*

4. Take care not to reinforce dependent behaviors. Encourage client to perform as independently as possible, and provide positive feedback. *Independent accomplishment and positive reinforcement enhance self-esteem and encourage repetition of desirable behaviors.*

5. Help client recognize some aspects of his or her life over which a measure of control is maintained. *Recognition of personal control, however minimal, diminishes the feeling of powerlessness and decreases the need for manipulation of others.*

6. Identify the stressor that precipitated the maladaptive coping. If a major life change has occurred, encourage client to express fears and feelings associated with the change. Assist client through the problem-solving process:
   a. Identify possible alternatives that indicate positive adaptation.
   b. Discuss benefits and consequences of each alternative.
   c. Select the most appropriate alternative.
   d. Implement the alternative.
   e. Evaluate the effectiveness of the alternative.
   f. Recognize areas of limitation, and make modifications. Request assistance with this process, if needed.

7. Provide positive reinforcement for application of adaptive coping skills and evidence of successful adjustment. *Positive reinforcement enhances self-esteem and encourages repetition of desirable behaviors.*

Outcome Criteria

1. Client is able to verbalize alternative, socially acceptable, and lifestyle-appropriate coping skills he or she plans to use in response to stress.
2. Client is able to solve problems and fulfill activities of daily living independently.
3. Client does not manipulate others for own gratification.

• RISK-PRONE HEALTH BEHAVIOR*

Definition: Impaired ability to modify lifestyle/behaviors in a manner that improves health status.

Possible Etiologies ("related to")

[Low self-esteem]
[Intense emotional state]
[Negative attitudes toward health behavior]
[Absence of intent to change behavior]
Multiple stressors
[Absence of social support for changed beliefs and practices]
[Disability or health status change requiring change in lifestyle]
[Lack of motivation to change behaviors]

Defining Characteristics ("evidenced by")

Minimizes health status change
Failure to achieve optimal sense of control
Failure to take action that prevents health problems
Demonstrates nonacceptance of health status change

Goals/Objectives

Short-term Goals

1. Client will discuss with primary nurse the kinds of lifestyle changes that will occur because of the change in health status.
2. With the help of primary nurse, client will formulate a plan of action for incorporating those changes into his or her lifestyle.
3. Client will demonstrate movement toward independence, considering change in health status.

---

* According to the NANDA International definition, this diagnosis is appropriate for the person with adjustment disorder only if the precipitating stressor is a change in health status.

Long-term Goal

Client will demonstrate competence to function independently to his or her optimal ability, considering change in health status, by time of discharge from treatment.

Interventions with *Selected Rationales*

1. Encourage client to talk about lifestyle prior to the change in health status. Discuss coping mechanisms that were used at stressful times in the past. *It is important to identify the client's strengths so that they may be used to facilitate adaptation to the change or loss that has occurred.*

2. Encourage client to discuss the change or loss and particularly to express anger associated with it. *Some individuals may not realize that anger is a normal stage in the grieving process. If it is not released in an appropriate manner, it may be turned inward on the self, leading to pathological depression.*

3. Encourage client to express fears associated with the change or loss, or alteration in lifestyle that the change or loss has created. *Change often creates a feeling of disequilibrium and the individual may respond with fears that are irrational or unfounded. He or she may benefit from feedback that corrects misperceptions about how life will be with the change in health status.*

4. Provide assistance with activities of daily living (ADLs) as required, but encourage independence to the limit that client's ability will allow. Give positive feedback for activities accomplished independently. *Independent accomplishments and positive feedback enhance self-esteem and encourage repetition of desired behaviors. Successes also provide hope that adaptive functioning is possible and decrease feelings of powerlessness.*

5. Help client with decision making regarding incorporation of change or loss into lifestyle. Identify problems that the change or loss is likely to create. Discuss alternative solutions, weighing potential benefits and consequences of each alternative. Support client's decision in the selection of an alternative. *The great amount of anxiety that usually accompanies a major lifestyle change often interferes with an individual's ability to solve problems and to make appropriate decisions. Client may need assistance with this process in an effort to progress toward successful adaptation.*

6. Use role-playing *to decrease anxiety* as client anticipates stressful situations that might occur in relation to the health status change. *Role-playing decreases anxiety and provides a feeling of security by providing client with a plan of action for responding in an appropriate manner when a stressful situation occurs.*

7. Ensure that client and family are fully knowledgeable regarding the physiology of the change in health status and its necessity for optimal wellness. Encourage them to ask questions, and provide printed material explaining the change to which they may refer following discharge. ***Increased knowledge enhances successful adaptation.***

8. Help client identify resources within the community from which he or she may seek assistance in adapting to the change in health status. Examples include self-help or support groups and public health nurse, counselor, or social worker. Encourage client to keep follow-up appointments with physician, or to call physician's office prior to follow-up date if problems or concerns arise.

Outcome Criteria

1. Client is able to perform ADLs independently.
2. Client is able to make independent decisions regarding lifestyle considering change in health status.
3. Client is able to express hope for the future with consideration of change in health status.

• COMPLICATED GRIEVING

Definition: A disorder that occurs after the death of a significant other [or any other loss of significance to the individual], in which the experience of distress accompanying bereavement fails to follow normative expectations and manifests in functional impairment.

Possible Etiologies ("related to")

[Real or perceived loss of any entity of value to the individual]
[Bereavement overload (cumulative grief from multiple unresolved losses)]
[Thwarted grieving response to a loss]
[Absence of anticipatory grieving]
[Feelings of guilt generated by ambivalent relationship with lost entity]

Defining Characteristics ("evidenced by")

[Verbal expression of distress at loss]
[Idealization of lost entity]
[Denial of loss]
[Excessive anger, expressed inappropriately]
[Developmental regression]
[Altered activities of daily living]

[Diminished sense of control]
[Persistent anxiety]
Depression

Goals/Objectives
Short-term Goal
By end of 1 week, client will express anger toward lost entity.
Long-term Goal
Client will be able to verbalize behaviors associated with the normal stages of grief and identify own position in grief process, while progressing at own pace toward resolution.

Interventions with *Selected Rationales*

1. Determine stage of grief in which client is fixed. Identify behaviors associated with this stage. *Accurate baseline assessment data are necessary to plan effective care for the grieving client.*
2. Develop trusting relationship with client. Show empathy and caring. Be honest and keep all promises. *Trust is the basis for a therapeutic relationship.*
3. Convey an accepting attitude so that the client is not afraid to express feelings openly. *An accepting attitude conveys to the client that you believe he or she is a worthwhile person. Trust is enhanced.*
4. Allow client to express anger. Do not become defensive if initial expression of anger is displaced on nurse or therapist. Help client explore angry feelings so that they may be directed toward the intended object or person. *Verbalization of feelings in a nonthreatening environment may help client come to terms with unresolved issues.*
5. Help client discharge pent-up anger through participation in large motor activities (e.g., brisk walks, jogging, physical exercises, volleyball, punching bag, exercise bike). *Physical exercise provides a safe and effective method for discharging pent-up tension.*
6. Explain to client the normal stages of grief and the behaviors associated with each stage. Help client to understand that feelings such as guilt and anger toward the lost entity are appropriate and acceptable during the grief process. *Knowledge of the acceptability of the feelings associated with normal grieving may help to relieve some of the guilt that these responses generate.*
7. Encourage client to review personal perception of the loss or change. With support and sensitivity, point out reality of the situation in areas where misrepresentations are expressed. *Client must give up an idealized perception and be able to*

accept both positive and negative aspects about the painful life change before the grief process is complete.

8. Communicate to client that crying is acceptable. Use of touch is therapeutic and appropriate with most clients. Knowledge of cultural influences specific to the client is important before employing this technique. *Touch is considered inappropriate in some cultures.*

9. Help client solve problems as he or she attempts to determine methods for more adaptive coping with the experienced loss. Provide positive feedback for strategies identified and decisions made. *Positive reinforcement enhances self-esteem and encourages repetition of desirable behaviors.*

10. Encourage client to reach out for spiritual support during this time in whatever form is desirable to him or her. Assess spiritual needs of client, and assist as necessary in the fulfillment of those needs. *Spiritual support can enhance successful adaptation to painful life experiences for some individuals.*

Outcome Criteria

1. Client is able to verbalize normal stages of grief process and behaviors associated with each stage.
2. Client is able to identify own position within the grief process and express honest feelings related to the lost entity.
3. Client is no longer manifesting exaggerated emotions and behaviors related to complicated grieving and is able to carry out ADLs independently.

● LOW SELF-ESTEEM

Definition: Negative self-evaluating/feelings about self or self-capabilities.

Possible Etiologies ("related to")

Repeated negative reinforcement
[Unmet dependency needs]
[Retarded ego development]
Repeated failures
[Personal or situational factors such as dysfunctional family system or absence of social support]

Defining Characteristics ("evidenced by")

Rejects positive feedback about self
Exaggerates negative feedback about self
[Nonparticipation in therapy]

Self-negating verbalizations
Evaluation of self as unable to deal with events or situations
Hesitant to try new things or situations [because of fear of failure]
[Projection of blame or responsibility for problems]
[Rationalization of personal failures]
[Hypersensitivity to slight or criticism]
[Grandiosity]
Lack of eye contact
[Manipulation of one staff member against another in an attempt to gain special privileges]
[Inability to form close, personal relationships]
[Degradation of others in an attempt to increase own feelings of self-worth]

Goals/Objectives

Short-term Goals

1. Client will discuss fear of failure with nurse within (realistic time period).
2. Client will verbalize things he or she likes about self within (realistic time period).

Long-term Goals

1. Client will exhibit increased feelings of self-worth as evidenced by verbal expression of positive aspects about self, past accomplishments, and future prospects.
2. Client will exhibit increased feelings of self-worth by setting realistic goals and trying to reach them, thereby demonstrating a decrease in fear of failure.

Interventions with *Selected Rationales*

1. Ensure that goals are realistic. It is important for client to achieve something, so plan for activities in which success is likely. *Success enhances self-esteem.*
2. Convey unconditional positive regard for the client. Promote understanding of your acceptance for him or her as a worthwhile human being. *Unconditional positive regard and acceptance promote trust and increase client's feelings of self-worth.*
3. Spend time with the client, both on a one-to-one basis and in group activities. *This conveys to client that you feel he or she is worth your time.*
4. Help client identify positive aspects of self and to develop plans for changing the characteristics he or she views as negative. *Individuals with low self-esteem often have difficulty recognizing their positive attributes. They may also lack problem-solving ability and require assistance to formulate a plan for implementing the desired changes.*

5. Encourage and support client in confronting the fear of failure by attending therapy activities and undertaking new tasks. Offer recognition of successful endeavors and positive reinforcement for attempts made. ***Recognition and positive reinforcement enhance self-esteem.***

6. Do not allow client to ruminate about past failures. Withdraw attention if he or she persists. ***Lack of attention to these behaviors may discourage their repetition. Client must focus on positive attributes if self-esteem is to be enhanced.***

7. Minimize negative feedback to client. Enforce limit-setting in matter-of-fact manner, imposing previously established consequences for violations. ***Negative feedback can be extremely threatening to a person with low self-esteem, possibly aggravating the problem. Consequences should convey unacceptability of the behavior, but not the person.***

8. Encourage independence in the performance of personal responsibilities, as well as in decision-making related to own self-care. Offer recognition and praise for accomplishments. ***The ability to perform self-care activities independently enhances self-esteem. Positive reinforcement encourages repetition of the desirable behavior.***

9. Help client increase level of self-awareness through critical examination of feelings, attitudes, and behaviors. Help him or her to understand that it is perfectly acceptable for one's attitudes and behaviors to differ from those of others as long as they do not become intrusive. ***As the client achieves self-awareness and self-acceptance, the need for judging the behavior of others will diminish.***

Outcome Criteria

1. Client verbalizes positive perception of self.
2. Client demonstrates ability to manage own self-care, make independent decisions, and use problem-solving skills.
3. Client sets goals that are realistic and works to achieve those goals without evidence of fear of failure.

• IMPAIRED SOCIAL INTERACTION

Definition: Insufficient or excessive quantity or ineffective quality of social exchange.

Possible Etiologies ("related to")

[Retarded ego development]
[Fixation in an earlier level of development]

[Negative role modeling]
Self-concept disturbance

Defining Characteristics ("evidenced by")

Discomfort in social situations
Inability to receive or communicate a satisfying sense of social engagement (e.g., belonging, caring, interest, shared history)
Use of unsuccessful social interaction behaviors
Dysfunctional interaction with others
[Exhibiting behaviors unacceptable for age, as defined by dominant cultural group]

Goals/Objectives

Short-term Goal

Client will develop trusting relationship with staff member within (realistic time period), seeking that staff member out for one-to-one interaction.

Long-term Goals

1. Client will be able to interact with others on a one-to-one basis with no indication of discomfort.
2. Client will voluntarily spend time with others in group activities demonstrating acceptable, age-appropriate behavior.

Interventions with *Selected Rationales*

1. Develop trusting relationship with client. Be honest; keep all promises; convey acceptance of person, separate from unacceptable behaviors ("It is not *you*, but your *behavior*, that is unacceptable.") *Unconditional acceptance of the client increases his or her feelings of self-worth.*
2. Offer to remain with client during initial interactions with others on the unit. *Presence of a trusted individual provides a feeling of security.*
3. Provide constructive criticism and positive reinforcement for efforts. *Positive reinforcement enhances self-esteem and encourages repetition of desirable behaviors.*
4. Confront client and withdraw attention when interactions with others are manipulative or exploitative. *Attention to the unacceptable behavior may reinforce it.*
5. Act as role model for client through appropriate interactions with him or her, other clients, and staff members. *Role modeling is one of the strongest forms of learning.*
6. Provide group situations for client. *It is through these group interactions, with positive and negative feedback from his or her peers, that client will learn socially acceptable behavior.*

Outcome Criteria

1. Client seeks out staff member for social as well as therapeutic interaction.
2. Client has formed and satisfactorily maintained one interpersonal relationship with another client.
3. Client willingly and appropriately participates in group activities.
4. Client verbalizes reasons for inability to form close interpersonal relationships with others in the past.

● RELOCATION STRESS SYNDROME*

Definition: Physiological and/or psychosocial disturbance following transfer from one environment to another.

Possible Etiologies ("related to")

Move from one environment to another
[Losses involved with decision to move]
Feelings of powerlessness
Lack of adequate support system
[Little or no preparation for the impending move]
Impaired psychosocial health [status]
Decreased [physical] health status

Defining Characteristics ("evidenced by")

Anxiety
Depression
Loneliness
Verbalizes unwillingness to move
Sleep disturbance
Increased physical symptoms
Dependency
Insecurity
Withdrawal
Anger; fear

Goals/Objectives
Short-term Goal

Client will verbalize at least one positive aspect regarding relocation to new environment within (realistic time period).

---

* This diagnosis would be appropriate for the individual with adjustment disorder if the precipitating stressor was relocation to a new environment.

Long-term Goal

Client will demonstrate positive adaptation to new environment, as evidenced by involvement in activities, expression of satisfaction with new acquaintances, and elimination of previously evident physical and psychological symptoms associated with the relocation (time dimension to be determined individually).

Interventions with *Selected Rationales*

1. Encourage individual to discuss feelings (concerns, fears, anger) regarding relocation. *Exploration of feelings with a trusted individual may help the individual perceive the situation more realistically and come to terms with the inevitable change.*
2. Encourage individual to discuss how the change will affect his or her life. Ensure that the individual is involved in decision-making and problem-solving regarding the move. *Taking responsibility for making choices regarding the relocation will increase feelings of control and decrease feelings of powerlessness.*
3. Help the individual identify positive aspects about the move. *Anxiety associated with the opposed relocation may interfere with the individual's ability to recognize anything positive about it. Assistance may be required.*
4. Help the individual identify resources within the new community from which assistance with various types of services may be obtained. *Because of anxiety and depression, the individual may not be able to identify these resources alone. Assistance with problem-solving may be required.*
5. Identify groups within the community that specialize in helping individuals adapt to relocation. Examples include Newcomers' Club, Welcome Wagon International, senior citizens' groups, and school and church organizations. *These groups offer support from individuals who may have encountered similar experiences. Adaptation may be enhanced by the reassurance, encouragement, and support of peers who exhibit positive adaptation to relocation stress.*
6. Refer individual or family for professional counseling if deemed necessary. *An individual who is experiencing complicated grieving over loss of previous residence may require therapy to achieve resolution of the problem. It may be that other unresolved issues are interfering with successful adaptation to the relocation.*

Outcome Criteria

1. The individual no longer exhibits signs of anxiety, depression, or somatic symptoms.

2. The individual verbalizes satisfaction with new environment.
3. The individual willingly participates in social and vocational activities within his or her new environment.

@ INTERNET REFERENCES

- Additional information about adjustment disorder may be located at the following websites:
  a. http://www.mentalhealth.com/rx/p23-aj01.html
  b. http://psyweb.com/Mdisord/jsp/adjd.jsp
  c. http://emedicine.medscape.com/article/292759-overview
  d. http://www.athealth.com/Consumer/disorders/Adjustment.html
  e. http://www.nlm.nih.gov/medlineplus/ency/article/000932.htm
  f. http://www.mayoclinic.com/health/adjustment-disorders/DS00584

Impulse Control Disorders

● BACKGROUND ASSESSMENT DATA

Impulse control disorders are characterized by a need or desire that must be satisfied immediately, regardless of the consequences. Many of the behaviors have adverse or even destructive consequences for the individuals affected, and seldom do these individuals know why they do what they do or why it is pleasurable.

The American Psychiatric Association (APA, 2000) *Diagnostic and Statistical Manual of Mental Disorders, Fourth Edition, Text Revision (DSM-IV-TR)* describes the essential features of impulse control disorders as follows:

1. The individual is unable to resist an impulse, drive, or temptation to act in a way that is harmful to the person or others.
2. The individual experiences an increasing sense of tension or arousal before committing the act and pleasure, gratification, or relief at the time of committing the act.
3. Afterward, he or she may experience regret, remorse, or embarrassment.

The *DSM-IV-TR* (APA, 2000) describes the following categories of impulse control disorders:

Intermittent Explosive Disorder

This disorder is characterized by episodes of loss of aggression control resulting in serious assaultive acts or destruction of property (APA, 2000). Some clients report changes in sensorium, such as confusion during an episode or amnesia for events that occurred during an episode. Symptoms usually appear suddenly without apparent provocation and terminate abruptly, lasting only minutes to a few hours, followed by feelings of genuine remorse and self-reproach about the behavior.

Kleptomania

"Kleptomania" is described by the *DSM-IV-TR* as "the recurrent failure to resist impulses to steal items not needed for personal use or for their monetary value" (APA, 2000, p. 667). Often the stolen items (for which the individual usually has enough money to pay) are given away, discarded, returned, or kept and hidden. The individual with kleptomania steals purely for the sake of stealing and for the sense of relief and gratification that follows an episode.

Pathological Gambling

The *DSM-IV-TR* defines "pathological gambling" as "persistent and recurrent maladaptive gambling behavior that disrupts personal, family, or vocational pursuits" (APA, 2000, p. 671). The preoccupation with gambling, and the impulse to gamble, intensifies when the individual is under stress. Many pathological gamblers exhibit characteristics associated with narcissism and grandiosity and often have difficulties with intimacy, empathy, and trust.

Pyromania

Pyromania is the inability to resist the impulse to set fires. The act itself is preceded by tension or affective arousal, and the individual experiences intense pleasure, gratification, or relief when setting the fires, witnessing their effects, or participating in their aftermath (APA, 2000). Motivation for the behavior is self-gratification, and even though some individuals with pyromania may take precautions to avoid apprehension, many are totally indifferent to the consequences of their behavior.

Trichotillomania

This disorder is defined by the *DSM-IV-TR* as "the recurrent pulling out of one's own hair that results in noticeable hair loss" (APA, 2000, p. 674). The impulse is preceded by an increasing sense of tension, and the individual experiences a sense of release or gratification from pulling out the hair.

Predisposing Factors to Impulse Control Disorders

1. **Physiological**
   a. *Genetics.* A familial tendency appears to be a factor in some cases of intermittent explosive disorder and pathological gambling.
   b. *Physical Factors.* Brain trauma or dysfunction and mental retardation have also been implicated in the predisposition to impulse control disorders.

2. **Psychosocial**
   a. ***Family Dynamics.*** Various dysfunctional family patterns have been suggested as contributors in the predisposition to impulse control disorders. These include the following:
      - Child abuse or neglect
      - Parental rejection or abandonment
      - Harsh or inconsistent discipline
      - Emotional deprivation
      - Parental substance abuse
      - Parental unpredictability

Symptomatology (Subjective and Objective Data)

1. Sudden inability to control violent, aggressive impulses
2. Aggressive behavior accompanied by confusion or amnesia
3. Feelings of remorse following aggressive behavior
4. Inability to resist impulses to steal
5. Increasing tension before committing the theft, followed by pleasure or relief during and following the act
6. Sometimes discards, returns, or hides stolen items
7. Inability to resist impulses to gamble
8. Preoccupation with ways to obtain money with which to gamble
9. Increasing tension that is relieved only by placing a bet
10. The need to gamble or loss of money interferes with social and occupational functioning
11. Inability to resist the impulse to set fires
12. Increasing tension that is relieved only by starting a fire
13. Inability to resist impulses to pull out one's own hair
14. Increasing tension followed by a sense of release or gratification from pulling out the hair
15. Hair-pulling may be accompanied by other types of self-mutilation (e.g., head-banging, biting, scratching)

Common Nursing Diagnoses and Interventions

(Interventions are applicable to various health-care settings, such as inpatient and partial hospitalization, community outpatient clinic, home health, and private practice.)

● RISK FOR OTHER-DIRECTED VIOLENCE

Definition: At risk for behaviors in which an individual demonstrates that he or she can be physically, emotionally, and/or sexually harmful to others.

Related/Risk Factors ("related to")

[Possible familial tendency]
[Dysfunctional family system, resulting in behaviors such as the
following:
    Child abuse or neglect
    Parental rejection or abandonment
    Harsh or inconsistent discipline
    Emotional deprivation
    Parental substance abuse
    Parental unpredictability]
    Body language (e.g., rigid posture, clenching of fists and
      jaw, hyperactivity, pacing, breathlessness, threatening
      stances)
    History of threats of violence [toward others or of destruc-
      tion to the property of others]
    Impulsivity
    Neurological impairment
    Cognitive impairment

Goals/Objectives

Short-term Goal

Client will recognize signs of increasing tension, anxiety, and
agitation, and report to staff (or others) for assistance with intervention (time dimension to be individually determined).

Long-term Goal

Client will not harm others or the property of others (time
dimension to be individually determined).

Interventions with *Selected Rationales*

1. Convey an accepting attitude toward the client. Feelings of
   rejection are undoubtedly familiar to him or her. Work on the
   development of trust. Be honest, keep all promises, and convey the message that it is not the *person* but the *behavior* that is
   unacceptable. *An attitude of acceptance promotes feelings of
   self-worth. Trust is the basis of a therapeutic relationship.*
2. Maintain low level of stimuli in client's environment (low
   lighting, few people, simple decor, low noise level). *A stimulating environment may increase agitation and promote
   aggressive behavior. Make the client's environment as safe
   as possible* by removing all potentially dangerous objects.
3. Help client identify the true object of his or her hostility.
   *Because of weak ego development, client may be unable to
   use ego defense mechanisms correctly. Helping him or her
   recognize this in a nonthreatening manner may help reveal
   unresolved issues so that they may be confronted.*
4. Staff should maintain and convey a calm attitude. *Anxiety
   is contagious and can be transferred from staff to client. A*

calm attitude provides the client with a feeling of safety and security.

5. Help client recognize the signs that tension is increasing and ways in which violence can be averted. *Activities that require physical exertion are helpful in relieving pent-up tension.*

6. Explain to the client that should explosive behavior occur, staff will intervene in whatever way is required (e.g., tranquilizing medication, restraints, isolation) to protect client and others. *This conveys to the client evidence of control over the situation and provides a feeling of safety and security.*

Outcome Criteria

1. Anxiety is maintained at a level at which client feels no need for aggression.
2. The client is able to verbalize the symptoms of increasing tension and adaptive ways of coping with it.
3. The client is able to inhibit the impulse for violence and aggression.

● RISK FOR SELF-MUTILATION

Definition: At risk for deliberate self-injurious behavior causing tissue damage with the intent of causing nonfatal injury to attain relief of tension.

Related/Risk Factors ("related to")

[Central nervous system trauma]
[Mental retardation]
[Early emotional deprivation]
[Parental rejection or abandonment]
[Child abuse or neglect]
[History of self-mutilative behaviors in response to increasing anxiety: hair-pulling, biting, head-banging, scratching]

Goals/Objectives
Short-term Goals

1. Client will cooperate with plan of behavior modification in an effort to respond more adaptively to stress (time dimension ongoing).
2. Client will not harm self.

Long-term Goal

Client will not harm self.

Interventions with *Selected Rationales*

1. Intervene to protect client when self-mutilative behaviors, such as head-banging or hair-pulling, become evident. *The nurse is responsible for ensuring client safety.*
2. A helmet may be used *to protect against head-banging*, hand mitts *to prevent hair-pulling*, and appropriate padding *to protect extremities from injury* during hysterical movements.
3. Try to determine if self-mutilative behaviors occur in response to increasing anxiety, and if so, to what the anxiety may be attributed. *Self-mutilative behaviors may be averted if the cause can be determined.*
4. Work on one-to-one basis with client *to establish trust.*
5. Assist with plan for behavior modification *in an effort to teach the client more adaptive ways of responding to stress.*
6. Encourage client to discuss feelings, particularly anger, *in an effort to confront unresolved issues and expose internalized rage that may be triggering self-mutilative behaviors.*
7. Offer self to client during times of increasing anxiety, *to provide feelings of security and decrease need for self-mutilative behaviors.*

Outcome Criteria

1. Anxiety is maintained at a level at which client feels no need for self-mutilation.
2. Client demonstrates ability to use adaptive coping strategies in the face of stressful situations.

● INEFFECTIVE COPING

Definition: Inability to form a valid appraisal of the stressors, inadequate choices of practiced responses, and/or inability to use available resources.

Possible Etiologies ("related to")

[Possible hereditary factors]
[Brain trauma or dysfunction]
[Mental retardation]
[Dysfunctional family system, resulting in behaviors such as the following:
    Child abuse or neglect
    Parental rejection or abandonment
    Harsh or inconsistent discipline
    Emotional deprivation
    Parental substance abuse
    Parental unpredictability]

Defining Characteristics ("evidenced by")

[Inability to control impulse of violence or aggression]
[Inability to control impulse to steal]
[Inability to control impulse to gamble]
[Inability to control impulse to set fires]
[Inability to control impulse to pull out own hair]
[Feeling of intense anxiety and tension that precedes, and is
relieved by, engaging in these impulsive behaviors]

Goals/Objectives

Short-term Goal

Client will verbalize adaptive ways to cope with stress by means
other than impulsive behaviors (time dimension to be individually determined).

Long-term Goal

Client will be able to delay gratification and use adaptive coping
strategies in response to stress (time dimension to be individually determined).

Interventions with *Selected Rationales*

1. Help client gain insight into his or her behaviors. Often these
   individuals rationalize to such an extent that they deny that
   what they have done is wrong. *Client must come to understand that certain behaviors will not be tolerated within the
   society and that severe consequences will be imposed on those
   individuals who refuse to comply. Client must WANT to
   become a productive member of society before he or she can
   be helped.*
2. Talk about past behaviors with client. Discuss behaviors that
   are acceptable by societal norms and those that are not. Help
   client identify ways in which he or she has exploited others.
   Encourage client to explore how he or she would feel if the
   circumstances were reversed. *An attempt may be made to
   enlighten the client to the sensitivity of others by promoting
   self-awareness in an effort to assist the client gain insight
   into his or her own behavior.*
3. Throughout relationship with client, maintain attitude of "It
   is not *you*, but your *behavior*, that is unacceptable." *An attitude
   of acceptance promotes feelings of dignity and self-worth.*
4. Work with client to increase the ability to delay gratification.
   Reward desirable behaviors, and provide immediate positive
   feedback. *Rewards and positive feedback enhance self-esteem
   and encourage repetition of desirable behaviors.*
5. Help client identify and practice more adaptive strategies for
   coping with stressful life situations. *The impulse to perform
   the maladaptive behavior may be so great that the client is
   unable to see any other alternatives to relieve stress.*

Outcome Criteria

1. Client is able to demonstrate techniques that may be used in response to stress to prevent resorting to maladaptive impulsive behaviors.
2. Client verbalizes understanding that behavior is unacceptable and accepts responsibility for own behavior.

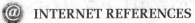 **INTERNET REFERENCES**

- Additional information about impulse control disorders may be located at the following websites:
  a. http://www.ncpgambling.org/
  b. http://www.gamblersanonymous.org/
  c. http://www.crescentlife.com/disorders/pyromania.htm
  d. http://www.biopsychiatry.com/klepto.htm
  e. http://www.enotes.com/medicine-encyclopedia/impulse-control-disorders
  f. http://emedicine.medscape.com/article/915057-overview
  g. http://emedicine.medscape.com/article/294626-overview

Chapter 15

Psychological Factors Affecting Medical Condition

● **BACKGROUND ASSESSMENT DATA**

The American Psychiatric Association (APA, 2000, p. 731) *Diagnostic and Statistical Manual of Mental Disorders, Fourth Edition, Text Revision (DSM-IV-TR)* identifies "psychological factors affecting medical condition" as "the presence of one or more specific psychological or behavioral factors that adversely affect a general medical condition." These factors can adversely affect the medical condition in several ways:

1. By influencing the course of the medical condition (i.e., contributing to the development or exacerbation of, or delayed recovery from, the medical condition).
2. By interfering with treatment of the medical condition.
3. By constituting an additional health risk for the individual (e.g., the individual who has peptic ulcers who continues to drink and smoke).

Several types of psychological factors are implicated by the *DSM-IV-TR* as those that can affect the general medical condition. They include:

1. Mental disorders (e.g., Axis I disorders, such as major depression).
2. Psychological symptoms (e.g., depressed mood or anxiety).
3. Personality traits or coping style (e.g., denial of the need for medical care).
4. Maladaptive health behaviors (e.g., smoking or overeating).
5. Stress-related physiological responses (e.g., tension headaches).
6. Other or unspecified psychological factors (e.g., interpersonal or cultural factors).

Defined

This diagnosis is indicated when there is evidence of a physical symptom(s) or a physical disorder that is adversely affected by psychological factors. The *DSM-IV-TR* (APA, 2000) states,

> Psychological and behavioral factors may affect the course of almost every major category of disease, including cardiovascular conditions, dermatological conditions, endocrinological conditions, gastrointestinal conditions, neoplastic conditions, neurological conditions, pulmonary conditions, renal conditions, and rheumatological conditions (p. 732).

This category differs from somatoform disorders and conversion disorders in that there is evidence of either demonstrable organic pathology (e.g., the inflammation associated with rheumatoid arthritis) or a known pathophysiological process (e.g., the cerebral vasodilation of migraine headaches).

Predisposing Factors

1. **Physiological**
   a. *Physical Factors.* Selye (1956) believed that psychophysiological disorders can occur when the body is exposed to prolonged stress, producing a number of physiological effects under direct control of the pituitary-adrenal axis. He also suggests that genetic predisposition influences which organ system will be affected and determines the type of psychophysiological disorder the individual will develop.

2. **Psychosocial**
   a. *Emotional Response Pattern.* It has been hypothesized that individuals exhibit specific physiological responses to certain emotions. For example, in response to the emotion of anger, one person may experience peripheral vasoconstriction, resulting in an increase in blood pressure. The same emotion, in another individual, may evoke the response of cerebral vasodilation, manifesting a migraine headache.
   b. *Personality Traits.* Various studies have suggested that individuals with specific personality traits are predisposed to certain disease processes. Although personality cannot account totally for the development of psychophysiological disorders, the literature has alluded to the following possible relationships:

Asthma	Dependent personality characteristics
Ulcers, hypertension	Repressed anger
Cancer	Depressive personality
Rheumatoid arthritis, ulcerative colitis	Self-sacrificing; suppressed anger
Migraine headaches	Compulsive and perfectionistic
Coronary heart disease	Aggressive and competitive

   c. *Learning Theory.* A third psychosocial theory considers the role of learning in the psychophysiological response to stress. If a child grows up observing the attention, increased dependency, or other secondary gain an individual receives because of the illness, such behaviors may be viewed as desirable responses and subsequently imitated by the child.

   d. *Theory of Family Dynamics.* This theory relates to the predisposition of those individuals who are members of dysfunctional family systems to use psychophysiological problems to cover up interpersonal conflicts. The anxiety in a dysfunctional family situation is shifted from the conflict to the ailing individual. Anxiety decreases, the conflict is avoided, and the person receives positive reinforcement for his or her symptoms. The situation appears more comfortable, but the real problem remains unresolved.

Symptomatology (Subjective and Objective Data)

1. Complaints of physical illness that can be substantiated by objective evidence of physical pathology or known pathophysiological process
2. Moderate to severe level of anxiety
3. Denial of emotional problems; client is unable to see a relationship between physical problems and response to stress
4. Use of physical illness as excuse for noncompliance with psychiatric treatment plan
5. Repressed anger or anger expressed inappropriately
6. Verbal hostility
7. Depressed mood
8. Low self-esteem
9. Dependent behaviors
10. Attention-seeking behaviors
11. Report (or other evidence) of numerous stressors occurring in person's life

Common Nursing Diagnoses and Interventions*

(Interventions are applicable to various health-care settings, such as inpatient and partial hospitalization, community outpatient clinic, home health, and private practice.)

● INEFFECTIVE COPING

Definition: Inability to form a valid appraisal of the stressors, inadequate choices of practiced responses, and/or inability to use available resources.

Possible Etiologies ("related to")

[Repressed anxiety]
[Inadequate support systems]
[Inadequate coping methods]
[Low self-esteem]
[Unmet dependency needs]
[Negative role modeling]
[Dysfunctional family system]

Defining Characteristics ("evidenced by")

[Initiation or exacerbation of physical illness (specify)]
[Denial of relationship between physical symptoms and emotional problems]
[Use of sick role for secondary gains]
Inability to meet role expectations
Inadequate problem-solving

Goals/Objectives

Short-term Goals

1. Within 1 week, client will verbalize understanding of correlation between emotional problems and physical symptoms.
2. Within 1 week, client will verbalize adaptive ways of coping with stressful situations.

---

* A number of nursing diagnoses common to specific physical disorders or symptoms could be used (e.g., pain, activity intolerance, impaired tissue integrity, diarrhea). For purposes of this chapter, only nursing diagnoses common to the general category are presented.

Long-term Goal

Client will achieve physical wellness and demonstrate the ability to prevent exacerbation of physical symptoms as a coping mechanism in response to stress.

Interventions with *Selected Rationales*

1. Perform thorough physical assessment *in order to determine specific care required for client's physical condition.* Monitor laboratory values, vital signs, intake and output, and other assessments necessary *to maintain an accurate, ongoing appraisal.*

2. Together with the client, identify goals of care and ways in which client believes he or she can best achieve those goals. Client may need assistance with problem-solving. *Personal involvement in his or her care provides a feeling of control and increases chances for positive outcomes.*

3. Encourage client to discuss current life situations that he or she perceives as stressful and the feelings associated with each. *Verbalization of true feelings in a nonthreatening environment may help client come to terms with unresolved issues.*

4. During client's discussion, note times during which a sense of powerlessness or loss of control over life situations emerges. Focus on these times and discuss ways in which the client may maintain a feeling of control. *A sense of self-worth develops and is maintained when an individual feels power over his or her own life situations.*

5. As client becomes able to discuss feelings more openly, assist him or her, in a nonthreatening manner, to relate certain feelings to the appearance of physical symptoms. *Client may be unaware of the relationship between physical symptoms and emotional problems.*

6. Discuss stressful times when physical symptoms did not appear and the adaptive coping strategies that were used during those situations. *Therapy is facilitated by considering areas of strength and using them to the client's benefit.*

7. Provide positive reinforcement for adaptive coping mechanisms identified or used. Suggest alternative coping strategies but allow client to determine which can most appropriately be incorporated into his or her lifestyle. *Positive reinforcement enhances self-esteem and encourages repetition of desirable behaviors. Client may require assistance with problem-solving but must be allowed and encouraged to make decisions independently.*

8. Help client to identify a resource within the community (friend, significant other, group) to use as a support system

for the expression of feelings. *A positive support system may help to prevent maladaptive coping through physical illness.*

Outcome Criteria

1. Client is able to demonstrate techniques that may be used in response to stress to prevent the occurrence or exacerbation of physical symptoms.
2. Client verbalizes an understanding of the relationship between emotional problems and physical symptoms.

• LOW SELF-ESTEEM

Definition: Negative self-evaluating/feelings about self or self-capabilities.

Possible Etiologies ("related to")

Repeated negative reinforcement
[Unmet dependency needs]
[Retarded ego development]
[Dysfunctional family system]

Defining Characteristics ("evidenced by")

Rejects positive feedback about self
[Nonparticipation in therapy]
Self-negating verbalizations
Evaluation of self as unable to deal with events
Hesitant to try new things or situations [because of fear of failure]
[Hypersensitive to slight or criticism]
Lack of eye contact
[Inability to form close, personal relationships]
[Degradation of others in an attempt to increase own feelings of self-worth]

Goals/Objectives

Short-term Goals

1. Client will discuss fear of failure with nurse within 3 days.
2. Client will verbalize aspects he or she likes about self within 5 days.

Long-term Goals

1. Client will exhibit increased feelings of self-worth as evidenced by verbal expression of positive aspects about self, past accomplishments, and future prospects.

2. Client will exhibit increased feelings of self-worth by setting realistic goals and trying to reach them, thereby demonstrating a decrease in fear of failure.

Interventions with *Selected Rationales*

1. Ensure that goals are realistic. It is important for client to achieve something, so plan activities in which success is likely. *Success increases self-esteem.*

2. Minimize amount of attention given to physical symptoms. Client must perceive self as a worthwhile person, separate and apart from the role of client. *Lack of attention may discourage use of undesirable behaviors.*

3. Promote your acceptance of client as a worthwhile person by spending time with him or her. Develop trust through one-to-one interactions, then encourage client to participate in group activities. Support group attendance with your presence until client feels comfortable attending alone. *The feeling of acceptance by others increases self-esteem.*

4. Ask client to make a written list of positive and negative aspects about self. Discuss each item on the list with client. Develop plans of change for the characteristics viewed as negative. Assist client in implementing the plans. Provide positive feedback for successful change. *Individuals with low self-esteem often have difficulty recognizing their positive attributes. They may also lack problem-solving skills and require assistance to formulate a plan for implementing the desired changes. Positive feedback enhances self-esteem and encourages repetition of desired behaviors.*

5. Avoid fostering dependence by "doing for" the client. Allow client to perform as independently as physical condition will permit. Offer recognition and praise for accomplishments. *The ability to perform self-care activities independently provides a feeling of self-control and enhances self-esteem. Positive reinforcement encourages repetition of the desirable behavior.*

6. Allow client to be an active participant in his or her therapy. Promote feelings of control or power by encouraging input into the decision-making regarding treatment and for planning discharge from treatment. Provide positive feedback for adaptive responses. *Control over own life experiences promotes feelings of self-worth.*

Outcome Criteria

1. Client verbalizes positive perception of self.
2. Client demonstrates ability to manage own self-care, make independent decisions, and use problem-solving skills.
3. Client sets goals that are realistic and works to achieve those goals without evidence of fear of failure.

● INEFFECTIVE ROLE PERFORMANCE

Definition: Patterns of behavior and self-expression that do not match the environmental context, norms, and expectations.

Possible Etiologies ("related to")

[Physical illness accompanied by real or perceived disabling symptoms]
[Unmet dependency needs]
[Dysfunctional family system]

Defining Characteristics ("evidenced by")

Change in self-perception of role
Change in [physical] capacity to resume role
[Assumption of dependent role]
Change in usual patterns of responsibility [because of conflict within dysfunctional family system]

Goals/Objectives

Short-term Goal

Client will verbalize understanding that physical symptoms interfere with role performance in order to fill an unmet need.

Long-term Goal

Client will be able to assume role-related responsibilities by time of discharge from treatment.

Interventions with *Selected Rationales*

1. Determine client's usual role within the family system. Identify roles of other family members. *An accurate database is required in order to formulate appropriate plan of care for the client.*
2. Assess specific disabilities related to role expectations. Assess relationship of disability to physical condition. *It is important to determine the realism of client's role expectations.*
3. Encourage client to discuss conflicts evident within the family system. Identify ways in which client and other family members have responded to these conflicts. *It is necessary to identify specific stressors, as well as adaptive and maladaptive responses within the system, before assistance can be provided in an effort to create change.*
4. Help client identify feelings associated with family conflict, the subsequent exacerbation of physical symptoms, and the accompanying disabilities. *Client may be unaware of the relationship between physical symptoms and emotional*

problems. An awareness of the correlation is the first step toward creating change.

5. Help client identify changes he or she would like to occur within the family system. Encourage family participation in the development of plans to effect positive change, and work to resolve the conflict for which the client's sick role provides relief. *Input from the individuals who will be directly involved in the change will increase the likelihood of a positive outcome.*

6. Allow all family members input into the plan for change: knowledge of benefits and consequences for each alternative, selection of appropriate alternatives, methods for implementation of alternatives, and an alternate plan in the event initial change is unsuccessful. *Family may require assistance with this problem-solving process.*

7. Ensure that client has accurate perception of role expectations within the family system. Use role-playing to practice areas associated with his or her role that client perceives as painful. *Repetition through practice may help to desensitize client to the anticipated distress.*

8. As client is able to see the relationship between exacerbation of physical symptoms and existing conflict, discuss more adaptive coping strategies that may be used to prevent interference with role performance during times of stress.

CLINICAL PEARL Coping strategies are very individual, and only the client knows what will work for him or her. The nurse may make suggestions and help the client practice through role-play, but the client alone must decide what will be adaptive in his or her personal situation. The nurse must be careful not to impose on the client ideas that the nurse thinks are more appropriate but which may not be adaptive for the client.

Outcome Criteria

1. Client is able to verbalize realistic perception of role expectations.
2. Client is physically able to assume role-related responsibilities.
3. Client and family are able to verbalize plan for attempt at conflict resolution.

● DEFICIENT KNOWLEDGE (PSYCHOLOGICAL FACTORS AFFECTING MEDICAL CONDITION)

Definition: Absence or deficiency of cognitive information related to a specific topic.

Possible Etiologies ("related to")

Lack of interest in learning
[Severe level of anxiety]
[Low self-esteem]
[Regression to earlier level of development]

Defining Characteristics ("evidenced by")

[Denial of emotional problems]
[Statements such as, "I don't know why the doctor put me on the psychiatric unit. I have a physical problem."]
[History of numerous exacerbations of physical illness]
[Noncompliance with psychiatric treatment]
Inappropriate or exaggerated behaviors (e.g., hysterical, hostile, agitated, apathetic)

Goals/Objectives
Short-term Goal

Client will cooperate with plan for teaching provided by primary nurse.

Long-term Goal

By time of discharge from treatment, client will be able to verbalize psychological factors affecting his or her medical condition.

Interventions with *Selected Rationales*

1. Assess client's level of knowledge regarding effects of psychological problems on the body. *An adequate database is necessary for the development of an effective teaching plan.*
2. Assess client's level of anxiety and readiness to learn. *Learning does not occur beyond the moderate level of anxiety.*
3. Discuss physical examinations and laboratory tests that have been conducted. Explain purpose and results of each. *Fear of the unknown may contribute to elevated level of anxiety. The client has the right to know about and accept or refuse any medical treatment.*
4. Explore client's feelings and fears. Go slowly. These feelings may have been suppressed or repressed for so long that their disclosure may be very painful. Be supportive. *Verbalization of feelings in a nonthreatening environment and with a trusting individual may help the client come to terms with unresolved issues.*
5. Have client keep a diary of appearance, duration, and intensity of physical symptoms. A separate record of situations that the client finds especially stressful should also be kept. *Comparison of these records may provide objective data from which to observe the relationship between physical symptoms and stress.*

6. Help client identify needs that are being met through the sick role. Together, formulate more adaptive means for fulfilling these needs. Practice by role-playing. *Repetition through practice serves to reduce discomfort in the actual situation.*

7. Provide instruction in assertiveness techniques, especially the ability to recognize the differences among passive, assertive, and aggressive behaviors and the importance of respecting the human rights of others while protecting one's own basic human rights. *These skills will preserve client's self-esteem while also improving his or her ability to form satisfactory interpersonal relationships.*

8. Discuss adaptive methods of stress management such as relaxation techniques, physical exercise, meditation, breathing exercises, and autogenics. *Use of these adaptive techniques may decrease appearance of physical symptoms in response to stress.*

Outcome Criteria

1. Client verbalizes an understanding of the relationship between psychological stress and exacerbation of physical illness.

2. Client demonstrates the ability to use adaptive coping strategies in the management of stress.

@ **INTERNET REFERENCES**

- Additional information about psychophysiological disorders discussed in this chapter may be located at the following websites:
  a. http://www.cancer.gov/
  b. http://www.cancer.org
  c. http://www.heart.org/HEARTORG/
  d. http://www.headaches.org/
  e. http://www.pslgroup.com/ASTHMA.HTM
  f. http://www.gastro.org/
  g. http://www.pslgroup.com/HYPERTENSION.HTM
  h. http://www.arthritis.org
  i. http://digestive.niddk.nih.gov/ddiseases/pubs/colitis/

Personality Disorders

● BACKGROUND ASSESSMENT DATA

The American Psychiatric Association (APA, 2000, p. 686) *Diagnostic and Statistical Manual of Mental Disorders, Fourth Edition, Text Revision (DSM-IV-TR)* describes personality *traits* as "enduring patterns of perceiving, relating to, and thinking about the environment and oneself that are exhibited in a wide range of social and personal contexts." A personality *disorder* is said to exist only when these traits become inflexible and maladaptive and cause either significant functional impairment or subjective distress.

The *DSM-IV-TR* groups the personality disorders into three clusters. They are coded on Axis II in the *DMS-IV-TR* Classification. These clusters, and the disorders classified under each, are described as follows:

1. **Cluster A:** Behaviors described as odd or eccentric
    a. Paranoid personality disorder
    b. Schizoid personality disorder
    c. Schizotypal personality disorder
2. **Cluster B:** Behaviors described as dramatic, emotional, or erratic
    a. Antisocial personality disorder
    b. Borderline personality disorder
    c. Histrionic personality disorder
    d. Narcissistic personality disorder
3. **Cluster C:** Behaviors described as anxious or fearful
    a. Avoidant personality disorder
    b. Dependent personality disorder
    c. Obsessive-compulsive personality disorder
    d. Passive-aggressive personality disorder

Note: The third edition of the *DSM* included passive-aggressive personality disorder in Cluster C. In the *DSM-IV-TR*, this disorder is included in the section on *Criteria Provided for Further Study.* For purposes of this text, passive-aggressive personality disorder is described with the cluster C disorders.

Categories of personality disorders described by the *DSM-IV-TR* include the following:

1. **Cluster A**
   a. ***Paranoid Personality Disorder.*** The essential feature is a pervasive and unwarranted suspiciousness and mistrust of people. There is a general expectation of being exploited or harmed by others in some way. Symptoms include guardedness in relationships with others, pathological jealousy, hypersensitivity, inability to relax, unemotionality, and lack of a sense of humor. These individuals are very critical of others but have much difficulty accepting criticism themselves.
   b. ***Schizoid Personality Disorder.*** This disorder is characterized by an inability to form close, personal relationships. Symptoms include social isolation; absence of warm, tender feelings for others; indifference to praise, criticism, or the feelings of others; and flat, dull affect (appears cold and aloof).
   c. ***Schizotypal Personality Disorder.*** This disorder is characterized by peculiarities of ideation, appearance, and behavior, and deficits in interpersonal relatedness that are not severe enough to meet the criteria for schizophrenia. Symptoms include magical thinking; ideas of reference; social isolation; illusions; odd speech patterns; aloof, cold, suspicious behavior; and undue social anxiety.
2. **Cluster B**
   a. ***Antisocial Personality Disorder.*** This disorder is characterized by a pattern of socially irresponsible, exploitative, and guiltless behavior, as evidenced by the tendency to fail to conform to the law, to sustain consistent employment, to exploit and manipulate others for personal gain, to deceive, and to fail to develop stable relationships. The individual must be at least 18 years of age and have a history of conduct disorder before the age of 15. (Symptoms of this disorder are identified later in this chapter, along with predisposing factors and nursing care.)
   b. ***Borderline Personality Disorder.*** The features of this disorder are described as marked instability in interpersonal relationships, mood, and self-image. The instability is significant to the extent that the individual seems to hover on the border between neurosis and psychosis. (Symptoms of this disorder are identified later in this chapter, along with predisposing factors and nursing care.)
   c. ***Histrionic Personality Disorder.*** The essential feature of this disorder is described by the *DSM-IV-TR* as a "pervasive pattern of excessive emotionality and attention-seeking

behavior" (APA, 2000, p. 711). Symptoms include exaggerated expression of emotions, incessant drawing of attention to oneself, overreaction to minor events, constantly seeking approval from others, egocentricity, vain and demanding behavior, extreme concern with physical appearance, and inappropriately sexually seductive appearance or behavior.

d. *Narcissistic Personality Disorder.* This disorder is characterized by a grandiose sense of self-importance; preoccupation with fantasies of success, power, brilliance, beauty, or ideal love; a constant need for admiration and attention; exploitation of others for fulfillment of own desires; lack of empathy; response to criticism or failure with indifference or humiliation and rage; and preoccupation with feelings of envy.

3. **Cluster C**
   a. *Avoidant Personality Disorder.* This disorder is characterized by social withdrawal brought about by extreme sensitivity to rejection. Symptoms include unwillingness to enter into relationships unless given unusually strong guarantees of uncritical acceptance; low self-esteem; and social withdrawal despite a desire for affection and acceptance. Depression and anxiety are common. Social phobia may be a complication of this disorder.

   b. *Dependent Personality Disorder.* Individuals with this disorder passively allow others to assume responsibility for major areas of life because of their inability to function independently. They lack self-confidence, are unable to make decisions, perceive themselves as helpless and stupid, possess fear of being alone or abandoned, and seek constant reassurance and approval from others.

   c. *Obsessive-Compulsive Personality Disorder.* This disorder is characterized by a pervasive pattern of perfectionism and inflexibility. Interpersonal relationships have a formal and serious quality, and others often perceive these individuals as stilted or "stiff." Other symptoms include difficulty expressing tender feelings, insistence that others submit to his or her way of doing things, excessive devotion to work and productivity to the exclusion of pleasure, indecisiveness, perfectionism, preoccupation with details, depressed mood, and being judgmental of self and others.

   d. *Passive-Aggressive Personality Disorder.* Characteristic of this disorder is a passive resistance to demands for adequate performance in both occupational and social functioning (APA, 2000). Symptoms include obstructionism, procrastination, stubbornness, intentional inefficiency, dawdling, "forgetfulness," criticism of persons in authority, dependency, and low self-esteem. Oppositional defiant disorder in childhood or adolescence is a predisposing factor.

Many of the behaviors associated with the various personality disorders may be manifested by clients with virtually every psychiatric diagnosis, as well as by those individuals described as "healthy." It is only when personality traits or styles repetitively interfere with an individual's ability to function within age-appropriate cultural and developmental expectations, disrupt interpersonal relationships, and distort a person's pattern of perception and thinking about the environment that a diagnosis of personality disorder is assigned.

Individuals with personality disorders may be encountered in all types of treatment settings. They are not often treated in acute care settings, but because of the instability of the borderline client, hospitalization is necessary from time to time. The individual with antisocial personality disorder also may be hospitalized as an alternative to imprisonment when a legal determination is made that psychiatric intervention may be helpful. Because of these reasons, suggestions for inpatient care of individuals with these disorders are included in this chapter; however, these interventions may be used in other types of treatment settings as well. Undoubtedly, these clients represent the ultimate challenge for the psychiatric nurse.

● BORDERLINE PERSONALITY DISORDER
Defined

This personality disorder is characterized by instability of affect, behavior, object relationships, and self-image. The term "borderline" came into being because these clients' emotionally unstable behavior seems to fall *on the border* between neurotic and psychotic. Transient psychotic symptoms appear during periods of extreme stress. The disorder is more commonly diagnosed in women than in men.

Predisposing Factors to Borderline Personality Disorder

1. **Physiological**
   a. *Biochemical.* Cummings and Mega (2003) have suggested a possible serotonergic defect in clients with borderline personality disorder. In positron emission tomography using α-[^{11}C]methyl-L-tryptophan (α-[^{11}C]MTrp), which reflects serotonergic synthesis capability, clients with borderline personality demonstrated significantly decreased α-[^{11}C]MTrp in medial frontal, superior temporal, and

striatal regions of the brain. Cummings and Mega (2003) stated:

These functional imaging studies support a medial and orbitofrontal abnormality that may promote the impulsive aggression demonstrated by patients with the borderline personality disorder (p. 230).

b. *Genetic.* The decrease in serotonin may also have genetic implications for borderline personality disorder. Sadock and Sadock (2007) report that depression is common in the family backgrounds of clients with borderline personality disorder. They stated:

These patients have more relatives with mood disorders than do control groups, and persons with borderline personality disorder often have mood disorder as well (p. 791).

2. **Psychosocial**
   a. *Childhood Trauma.* Studies have shown that many individuals with borderline personality disorder were reared in families with chaotic environments. Lubit and Finley-Belgrad (2008) stated, "Risk factors [for borderline personality disorder] include family environments characterized by trauma, neglect, and/or separation; exposure to sexual and physical abuse; and serious parental psychopathology such as substance abuse and antisocial personality disorder." From 40% to 71% of borderline personality disorder clients report having been sexually abused, usually by a noncaregiver (National Institute of Mental Health [NIMH], 2009). In some instances, this disorder has been likened to posttraumatic stress disorder in response to childhood trauma and abuse. Oldham and associates (2006) stated:

   Even when full criteria for comorbid PTSD are not present, patients with borderline personality disorder may experience PTSD-like symptoms. For example, symptoms such as intrusion, avoidance, and hyperarousal may emerge during psychotherapy. Awareness of the trauma-related nature of these symptoms can facilitate both psychotherapeutic and pharmacological efforts in symptom relief (p. 1267).

   b. *Theory of Object Relations.* This theory suggests that the basis for borderline personality lies in the ways the child relates to the mother and does not separate from her. Mahler and associates (1975) define this process in a series of phases described as follows:
   • **Phase 1 (Birth to 1 month), Autistic Phase.** Most of the infant's time is spent in a half-waking, half-sleeping state. The main goal is fulfillment of needs for survival and comfort.

- **Phase 2 (1 to 5 months), Symbiotic Phase.** A type of psychic fusion of mother and child. The child views the self as an extension of the parenting figure, although there is a developing awareness of external sources of need fulfillment.
- **Phase 3 (5 to 10 months), Differentiation Phase.** The child is beginning to recognize that there is separateness between the self and the parenting figure.
- **Phase 4 (10 to 16 months), Practicing Phase.** This phase is characterized by increased locomotor functioning and the ability to explore the environment independently. A sense of separateness of the self is increased.
- **Phase 5 (16 to 24 months), Rapprochement Phase.** Awareness of separateness of the self becomes acute. This is frightening to the child, who wants to regain some lost closeness but not return to symbiosis. The child wants the mother there as needed for "emotional refueling" and to maintain feelings of security.
- **Phase 6 (24 to 36 months), On the Way to Object Constancy Phase.** In this phase, the child completes the individuation process and learns to relate to objects in an effective, constant manner. A sense of separateness is established, and the child is able to internalize a sustained image of the loved object or person when out of sight. Separation anxiety is resolved.

The theory of object relations suggests that the individual with borderline personality is fixed in the rapprochement phase of development. This fixation occurs when the mother begins to feel threatened by the increasing autonomy of her child and so withdraws her emotional support during those times *or* she may instead reward clinging, dependent behaviors. In this way, the child comes to believe that

"To grow up and be independent = a 'bad' child."
"To stay immature and dependent = a 'good' child."
"Mom withholds nurturing from 'bad' child."

Consequently, the child develops a deep fear of abandonment that persists into adulthood. In addition, because object constancy is never achieved, the child continues to view objects (people) as parts—either good or bad. This is called splitting, a primary defense mechanism of borderline personality.

Symptomatology (Subjective and Objective Data)

Individuals with borderline personality always seem to be in a state of crisis. Their affect is one of extreme intensity and their behavior reflects frequent changeability. These changes can occur within days, hours, or even minutes. Often these individuals exhibit a single, dominant affective tone, such as depression, which may give way periodically to anxious agitation or inappropriate outbursts of anger.

Common symptoms include the following:

1. **Chronic depression**. Depression is so common in clients with this disorder that before the inclusion of borderline personality disorder in the *DSM*, many of these clients were diagnosed as depressed. Depression occurs in response to feelings of abandonment by the mother in early childhood (see "Predisposing Factors"). Underlying the depression is a sense of rage that is sporadically turned inward on the self and externally on the environment. Seldom is the individual aware of the true source of these feelings until well into long-term therapy.

2. **Inability to be alone.** Because of this chronic fear of abandonment, clients with borderline personality disorder have little tolerance for being alone. They prefer a frantic search for companionship, no matter how unsatisfactory, to sitting with feelings of loneliness, emptiness, and boredom (Sadock & Sadock, 2007).

3. **Clinging and distancing.** The client with borderline personality disorder commonly exhibits a pattern of interaction with others that is characterized by clinging and distancing behaviors. When clients are clinging to another individual, they may exhibit helpless, dependent, or even childlike behaviors. They overidealize a single individual with whom they want to spend all their time, with whom they express a frequent need to talk, or from whom they seek constant reassurance. Acting-out behaviors, even self-mutilation, may result when they cannot be with this chosen individual. Distancing behaviors are characterized by hostility, anger, and devaluation of others, arising from a feeling of discomfort with closeness. Distancing behaviors also occur in response to separations, confrontations, or attempts to limit certain behaviors. Devaluation of others is manifested by discrediting or undermining their strengths and personal significance.

4. **Splitting.** Splitting is a primitive ego defense mechanism that is common in people with borderline personality disorder. It arises from their lack of achievement of object constancy and is manifested by an inability to integrate and accept both positive and negative feelings. In their view, people—including themselves—and life situations are either all good or all bad.

5. **Manipulation.** In their efforts to prevent the separation they so desperately fear, clients with this disorder become masters of manipulation. Virtually any behavior becomes an acceptable means of achieving the desired result: relief from

separation anxiety. Playing one individual against another is a common ploy to allay these fears of abandonment.

6. **Self-destructive behaviors.** Repetitive, self-mutilative behaviors, such as cutting, scratching, and burning, are classic manifestations of borderline personality disorder. Although these acts can be fatal, most commonly they are manipulative gestures designed to elicit a rescue response from significant others. Suicide attempts are not uncommon and often result from feelings of abandonment following separation from a significant other.

7. **Impulsivity.** Individuals with borderline personality disorder have poor impulse control based on primary process functioning. Impulsive behaviors associated with borderline personality disorder include substance abuse, gambling, promiscuity, reckless driving, and binging and purging (APA, 2000). Many times these acting-out behaviors occur in response to real or perceived feelings of abandonment.

8. **Feelings of unreality.** Transient episodes of extreme stress can precipitate periods of dissociation in the individual with borderline personality disorder.

9. **Rage reactions.** Difficulty controlling anger.

Common Nursing Diagnoses and Interventions

(Interventions are applicable to various health-care settings, such as inpatient and partial hospitalization, community outpatient clinic, home health, and private practice.)

● RISK FOR SELF-MUTILATION/ RISK FOR SELF-DIRECTED OR OTHER-DIRECTED VIOLENCE

Definition: At risk for deliberate self-injurious behavior causing tissue damage with the intent of causing nonfatal injury to attain relief of tension. At risk for behaviors in which an individual demonstrates that he or she can be physically, emotionally, and/or sexually harmful either to self or to others.

Related/Risk Factors ("related to")

[Extreme fears of abandonment]
[Feelings of unreality]
[Depressed mood]
[Use of suicidal gestures for manipulation of others]
[Unmet dependency needs]
Low self-esteem
[Unresolved grief]

[Rage reactions]

[Physically self-damaging acts (cutting, burning, drug overdose, etc.)]

Body language (e.g., rigid posture, clenching of fists and jaw, hyperactivity, pacing, breathlessness, threatening stances)

History or threats of violence toward self or others or of destruction to the property of others

Impulsivity

Suicidal ideation, plan, available means

History of suicide attempts

Goals/Objectives

Short-term Goals

1. Client will seek out staff member if feelings of harming self or others emerge.
2. Client will not harm self or others.

Long-term Goal

Client will not harm self or others.

Interventions with *Selected Rationales*

1. Observe client's behavior frequently. Do this through routine activities and interactions; avoid appearing watchful and suspicious. *Close observation is required so that intervention can occur if required to ensure client's (and others') safety.*
2. Secure a verbal contract from client that he or she will seek out a staff member when the urge for self-mutilation is experienced. *Discussing feelings of self-harm with a trusted individual provides some relief to the client. A contract gets the subject out in the open and places some of the responsibility for his or her safety with the client. An attitude of acceptance of the client as a worthwhile individual is conveyed.*
3. If self-mutilation occurs, care for the client's wounds in a matter-of-fact manner. Do not give positive reinforcement to this behavior by offering sympathy or additional attention. *Lack of attention to the maladaptive behavior may decrease repetition of its use.*
4. Encourage client to talk about feelings he or she was having just prior to this behavior. *To problem-solve the situation with the client, knowledge of the precipitating factors is important.*
5. Act as a role model for appropriate expression of angry feelings and give positive reinforcement to the client when attempts to conform are made. *It is vital that the client express angry feelings, because suicide and other self-destructive behaviors are often viewed as a result of anger turned inward on the self.*
6. Remove all dangerous objects from the client's environment. *Client safety is a nursing priority.*

7. Try to redirect violent behavior with physical outlets for the client's anxiety (e.g., punching bag, jogging). *Physical exercise is a safe and effective way of relieving pent-up tension.*

8. Have sufficient staff available to indicate a show of strength to the client if necessary. *This conveys to the client evidence of control over the situation and provides some physical security for staff.*

9. Administer tranquilizing medications as ordered by physician or obtain an order if necessary. Monitor the client for effectiveness of the medication and for the appearance of adverse side effects. *Tranquilizing medications such as anxiolytics or antipsychotics may have a calming effect on the client and may prevent aggressive behaviors.*

10. Use of mechanical restraints or isolation room may be required if less restrictive interventions are unsuccessful. Follow policy and procedure prescribed by the institution in executing this intervention. The Joint Commission (formerly the Joint Commission on Accreditation of Healthcare Organizations [JCAHO]) requires that an in-person evaluation (by a physician, clinical psychologist, or other licensed independent practitioner responsible for the care of the patient) be conducted within 1 hour of initiating restraint or seclusion (The Joint Commission, 2010). The physician must reevaluate and issue a new order for restraints every 4 hours for adults and every 1 to 2 hours for children and adolescents.

11. Observe the client in restraints every 15 minutes (or according to institutional policy). Ensure that circulation to extremities is not compromised (check temperature, color, pulses). Assist the client with needs related to nutrition, hydration, and elimination. Position the client so that comfort is facilitated and aspiration can be prevented. *Client safety is a nursing priority.*

12. May need to assign staff on a one-to-one basis if warranted by acuity of the situation. *Clients with borderline personality disorder have extreme fear of abandonment; leaving them alone at such a time may cause an acute rise in level of anxiety and agitation.*

Outcome Criteria

1. Client has not harmed self or others.
2. Anxiety is maintained at a level in which client feels no need for aggression.
3. Client denies any ideas of self-harm.
4. Client verbalizes community support systems from which assistance may be requested when personal coping strategies are unsuccessful.

● ANXIETY (SEVERE TO PANIC)

Definition: Vague uneasy feeling of discomfort or dread accompanied by an autonomic response (the source often nonspecific or unknown to the individual); a feeling of apprehension caused by anticipation of danger. It is an alerting signal that warns of impending danger and enables the individual to take measures to deal with threat.

Possible Etiologies ("related to")

Threat to self-concept

Unmet needs

[Extreme fear of abandonment]

Unconscious conflicts [associated with fixation in earlier level of development]

Defining Characteristics ("evidenced by")

[Transient psychotic symptoms in response to severe stress, manifested by disorganized thinking, confusion, altered communication patterns, disorientation, misinterpretation of the environment]

[Excessive use of projection (attributing own thoughts and feelings to others)]

[Depersonalization (feelings of unreality)]

[Derealization (a feeling that the environment is unreal)]

[Acts of self-mutilation in an effort to find relief from feelings of unreality]

Goals/Objectives

Short-term Goal

Client will demonstrate use of relaxation techniques to maintain anxiety at manageable level.

Long-term Goal

Client will be able to recognize events that precipitate anxiety and intervene to prevent disabling behaviors.

Interventions with *Selected Rationales*

1. Symptoms of depersonalization often occur at the panic level of anxiety. Clients with borderline personality disorder often resort to cutting or other self-mutilating acts in an effort to relieve the anxiety. Being able to feel pain or see blood is a reassurance of existence to the person. If injury occurs, care for the wounds in a matter-of-fact manner without providing reinforcement for this behavior. ***Lack of reinforcement may discourage repetition of the maladaptive behavior.***

2. During periods of panic anxiety, stay with the client and provide reassurance of safety and security. Orient client to the reality of the situation. *Client comfort and safety are nursing priorities.*

3. Administer tranquilizing medications as ordered by physician, or obtain order if necessary. Monitor client for effectiveness of the medication as well as for adverse side effects. *Antianxiety medications (e.g., lorazepam, chlordiazepoxide, alprazolam) provide relief from the immobilizing effects of anxiety and facilitate client's cooperation with therapy.*

4. Correct misinterpretations of the environment as expressed by client. *Confronting misinterpretations honestly, with a caring and accepting attitude, provides a therapeutic orientation to reality and preserves the client's feelings of dignity and self-worth.*

5. Encourage the client to talk about true feelings. Help him or her recognize ownership of these feelings rather than projecting them onto others in the environment. *Exploration of feelings with a trusted individual may help the client perceive the situation more realistically and come to terms with unresolved issues.*

6. Help client work toward achievement of object constancy. Client may feel totally abandoned when nurse or therapist leaves at shift change or at end of therapy session. There may even be feelings that the therapist ceases to exist. Leaving a signed note or card with the client for reassurance may help. It is extremely important for more than one nurse to develop a therapeutic relationship with the borderline client. It is also necessary that staff maintain open communication and consistency in the provision of care for these individuals. *Individuals with borderline personality disorder have a tendency to cling to one staff member, if allowed, transferring their maladaptive dependency to that individual. This dependency can be avoided if the client is able to establish therapeutic relationships with two or more staff members who encourage independent self-care activities.*

Outcome Criteria

1. Client is able to verbalize events that precipitate anxiety and demonstrate techniques for its reduction.
2. Client manifests no symptoms of depersonalization.
3. Client interprets the environment realistically.

● COMPLICATED GRIEVING

Definition: A disorder that occurs after the death of a significant other [or any other loss of significance to the individual], in which the experience of distress accompanying bereavement fails to follow normative expectations and manifests in functional impairment.

Possible Etiologies ("related to")

[Maternal deprivation during rapprochement phase of development (internalized as a loss, with fixation in the anger stage of the grieving process)]

Defining Characteristics ("evidenced by")

Persistent emotional distress
[Anger]
[Internalized rage]
Depression
[Labile affect]
[Extreme fear of being alone (fear of abandonment)]
[Acting-out behaviors, such as sexual promiscuity, suicidal gestures, temper tantrums, substance abuse]
[Difficulty expressing feelings]
[Altered activities of daily living]
[Reliving of past experiences with little or no reduction of intensity of the grief]
[Feelings of inadequacy; dependency]

Goals/Objectives

Short-term Goal

Client will discuss with nurse or therapist maladaptive patterns of expressing anger.

Long-term Goal

Client will be able to identify the true source of angry feelings, accept ownership of these feelings, and express them in a socially acceptable manner, in an effort to satisfactorily progress through the grieving process.

Interventions with *Selected Rationales*

1. Convey an accepting attitude—one that creates a nonthreatening environment for the client to express feelings. Be honest and keep all promises. *An accepting attitude conveys to the client that you believe he or she is a worthwhile person. Trust is enhanced.*
2. Identify the function that anger, frustration, and rage serve for the client. Allow the client to express these feelings within reason. *Verbalization of feelings in a nonthreatening environment may help the client come to terms with unresolved issues.*
3. Encourage client to discharge pent-up anger through participation in large motor activities (e.g., brisk walks, jogging,

physical exercises, volleyball, punching bag, exercise bike). *Physical exercise provides a safe and effective method for discharging pent-up tension.*

4. Explore with client the true source of the anger. This is painful therapy that often leads to regression as the client deals with the feelings of early abandonment. It seems that sometimes the client must "get worse before he or she can get better." *Reconciliation of the feelings associated with this stage is necessary before progression through the grieving process can continue.*

5. As anger is displaced onto the nurse or therapist, caution must be taken to guard against the negative effects of countertransference. *These are very difficult clients who have the capacity for eliciting a whole array of negative feelings from the therapist. The existence of negative feelings by the nurse or therapist must be acknowledged, but they must not be allowed to interfere with the therapeutic process.*

6. Explain the behaviors associated with the normal grieving process. Help the client to recognize his or her position in this process. *Knowledge of the acceptability of the feelings associated with normal grieving may help to relieve some of the guilt that these responses generate.*

7. Help client understand appropriate ways of expressing anger. Give positive reinforcement for behaviors used to express anger appropriately. Act as a role model. *Positive reinforcement enhances self-esteem and encourages repetition of desirable behaviors. It is appropriate to let the client know when he or she has done something that has generated angry feelings in you. Role-modeling ways to express anger in an appropriate manner is a powerful learning tool.*

8. Set limits on acting-out behaviors and explain consequences of violation of those limits. Be supportive, yet consistent and firm, in caring for this client. *Client lacks sufficient self-control to limit maladaptive behaviors, so assistance is required from staff. Without consistency on the part of all staff members working with this client, a positive outcome will not be achieved.*

Outcome Criteria

1. Client is able to verbalize how anger and acting-out behaviors are associated with maladaptive grieving.
2. Client is able to discuss the original source of the anger and demonstrates socially acceptable ways of expressing the emotion.

• IMPAIRED SOCIAL INTERACTION

Definition: Insufficient or excessive quantity or ineffective quality of social exchange.

Possible Etiologies ("related to")

[Fixation in rapprochement phase of development]
[Extreme fears of abandonment and engulfment]
[Lack of personal identity]

Defining Characteristics ("evidenced by")

[Alternating clinging and distancing behaviors]
[Inability to form satisfactory intimate relationship with another person]
Use of unsuccessful social interaction behaviors
[Use of primitive dissociation (splitting) in their relationships (viewing others as all good or all bad)]

Goals/Objectives

Short-term Goal

Client will discuss with nurse or therapist behaviors that impede the development of satisfactory interpersonal relationships.

Long-term Goals

1. Client will interact with others in the therapy setting in both social and therapeutic activities without difficulty by time of discharge from treatment.
2. Client will display no evidence of splitting or clinging and distancing behaviors in relationships by time of discharge from treatment.

Interventions with *Selected Rationales*

1. Encourage client to examine these behaviors (to recognize that they are occurring). *Client may be unaware of splitting or of clinging and distancing pattern of interaction with others.*
2. Help client realize that you will be available, without reinforcing dependent behaviors. *Knowledge of your availability may provide needed security for the client.*
3. Give positive reinforcement for independent behaviors. *Positive reinforcement enhances self-esteem and encourages repetition of desirable behaviors.*
4. Rotate staff who work with the client in order to avoid client's developing dependence on particular staff members. *Client must learn to relate to more than one staff member in an*

effort to decrease use of splitting and to diminish fears of abandonment.

CLINICAL PEARL Recognize when the client is playing one staff member against another. Remember that splitting is a primary defense mechanism of these individuals, and the impressions they have of others as either "good" or "bad" are a manifestation of this defense. Do not listen as the client tries to degrade other staff members. Suggest that the client discuss the problem directly with the staff person involved.

5. Explore with client feelings that relate to fears of abandonment and engulfment. Help client understand that clinging and distancing behaviors are engendered by these fears. *Exploration of feelings with a trusted individual may help client come to terms with unresolved issues.*
6. Help client understand how these behaviors interfere with satisfactory relationships. *Client may be unaware of others' perception of him or her and why these behaviors are not acceptable to others.*
7. Assist the client to work toward achievement of object constancy. Be available, without promoting dependency. *This may help client resolve fears of abandonment and develop the ability to establish satisfactory intimate relationships.*

Outcome Criteria

1. Client is able to interact with others in both social and therapeutic activities in a socially acceptable manner.
2. Client does not use splitting or clinging and distancing behaviors in relationships and is able to relate the use of these behaviors to failure of past relationships.

● DISTURBED PERSONAL IDENTITY

Definition: Inability to maintain an integrated and complete perception of self.

Possible Etiologies ("related to")

[Failure to complete tasks of separation/individuation stage of development]
[Underdeveloped ego]
[Unmet dependency needs]
[Absence of, or rejection by, parental sex-role model]

Defining Characteristics ("evidenced by")

[Excessive use of projection]
[Vague self-image]

[Unable to tolerate being alone]
[Feelings of depersonalization and derealization]
[Self-mutilation (cutting, burning) to validate existence of self]
Gender confusion
Feelings of emptiness
Uncertainties about goals and values

Goals/Objectives
Short-term Goal
Client will describe characteristics that make him or her a unique individual.

Long-term Goal
Client will be able to distinguish own thoughts, feelings, behaviors, and image from those of others, as the initial step in the development of a healthy personal identity.

Interventions with *Selected Rationales*

1. Help client recognize the reality of his or her separateness. Do not attempt to translate client's thoughts and feelings into words. *Because of the blurred ego boundaries, client may believe you can read his or her mind.* For this reason, caution should be taken in the use of empathetic understanding. For example, avoid statements such as, "I know how you must feel about that."

2. Help client recognize separateness from nurse by clarifying which behaviors and feelings belong to whom. If deemed appropriate, allow client to touch your hand or arm. *Touch and physical presence provide reality for the client and serve to strengthen weak ego boundaries.*

3. Encourage client to discuss thoughts and feelings. Help client recognize ownership of these feelings rather than projecting them onto others in the environment. *Verbalization of feelings in a nonthreatening environment may help client come to terms with unresolved issues.*

4. Confront statements that project client's feelings onto others. Ask client to validate that others possess those feelings. The expression of *reasonable doubt* as a therapeutic technique may be helpful ("I find that hard to believe").

5. If the problem is with gender identity, ask the client to describe his or her perception of appropriate male and female behaviors. Provide information about role behaviors and sex education, if necessary. Convey acceptance of the person regardless of preferred identity. *Client may require clarification of distorted ideas or misinformation. An attitude of acceptance reinforces client's feelings of self-worth.*

6. Always call client by his or her name. If client experiences feelings of depersonalization or derealization, orientation to the environment and correction of misperceptions may be helpful. *These interventions help to preserve client's feelings of dignity and self-worth.*

7. Help client understand that there are more adaptive ways of validating his or her existence than self-mutilation. Contract with the client to seek out staff member when these feelings occur. *A contract gets the subject out in the open and places some of the responsibility for his or her safety with the client. Client safety is a nursing priority.*

8. Work with client to clarify values. Discuss beliefs, attitudes, and feelings underlying his or her behaviors. Help client to identify those values that have been (or are intended to be) incorporated as his or her own. Care must be taken by the nurse to avoid imposing his or her own value system on the client. *Because of underdeveloped ego and fixation in early developmental level, client may not have established own value system. In order to accomplish this, ownership of beliefs and attitudes must be identified and clarified.*

9. Use of photographs of the client may help to establish or clarify ego boundaries. *Photographs may help to increase client's awareness of self as separate from others.*

10. Alleviate anxiety by providing assurance to client that he or she will not be left alone. *Early childhood traumas may predispose borderline clients to extreme fears of abandonment.*

11. Use of touch is sometimes therapeutic in identity confirmation. Before this technique is used, however, assess cultural influences and degree of trust. *Touch and physical presence provide reality for the client and serve to strengthen weak ego boundaries.*

Outcome Criteria

1. Client is able to distinguish between own thoughts and feelings and those of others.
2. Client claims ownership of those thoughts and feelings and does not use projection in relationships with others.
3. Client has clarified own feelings regarding sexual identity.

● LOW SELF-ESTEEM

Definition: Negative self-evaluating/feelings about self or self-capabilities.

Possible Etiologies ("related to")

[Lack of positive feedback]
[Unmet dependency needs]
[Retarded ego development]
[Repeated negative feedback, resulting in diminished self-worth]
[Dysfunctional family system]
[Fixation in earlier level of development]

Defining Characteristics ("evidenced by")

[Difficulty accepting positive reinforcement]
[Self-destructive behavior]
[Frequent use of derogatory and critical remarks against the self]
Lack of eye contact
[Manipulation of one staff member against another in an attempt to gain special privileges]
[Inability to form close, personal relationships]
[Inability to tolerate being alone]
[Degradation of others in an attempt to increase own feelings of self-worth]
Hesitancy to try new things or situations [because of fear of failure]

Goals/Objectives

Short-term Goals

1. Client will discuss fear of failure with nurse or therapist.
2. Client will verbalize things he or she likes about self.

Long-term Goals

1. Client will exhibit increased feelings of self-worth as evidenced by verbal expression of positive aspects about self, past accomplishments, and future prospects.
2. Client will exhibit increased feelings of self-worth by setting realistic goals and trying to reach them, thereby demonstrating a decrease in fear of failure.

Interventions with *Selected Rationales*

1. Ensure that goals are realistic. It is important for client to achieve something, so plan for activities in which success is likely. *Success increases self-esteem.*
2. Convey unconditional positive regard for client. Promote understanding of your acceptance for him or her as a worthwhile human being. *Acceptance by others increases feelings of self-worth.*
3. Set limits on manipulative behavior. Identify the consequences for violation of those limits. Minimize negative feedback to

the client. Enforce the limits and impose the consequences for violations in a matter-of-fact manner. Consistency among all staff members is essential. *Negative feedback can be extremely threatening to a person with low self-esteem and possibly aggravate the problem. Consequences should convey unacceptability of the* **behavior** *but not the* **person.**

4. Encourage independence in the performance of personal responsibilities, as well as in decision-making related to client's self-care. Offer recognition and praise for accomplishments. *Positive reinforcement enhances self-esteem and encourages repetition of desirable behaviors.*

5. Help client increase level of self-awareness through critical examination of feelings, attitudes, and behaviors. *Self-exploration in the presence of a trusted individual may help the client come to terms with unresolved issues.*

6. Help client identify positive self-attributes as well as those aspects of the self he or she finds undesirable. Discuss ways to effect change in these areas. *Individuals with low self-esteem often have difficulty recognizing their positive attributes. They may also lack problem-solving ability and require assistance to formulate a plan for implementing the desired changes.*

7. Discuss client's future. Assist client in the establishment of short-term and long-term goals. What are his or her strengths? How can he or she best use those strengths to achieve those goals? Encourage client to perform at a level realistic to his or her ability. Offer positive reinforcement for decisions made.

Outcome Criteria

1. Client verbalizes positive aspects about self.
2. Client demonstrates ability to make independent decisions regarding management of own self-care.
3. Client expresses some optimism and hope for the future.
4. Client sets realistic goals for self and demonstrates willingness to reach them.

● ANTISOCIAL PERSONALITY DISORDER
Defined

Antisocial personality disorder is characterized by a pattern of antisocial behavior that began before the age of 15. These behaviors violate the rights of others, and individuals with this disorder display no evidence of guilt feelings at having done so. There is often a long history of involvement with law-enforcement agencies. Substance abuse is not uncommon. The disorder is more frequently diagnosed in men than in women. Individuals with antisocial personalities are often labeled *sociopathic* or *psychopathic* in the lay literature.

Predisposing Factors to Antisocial Personality Disorder

1. **Physiological**
   a. *Genetics.* The *DSM-IV-TR* reports that antisocial personality is more common among first-degree biological relatives of those with the disorder than among the general population (APA, 2000). Twin and adoptive studies have implicated the role of genetics in antisocial personality disorder (Skodol & Gunderson, 2008). These studies of families of individuals with antisocial personality show higher numbers of relatives with antisocial personality or alcoholism than are found in the general population. Additional studies have shown that children of parents with antisocial behavior are more likely to be diagnosed as antisocial personality, even when they are separated at birth from their biological parents and reared by individuals without the disorder.
   b. *Temperament.* Characteristics associated with temperament in the newborn may be significant in the predisposition to antisocial personality. Parents who bring their children with behavior disorders to clinics often report that the child displayed temper tantrums from infancy and would become furious when awaiting a bottle or a diaper change. As these children mature, they commonly develop a bullying attitude toward other children. Parents report that they are undaunted by punishment and generally quite unmanageable. They are daring and foolhardy in their willingness to chance physical harm, and they seem unaffected by pain.

2. **Psychosocial**
   a. *Theories of Family Dynamics.* Antisocial personality disorder frequently arises from a chaotic home environment. Parental deprivation during the first 5 years of life appears to be a critical predisposing factor in the development of antisocial personality disorder. Separation due to parental delinquency appears to be more highly correlated with the disorder than is parental loss from other causes. The presence or intermittent appearance of inconsistent impulsive parents, not the loss of a consistent parent, is environmentally *most* damaging.

   Studies have shown that individuals with antisocial personality disorder often have been severely physically abused in childhood. The abuse contributes to the development of antisocial behavior in several ways. First, it provides a model for behavior. Second, it may result in injury to the child's central nervous system, thereby impairing the child's ability to function appropriately. Finally, it engenders rage in the victimized child, which is then displaced onto others in the environment.

Disordered family functioning has been implicated as an important factor in determining whether an individual develops antisocial personality (Hill, 2003; Skodol & Gunderson, 2008; Ramsland, 2009). The following circumstances may be influential in the predisposition to the disorder:
- Absence of parental discipline
- Extreme poverty
- Removal from the home
- Growing up without parental figures of both genders
- Erratic and inconsistent methods of discipline
- Being "rescued" each time they are in trouble (never having to suffer the consequences of their own behavior)
- Maternal deprivation

Symptomatology (Subjective and Objective Data)

1. Extremely low-self esteem (abuses other people in an attempt to validate his or her own superiority)
2. Inability to sustain satisfactory job performance
3. Inability to function as a responsible parent
4. Failure to follow social and legal norms; repeated performance of antisocial acts that are grounds for arrest (whether arrested or not)
5. Inability to develop satisfactory, enduring, intimate relationship with a sexual partner
6. Aggressive behaviors; repeated physical fights; spouse or child abuse
7. Extreme impulsivity
8. Repeated lying for personal benefit
9. Reckless driving; driving while intoxicated
10. Inability to learn from punishment
11. Lack of guilt or remorse felt in response to exploitation of others
12. Difficulty with interpersonal relationships
13. Social extroversion; stimulation through interaction with and abuse of others
14. Repeated failure to honor financial obligations

● COMMON NURSING DIAGNOSES AND INTERVENTIONS

(Interventions are applicable to various health-care settings, such as inpatient and partial hospitalization, community outpatient clinic, home health, and private practice.)

● RISK FOR OTHER-DIRECTED VIOLENCE

Definition: At risk for behaviors in which an individual demonstrates that he or she can be physically, emotionally, and/or sexually harmful to others.

Related/Risk Factors ("related to")

[Rage reactions]
History of witnessing family violence
Neurological impairment (e.g., positive electroencephalogram)
[Suspiciousness of others]
[Interruption of client's attempt to fulfill own desires]
[Inability to tolerate frustration]
[Learned behavior within client's subculture]
[Vulnerable self-esteem]
Body language (e.g., rigid posture, clenching of fists and jaw, hyperactivity, pacing, breathlessness, threatening stances)
[History or threats of violence toward self or others or of destruction to the property of others]
Impulsivity
Availability of weapon(s)
[Substance abuse or withdrawal]
[Provocative behavior: Argumentative, dissatisfied, overreactive, hypersensitive]
History of childhood abuse

Goals/Objectives
Short-term Goals
1. Client will discuss angry feelings and situations that precipitate hostility.
2. Client will not harm others.

Long-term Goal
Client will not harm others.

Interventions with *Selected Rationales*
1. Convey an accepting attitude toward this client. Feelings of rejection are undoubtedly familiar to him or her. Work on development of trust. Be honest, keep all promises, and convey the message to the client that it is not *him* or *her*, but the *behavior* that is unacceptable. ***An attitude of acceptance promotes feelings of self-worth. Trust is the basis of a therapeutic relationship.***

2. Maintain low level of stimuli in client's environment (low lighting, few people, simple decor, low noise level). *A stimulating environment may increase agitation and promote aggressive behavior.*

3. Observe client's behavior frequently. Do this through routine activities and interactions; avoid appearing watchful and suspicious. *Close observation is required so that intervention can occur if needed to ensure client's (and others') safety.*

4. Remove all dangerous objects from client's environment. *Client safety is a nursing priority.*

5. Help client identify the true object of his or her hostility (e.g., "You seem to be upset with..."). *Because of weak ego development, client may be misusing the defense mechanism of displacement. Helping him or her recognize this in a nonthreatening manner may help reveal unresolved issues so that they may be confronted.*

6. Encourage client to gradually verbalize hostile feelings. *Verbalization of feelings in a nonthreatening environment may help client come to terms with unresolved issues.*

7. Explore with client alternative ways of handling frustration (e.g., large motor skills that channel hostile energy into socially acceptable behavior). *Physically demanding activities help to relieve pent-up tension.*

8. Staff should maintain and convey a calm attitude toward client. *Anxiety is contagious and can be transferred from staff to client. A calm attitude provides client with a feeling of safety and security.*

9. Have sufficient staff available to present a show of strength to client if necessary. *This conveys to the client evidence of control over the situation and provides some physical security for staff.*

10. Administer tranquilizing medications as ordered by physician or obtain an order if necessary. Monitor client for effectiveness of the medication as well as for appearance of adverse side effects. *Antianxiety agents (e.g., lorazepam, chlordiazepoxide, oxazepam) produce a calming effect and may help to allay hostile behaviors.* (NOTE: Medications are often not prescribed for clients with antisocial personality disorder because of these individuals' strong susceptibility to addictions.)

11. If client is not calmed by "talking down" or by medication, use of mechanical restraints may be necessary. Be sure to have sufficient staff available to assist. Follow protocol established by the institution in executing this intervention. The Joint Commission requires that and in-person evaluation by a licensed independent practitioner be conducted within 1 hour of initiating restraint or seclusion. The physician must reevaluate and issue a new order for restraints

every 4 hours for adults age 18 and older. Never use restraints as a punitive measure but rather as a protective measure for a client who is out of control.
12. Observe client in restraints every 15 minutes (or according to institutional policy). Ensure that circulation to extremities is not compromised (check temperature, color, pulses). Assist client with needs related to nutrition, hydration, and elimination. Position client so that comfort is facilitated and aspiration can be prevented. ***Client safety is a nursing priority.***

Outcome Criteria

1. Client is able to rechannel hostility into socially acceptable behaviors.
2. Client is able to discuss angry feelings and verbalize ways to tolerate frustration appropriately.

● INEFFECTIVE COPING

Definition: Inability to form a valid appraisal of the stressors, inadequate choices of practiced responses, and/or inability to use available resources.

Possible Etiologies ("related to")

[Inadequate support systems]
[Inadequate coping method]
[Underdeveloped ego]
[Underdeveloped superego]
[Dysfunctional family system]
[Negative role modeling]
[Absent, erratic, or inconsistent methods of discipline]
[Extreme poverty]

Defining Characteristics ("evidenced by")

[Disregard for societal norms and laws]
[Absence of guilt feelings]
[Inability to delay gratification]
[Extreme impulsivity]
[Inability to learn from punishment]

Goals/Objectives
Short-term Goal

Within 24 hours after admission, client will verbalize understanding of the rules and regulations of the treatment setting and the consequences for violation of them.

Long-term Goal
Client will be able to cope more adaptively by delaying gratification of own desires and following rules and regulations of the treatment setting by time of discharge.

Interventions with *Selected Rationales*

1. From the onset, client should be made aware of which behaviors will not be accepted in the treatment setting. Explain consequences of violation of the limits. Consequences must involve something of value to the client. All staff must be consistent in enforcing these limits. Consequences should be administered in a matter-of-fact manner immediately after the infraction. *Because client cannot (or will not) impose own limits on maladaptive behaviors, these behaviors must be delineated and enforced by staff. Undesirable consequences may help to decrease repetition of these behaviors.*

2. Do not attempt to coax or convince client to do the "right thing." Do not use the words "You should (or shouldn't)…"; instead, use "You will be expected to… ." The ideal would be for this client to eventually internalize societal norms, beginning with this step-by-step, "either/or" approach on the unit (*either* you do [don't do] this, *or* this will occur). *Explanations must be concise, concrete, and clear, with little or no capacity for misinterpretation.*

3. Provide positive feedback or reward for acceptable behaviors. *Positive reinforcement enhances self-esteem and encourages repetition of desirable behaviors.*

4. *In an attempt to assist client to delay gratification,* begin to increase the length of time requirement for acceptable behavior in order to achieve the reward. For example, 2 hours of acceptable behavior may be exchanged for a telephone call; 4 hours of acceptable behavior for 2 hours of television; 1 day of acceptable behavior for a recreational therapy bowling activity; 5 days of acceptable behavior for a weekend pass.

5. A milieu unit provides an appropriate environment for the client with antisocial personality. *The democratic approach, with specific rules and regulations, community meetings, and group therapy sessions, emulates the type of societal situation in which the client must learn to live. Feedback from peers is often more effective than confrontation from an authority figure. The client learns to follow the rules of the group as a positive step in the progression toward internalizing the rules of society.*

6. Help client gain insight into own behavior. Often, these individuals rationalize to such an extent that they deny that their behavior is inappropriate. (For example, "The owner of this store has so much money, he'll never miss the little bit I take.

He has everything, and I have nothing. It's not fair! I deserve to have some of what he has.") *Client must come to understand that certain behaviors will not be tolerated within the society and that severe consequences will be imposed on those individuals who refuse to comply. Client must want to become a productive member of society before he or she can be helped.*

7. Talk about past behaviors with client. Discuss which behaviors are acceptable by societal norms and which are not. Help client identify ways in which he or she has exploited others. Encourage client to explore how he or she would feel if the circumstances were reversed. *An attempt may be made to enlighten the client to the sensitivity of others by promoting self-awareness in an effort to help the client gain insight into his or her own behavior.*

8. Throughout relationship with client, maintain attitude of "It is not *you*, but your *behavior*, that is unacceptable." *An attitude of acceptance promotes feelings of dignity and self-worth.*

Outcome Criteria

1. Client follows rules and regulations of the milieu environment.
2. Client is able to verbalize which of his or her behaviors are not acceptable.
3. Client shows regard for the rights of others by delaying gratification of own desires when appropriate.

● DEFENSIVE COPING

Definition: Repeated projection of falsely positive self-evaluation based on a self-protective pattern that defends against underlying perceived threats to positive self-regard.

Possible Etiologies ("related to")

[Low self-esteem]
[Retarded ego development]
[Underdeveloped superego]
[Negative role models]
[Lack of positive feedback]
[Absent, erratic, or inconsistent methods of discipline]
[Dysfunctional family system]

Defining Characteristics ("evidenced by")

Denial of obvious problems or weaknesses
Projection of blame or responsibility

Rationalization of failures
Hypersensitivity to criticism
Grandiosity
Superior attitude toward others
Difficulty establishing or maintaining relationships
Hostile laughter or ridicule of others
Difficulty in perception of reality testing
Lack of follow-through or participation in treatment or therapy

Goals/Objectives

Short-term Goal

Client will verbalize personal responsibility for difficulties experienced in interpersonal relationships within (time period reasonable for client).

Long-term Goal

Client will demonstrate ability to interact with others without becoming defensive, rationalizing behaviors, or expressing grandiose ideas.

Interventions with *Selected Rationales*

1. Recognize and support basic ego strengths. *Focusing on positive aspects of the personality may help to improve self-concept.*
2. Encourage client to recognize and verbalize feelings of inadequacy and need for acceptance from others, and how these feelings provoke defensive behaviors, such as blaming others for own behaviors. *Recognition of the problem is the first step in the change process toward resolution.*
3. Provide immediate, matter-of-fact, nonthreatening feedback for unacceptable behaviors. *Client may lack knowledge about how he or she is being perceived by others. Providing this information in a nonthreatening manner may help to eliminate these undesirable behaviors.*
4. Help client identify situations that provoke defensiveness and practice through role-playing more appropriate responses. *Role-playing provides confidence to deal with difficult situations when they actually occur.*
5. Provide immediate positive feedback for acceptable behaviors. *Positive feedback enhances self-esteem and encourages repetition of desirable behaviors.*
6. Help client set realistic, concrete goals and determine appropriate actions to meet those goals. *Success increases self-esteem.*
7. Evaluate with client the effectiveness of the new behaviors and discuss any modifications for improvement. *Because of*

limited problem-solving ability, assistance may be required to reassess and develop new strategies in the event that certain of the new coping methods prove ineffective.

Outcome Criteria

1. Client verbalizes and accepts responsibility for own behavior.
2. Client verbalizes correlation between feelings of inadequacy and the need to defend the ego through rationalization and grandiosity.
3. Client does not ridicule or criticize others.
4. Client interacts with others in group situations without taking a defensive stance.

● **LOW SELF-ESTEEM**

Definition: Negative self-evaluating/feelings about self or self-capabilities.

Possible Etiologies ("related to")

[Lack of positive feedback]

[Unmet dependency needs]

[Retarded ego development]

[Repeated negative feedback, resulting in diminished self-worth]

[Dysfunctional family system]

[Absent, erratic, or inconsistent parental discipline]

[Extreme poverty]

[History of childhood abuse]

Defining Characteristics ("evidenced by")

[Denial of problems obvious to others]

[Projection of blame or responsibility for problems]

[Grandiosity]

[Aggressive behavior]

[Frequent use of derogatory and critical remarks against others]

[Manipulation of one staff member against another in an attempt to gain special privileges]

[Inability to form close, personal relationships]

Goals/Objectives

Short-term Goal

Client will verbalize an understanding that derogatory and critical remarks against others reflects feelings of self-contempt.

Long-term Goal

Client will experience an increase in self-esteem, as evidenced by verbalizations of positive aspects of self and the lack of manipulative behaviors toward others.

Interventions with *Selected Rationales*

1. Ensure that goals are realistic. It is important for client to achieve something, so plan for activities in which success is likely. *Success increases self-esteem.*
2. Identify ways in which client is manipulating others. Set limits on manipulative behavior. *Because client is unable (or unwilling) to limit own maladaptive behaviors, assistance is required from staff.*
3. Explain consequences of manipulative behavior. All staff must be consistent and follow through with consequences in a matter-of-fact manner. *From the onset, client must be aware of the outcomes his or her maladaptive behaviors will effect. Without consistency of follow-through from all staff, a positive outcome cannot be achieved.*
4. Encourage client to talk about his or her behavior, the limits, and consequences for violation of those limits. *Discussion of feelings regarding these circumstances may help the client achieve some insight into his or her situation.*
5. Discuss how manipulative behavior interferes with formation of close, personal relationships. *Client may be unaware of others' perception of him or her and of why these behaviors are not acceptable to others.*
6. Help client identify more adaptive interpersonal strategies. Provide positive feedback for nonmanipulative behaviors. *Client may require assistance with solving problems. Positive reinforcement enhances self-esteem and encourages repetition of desirable behaviors.*
7. Encourage client to confront the fear of failure by attending therapy activities and undertaking new tasks. Offer recognition of successful endeavors.
8. Help client identify positive aspects of the self and develop ways to change the characteristics that are socially unacceptable. *Individuals with low self-esteem often have difficulty recognizing their positive attributes. They may also lack problem-solving ability and require assistance to formulate a plan for implementing the desired changes.*
9. Minimize negative feedback to client. Enforce limit-setting in a matter-of-fact manner, imposing previously established consequences for violations. *Negative feedback can be extremely threatening to a person with low self-esteem, possibly aggravating the problem. Consequences should convey unacceptability of the behavior but not the person.*

10. Encourage independence in the performance of personal responsibilities and in decision-making related to own self-care. Offer recognition and praise for accomplishments. *Positive reinforcement enhances self-esteem and encourages repetition of desirable behaviors.*

11. Help client increase level of self-awareness through critical examination of feelings, attitudes, and behaviors. Help client understand that it is perfectly acceptable for attitudes and behaviors to differ from those of others, as long as they do not become intrusive. *As the client becomes more aware and accepting of himself or herself, the need for judging the behavior of others will diminish.*

12. Teach client assertiveness techniques, especially the ability to recognize the differences among passive, assertive, and aggressive behaviors and the importance of respecting the human rights of others while protecting one's own basic human rights. *These techniques increase self-esteem while enhancing the ability to form satisfactory interpersonal relationships.*

Outcome Criteria
1. Client verbalizes positive aspects about self.
2. Client does not manipulate others in an attempt to increase feelings of self-worth.
3. Client considers the rights of others in interpersonal interactions.

● IMPAIRED SOCIAL INTERACTION

Definition: Insufficient or excessive quantity or ineffective quality of social exchange.

Possible Etiologies ("related to")
Self-concept disturbance
[Unmet dependency needs]
[Retarded ego development]
[Retarded superego development]
[Negative role-modeling]
Knowledge deficit about ways to enhance mutuality

Defining Characteristics ("evidenced by")
Discomfort in social situations
Inability to receive or communicate a satisfying sense of social engagement (e.g., belonging, caring, interest, shared history)
Use of unsuccessful social interaction behaviors

Dysfunctional interaction with others

[Exploitation of others for the fulfillment of own desires]

[Inability to develop satisfactory, enduring, intimate relationship with a sexual partner]

[Physical and verbal hostility toward others when fulfillment of own desires is thwarted]

Goals/Objectives

Short-term Goal

Client will develop satisfactory relationship (no evidence of manipulation or exploitation) with nurse or therapist within 1 week.

Long-term Goal

Client will interact appropriately with others, demonstrating concern for the needs of others as well as for his or her own needs, by time of discharge from treatment.

Interventions with *Selected Rationales*

1. Develop therapeutic rapport with client. Establish trust by always being honest; keep all promises; convey acceptance of person, separate from unacceptable behaviors ("It is not *you*, but your *behavior*, that is unacceptable.") *An attitude of acceptance promotes feelings of self-worth. Trust is the basis of a therapeutic relationship.*

2. Offer to remain with client during initial interactions with others. *Presence of a trusted individual increases feelings of security during uncomfortable situations.*

3. Provide constructive criticism and positive reinforcement for efforts. *Positive feedback enhances self-esteem and encourages repetition of desirable behaviors.*

4. Confront client as soon as possible when interactions with others are manipulative or exploitative. Establish consequences for unacceptable behavior, and always follow through. *Because of the strong id influence on client's behavior, he or she should receive immediate feedback when behavior is unacceptable. Consistency in enforcing the consequences is essential if positive outcomes are to be achieved. Inconsistency creates confusion and encourages testing of limits.*

5. Act as a role model for client through appropriate interactions with him or her and with others. *Role-modeling is a powerful and effective form of learning.*

6. Provide group situations for client. *It is through these group interactions with positive and negative feedback from his or her peers that client will learn socially acceptable behavior.*

Outcome Criteria

1. Client willingly and appropriately participates in group activities.
2. Client has satisfactorily established and maintained one interpersonal relationship with nurse or therapist, without evidence of manipulation or exploitation.
3. Client demonstrates ability to interact appropriately with others, showing respect for self and others.
4. Client is able to verbalize reasons for inability to form close interpersonal relationships with others in the past.

● DEFICIENT KNOWLEDGE (SELF-CARE ACTIVITIES TO ACHIEVE AND MAINTAIN OPTIMAL WELLNESS)

Definition: Absence or deficiency of cognitive information related to a specific topic.

Possible Etiologies ("related to")

Lack of interest in learning
[Low self-esteem]
[Denial of need for information]
[Denial of risks involved with maladaptive lifestyle]
Unfamiliarity with information sources

Defining Characteristics ("evidenced by")

[History of substance abuse]
[Statement of lack of knowledge]
[Statement of misconception]
[Request for information]
[Demonstrated lack of knowledge regarding basic health practices]
[Reported or observed inability to take the responsibility for meeting basic health practices in any or all functional pattern areas]
[History of lack of health-seeking behavior]
Inappropriate or exaggerated behaviors (e.g., hysterical, hostile, agitated, apathetic)

Goals/Objectives

Short-term Goal

Client will verbalize understanding of knowledge required to fulfill basic health needs following implementation of teaching plan.

Long-term Goal

Client will be able to demonstrate skills learned for fulfillment of basic health needs by time of discharge from therapy.

Interventions with *Selected Rationales*

1. Assess client's level of knowledge regarding positive self-care practices. *An adequate database is necessary for the development of an effective teaching plan.*

2. Assess client's level of anxiety and readiness to learn. *Learning does not occur beyond the moderate level of anxiety.*

3. Determine method of learning most appropriate for client (e.g., discussion, question and answer, use of audio or visual aids, oral, written). Be sure to consider level of education and development. *Teaching will be ineffective if presented at a level or by a method inappropriate to the client's ability to learn.*

4. Develop teaching plan, including measurable objectives for the learner. Provide information regarding healthful strategies for activities of daily living as well as about harmful effects of substance abuse on the body. Include suggestions for community resources to assist client when adaptability is impaired. *Client needs this information to promote effective health maintenance.*

5. Include significant others in the learning activity, if possible. *Input from individuals who are directly involved in the potential change increases the likelihood of a positive outcome.*

6. Implement teaching plan at a time that facilitates, and in a place that is conducive to, optimal learning (e.g., in the evening when family members visit; in an empty, quiet classroom or group therapy room). *Learning is enhanced by an environment with few distractions.*

7. Begin with simple concepts and progress to the more complex. *Retention is increased if introductory material is easy to understand.*

8. Provide activities for client and significant others in which to actively participate during the learning exercise. *Active participation increases retention.*

9. Ask client and significant others to demonstrate knowledge gained by verbalizing information regarding positive self-care practices. *Verbalization of knowledge gained is a measurable method of evaluating the teaching experience.*

10. Provide positive feedback for participation, as well as for accurate demonstration of knowledge gained. *Positive feedback enhances self-esteem and encourages repetition of desirable behaviors.*

Outcome Criteria

1. Client is able to verbalize information regarding positive self-care practices.
2. Client is able to verbalize available community resources for obtaining knowledge about and help with deficits related to health care.

@ INTERNET REFERENCES

- Additional information about personality disorders may be located at the following websites:
  - a. http://www.mentalhealth.com/dis/p20-pe04.html
  - b. http://www.mentalhealth.com/dis/p20-pe08.html
  - c. http://www.mentalhealth.com/dis/p20-pe05.html
  - d. http://www.mentalhealth.com/dis/p20-pe09.html
  - e. http://www.mentalhealth.com/dis/p20-pe06.html
  - f. http://www.mentalhealth.com/dis/p20-pe07.html
  - g. http://www.mentalhealth.com/dis/p20-pe10.html
  - h. http://www.mentalhealth.com/dis/p20-pe01.html
  - i. http://www.mentalhealth.com/dis/p20-pe02.html
  - j. http://www.mentalhealth.com/dis/p20-pe03.html
  - k. http://www.mentalhealth.com/p13.html#Per

Movie Connections

Taxi Driver (schizoid personality) • *One Flew Over the Cuckoo's Nest (antisocial)* • *The Boston Strangler (antisocial)* • *Just Cause (antisocial)* • *The Dream Team (antisocial)* • *Goodfellas (antisocial)* • *Fatal Attraction (borderline)* • *Play Misty for Me (borderline)* • *Girl, Interrupted (borderline)* • *Gone With the Wind (histrionic)* • *Wall Street (narcissistic)* • *The Odd Couple (obsessive-compulsive)* • *As Good As It Gets (obsessive-compulsive)*

UNIT THREE

SPECIAL TOPICS IN PSYCHIATRIC/MENTAL HEALTH NURSING

C HAPTER 17

Problems Related to Abuse or Neglect

● **BACKGROUND ASSESSMENT DATA**
Categories of Abuse and Neglect
Physical Abuse of a Child
Physical abuse of a child includes "any nonaccidental physical injury (ranging from minor bruises to severe fractures or death) as a result of punching, beating, kicking, biting, burning, shaking, throwing, stabbing, choking, hitting (with a hand, stick, strap, or other object), burning, or otherwise harming a child, that is inflicted by a parent, caregiver, or other person who has responsibility for the child" (Child Welfare Information Gateway [CWIG], 2008). The most obvious way to detect it is by outward physical signs. However, behavioral indicators may also be evident.

Sexual Abuse of a Child
This category is defined as "employment, use, persuasion, inducement, enticement, or coercion of any child to engage in, or assist any other person to engage in, any sexually explicit conduct or any simulation of such conduct for the purpose of producing any visual depiction of such conduct; or the rape, and in

cases of caretaker or inter-familial relationships, statutory rape, molestation, prostitution, or other form of sexual exploitation of children, or incest with children" (CWIG, 2008). **Incest** is the occurrence of sexual contacts or interaction between, or sexual exploitation of, close relatives, or between participants who are related to each other by a kinship bond that is regarded as a prohibition to sexual relations (e.g., caretakers, stepparents, stepsiblings) (Sadock & Sadock, 2007).

Neglect of a Child

Physical neglect of a child includes refusal of or delay in seeking health care, abandonment, expulsion from the home or refusal to allow a runaway to return home, and inadequate supervision. *Emotional neglect* refers to a chronic failure by the parent or caretaker to provide the child with the hope, love, and support necessary for the development of a sound, healthy personality.

Physical Abuse of an Adult

Physical abuse of an adult may be defined as behavior used with the intent to cause harm and to establish power and control over another person. It may include slaps, punches, biting, hair-pulling, choking, kicking, stabbing or shooting, or forcible restraint.

Sexual Abuse of an Adult

Sexual abuse of an adult may be defined as the expression of power and dominance by means of sexual violence, most commonly by men over women, although men may also be victims of sexual assault. Sexual assault is identified by the use of force and executed against the person's will.

Predisposing Factors (that Contribute to Patterns of Abuse)

1. **Physiological**
   a. *Neurophysiological Influences.* Various components of the neurological system in both humans and animals have been implicated in both the facilitation and inhibition of aggressive impulses. Areas of the brain that may be involved include the temporal lobe, the limbic system, and the amygdaloid nucleus (Tardiff, 2003).
   b. *Biochemical Influences.* Studies show that various neurotransmitters—in particular norepinephrine, dopamine, and serotonin—may play a role in the facilitation and inhibition of aggressive impulses (Hollander, Berlin, & Stein, 2008).
   c. *Genetic Influences.* Some studies have implicated heredity as a component in the predisposition to aggressive behavior. Both direct genetic links and the genetic karyotype

XYY have been investigated as possibilities. Evidence remains inconclusive.

   d. ***Disorders of the Brain.*** Various disorders of the brain including tumors, trauma, and certain diseases (e.g., encephalitis and epilepsy) have been implicated in the predisposition to aggressive behavior.

2. **Psychosocial**
   a. ***Psychodynamic Theory.*** The psychodynamic theorists imply that unmet needs for satisfaction and security result in an underdeveloped ego and a weak superego. It is thought that when frustration occurs, aggression and violence supply this individual with a dose of power and prestige that boosts the self-image and validates a significance to his or her life that is lacking. The immature ego cannot prevent dominant id behaviors from occurring, and the weak superego is unable to produce feelings of guilt.
   b. ***Learning Theory.*** This theory postulates that aggressive and violent behaviors are learned from prestigious and influential role models. Individuals who were abused as children or whose parents disciplined with physical punishment are more likely to behave in a violent manner as adults (Tardiff, 2003).
   c. ***Societal Influences.*** Social scientists believe that aggressive behavior is primarily a product of one's culture and social structure. Societal influences may contribute to violence when individuals believe that their needs and desires cannot be met through conventional means, and they resort to delinquent behaviors in an effort to obtain desired ends.

Symptomatology (Subjective and Objective Data)

1. Signs of physical abuse may include the following:
   a. Bruises over various areas of the body. They may present with different colors of bluish-purple to yellowish-green (indicating various stages of healing).
   b. Bite marks, skin welts, burns.
   c. Fractures, scars, serious internal injuries, brain damage.
   d. Lacerations, abrasions, or unusual bleeding.
   e. Bald spots indicative of severe hair pulling.
   f. In a child, regressive behaviors (such as thumb sucking and enuresis) are common.
   g. Extreme anxiety and mistrust of others.
2. Signs of neglect of a child may include the following:
   a. Soiled clothing that does not fit and may be inappropriate for the weather.
   b. Poor hygiene.

    c. Always hungry, with possible signs of malnutrition (e.g., emaciated with swollen belly).

    d. Listless and tired much of the time.

    e. Unattended medical problems.

    f. Social isolation; unsatisfactory peer relationships.

    g. Poor school performance and attendance record.

3. Signs of sexual abuse of a child include the following:

    a. Frequent urinary infections.

    b. Difficulty or pain in walking or sitting.

    c. Rashes or itching in the genital area; scratching the area a great deal or fidgeting when seated.

    d. Frequent vomiting.

    e. Seductive behavior; compulsive masturbation; precocious sex play.

    f. Excessive anxiety and mistrust of others.

    g. Sexually abusing another child.

4. Signs of sexual abuse of an adult include the following (Burgess, 2009):

    a. Contusions and abrasions about various parts of the body.

    b. Headaches, fatigue, sleep-pattern disturbances.

    c. Stomach pains, nausea, and vomiting.

    d. Vaginal discharge and itching, burning on urination, rectal bleeding and pain.

    e. Rage, humiliation, embarrassment, desire for revenge, self-blame.

    f. Fear of physical violence and death.

Common Nursing Diagnoses and Interventions

(Interventions are applicable to various health-care settings, such as inpatient and partial hospitalization, community outpatient clinic, home health, and private practice.)

● RAPE-TRAUMA SYNDROME

Definition: Sustained maladaptive response to a forced, violent sexual penetration against the victim's will and consent.

Possible Etiologies ("related to")

[Having been the victim of sexual violence executed with the use of force and against one's personal will and consent]

Defining Characteristics ("evidenced by")

Disorganization

Change in relationships

Confusion
Physical trauma (e.g., bruising, tissue irritation)
Suicide attempts
Denial; guilt
Paranoia; humiliation, embarrassment
Aggression; muscle tension and/or spasms
Mood swings
Dependence
Powerlessness; helplessness
Nightmares and sleep disturbances
Sexual dysfunction
Revenge; phobias
Loss of self-esteem
Impaired decision-making
Substance abuse; depression
Anger; anxiety; agitation
Shame; shock; fear

Goals/Objectives
Short-term Goal
The client's physical wounds will heal without complication.

Long-term Goal
The client will begin a healthy grief resolution, initiating the process of physical and psychological healing (time to be individually determined).

Interventions with *Selected Rationales*

1. It is important to communicate the following to the victim of sexual assault:
   a. You are safe here.
   b. I'm sorry that it happened.
   c. I'm glad that you survived.
   d. It's not your fault. No one deserves to be treated this way.
   e. You did the best that you could.
   The woman who has been sexually assaulted fears for her life and must be reassured of her safety. She may also be overwhelmed with self-doubt and self-blame, and these statements instill trust and validate self-worth.
2. Explain every assessment procedure that will be conducted and why. Ensure that data collection is conducted in a caring, nonjudgmental manner *to decrease fear and anxiety and increase trust.*
3. Ensure that the client has adequate privacy for all immediate post-crisis interventions. Try to have as few people as possible providing the immediate care or collecting immediate

evidence. *The post-trauma client is extremely vulnerable. Additional people in the environment increase this feeling of vulnerability and may escalate anxiety.*

4. Encourage the client to give an account of the assault. Listen, but do not probe. *Nonjudgmental listening provides an avenue for catharsis that the client needs to begin healing. A detailed account may be required for legal follow-up, and a caring nurse, as client advocate, may help to lessen the trauma of evidence collection.*

5. Discuss with the client whom to call for support or assistance. Provide information about referrals for aftercare. *Because of severe anxiety and fear, client may need assistance from others during this immediate postcrisis period. Provide referral information in writing for later reference (e.g., psychotherapist, mental health clinic, community advocacy group).*

Outcome Criteria

1. Client is no longer experiencing panic anxiety.
2. Client demonstrates a degree of trust in the primary nurse.
3. Client has received immediate attention to physical injuries.
4. Client has initiated behaviors consistent with the grief response.

● POWERLESSNESS

Definition: Perception that one's own action will not significantly affect an outcome; a perceived lack of control over a current situation or immediate happening.

Possible Etiologies ("related to")

Lifestyle of helplessness
[Low self-esteem]
[Living with, or in a long-term relationship with, an individual who victimizes by inflicting physical pain or injury with the intent to cause harm, and continues to do so over a long period of time]
[Lack of support network of caring others]
[Lack of financial independence]

Defining Characteristics ("evidenced by")

Verbal expressions of having no control [or influence] over situation or outcome
Reluctance to express true feelings
Passivity
[Verbalizations of abuse]

[Lacerations over areas of body]
[Fear for personal and children's safety]
[Verbalizations of no way to get out of relationship]

Goals/Objectives

Short-term Goal

Client will recognize and verbalize choices that are available, thereby perceiving some control over life situation (time dimension to be individually determined).

Long-term Goal

Client will exhibit control over life situation by making decision about what to do regarding living with cycle of abuse (time dimension to be individually determined).

Interventions with *Selected Rationales*

1. In collaboration with physician, ensure that all physical wounds, fractures, and burns receive immediate attention. Take photographs if the victim will permit. *Client safety is a nursing priority. Photographs may be called in as evidence if charges are filed.*

2. Take the client to a private area to do the interview. *If the client is accompanied by the person who did the battering, she or he is not likely to be truthful about the injuries.*

3. If she has come alone or with her children, assure her of her safety. (Author's note: *Female gender is used here because most intimate partner violence [IPV] is directed by men toward women— although it is understood that men are also victims of IPV.)* Encourage her to discuss the battering incident. Ask questions about whether this has happened before, whether the abuser takes drugs, whether the woman has a safe place to go, and whether she is interested in pressing charges. *Some women will attempt to keep secret how their injuries occurred in an effort to protect the partner or because they are fearful that the partner will kill them if they tell.*

4. Ensure that "rescue" efforts are not attempted by the nurse. Offer support, but remember that the final decision must be made by the client. *Making her own decision will give the client a sense of control over her life situation. Imposing judgments and giving advice are nontherapeutic.*

5. Stress to the victim the importance of safety. She must be made aware of the variety of resources that are available to her. These may include crisis hotlines, community groups for women who have been abused, shelters, counseling services, and information regarding the victim's rights in the civil and criminal justice system. Following a discussion of these available resources, the woman may choose for herself. If her

decision is to return to the marriage and home, this choice also must be respected. *Knowledge of available choices can serve to decrease the victim's sense of powerlessness, but true empowerment comes only when she chooses to use that knowledge for her own benefit.*

Outcome Criteria
1. Client has received immediate attention to physical injuries.
2. Client verbalizes assurance of her immediate safety.
3. Client discusses life situation with primary nurse.
4. Client is able to verbalize choices available to her from which she may receive assistance.

● RISK FOR DELAYED DEVELOPMENT

Definition: At risk for delay of 25% or more in one or more of the areas of social or self-regulatory behavior, or in cognitive, language, gross or fine motor skills.

Related/Risk Factors ("related to")
[The infliction by caretakers of physical or sexual abuse, usually occurring over an extended period of time]
[Ignoring the child's basic physiological needs]
[Indifference to the child]
[Ignoring the child's presence]
[Ignoring the child's social, educational, recreational, and developmental needs]

Goals/Objectives
Short-term Goal
Client will develop trusting relationship with nurse and report how evident injuries were sustained (time dimension to be individually determined).

Long-term Goal
Client will demonstrate behaviors consistent with age-appropriate growth and development.

Interventions with *Selected Rationales*
1. Perform complete physical assessment of the child. Take particular note of bruises (in various stages of healing), lacerations, and client complaints of pain in specific areas. Do not overlook or discount the possibility of sexual abuse. Assess for nonverbal signs of abuse: aggressive conduct, excessive fears, extreme hyperactivity, apathy, withdrawal, age-inappropriate

behaviors. *An accurate and thorough physical assessment is required in order to provide appropriate care for the client.*

2. Conduct an in-depth interview with the parent or adult who accompanies the child. *Consider:* If the injury is being reported as an accident, is the explanation reasonable? Is the injury consistent with the explanation? Is the injury consistent with the child's developmental capabilities? *Fear of imprisonment or loss of child custody may place the abusive parent on the defensive. Discrepancies may be evident in the description of the incident, and lying to cover up involvement is a common defense that may be detectable in an in-depth interview.*

3. Use games or play therapy to gain child's trust. Use these techniques to assist in describing his or her side of the story. *Establishing a trusting relationship with an abused child is extremely difficult. The child may not even want to be touched. These types of play activities can provide a non-threatening environment that may enhance the child's attempt to discuss these painful issues.*

4. Determine whether the nature of the injuries warrants reporting to authorities. Specific state statutes must enter into the decision of whether to report suspected child abuse. Individual state statues regarding what constitutes child abuse and neglect may be found at http://www.childwelfare. gov/systemwide/laws_policies/state/. *A report is commonly made if there is reason to suspect that a child has been injured as a result of physical, mental, emotional, or sexual abuse. "Reason to suspect" exists when there is evidence of a discrepancy or inconsistency in explaining a child's injury. Most states require that the following individuals report cases of suspected child abuse: all health-care workers, all mental health therapists, teachers, child-care providers, firefighters, emergency medical services personnel, and law enforcement personnel. Reports are made to the Department of Health and Human Services or a law enforcement agency.*

Outcome Criteria

1. Client has received immediate attention to physical injuries.
2. Client demonstrates trust in primary nurse by discussing abuse through the use of play therapy.
3. Client is demonstrating a decrease in regressive behaviors.

@ INTERNET REFERENCES

- Additional information related to child abuse may be located at the following websites:
  a. http://www.childwelfare.gov
  b. http://endabuse.org/

    c. http://www.child-abuse.com
    d. http://www.nlm.nih.gov/medlineplus/childabuse.html
- Additional information related to sexual assault may be located at the following websites:
    a. http://www.vaw.umn.edu/
    b. http://www.nlm.nih.gov/medlineplus/rape.html
- Additional information related to intimate partner violence may be located at the following websites:
    a. http://www.ndvh.org/
    b. http://home.cybergrrl.com/dv/book/toc.html
    c. http://www.crisis-support.org/
    d. http://www.ama-assn.org/ama/no-index/about-ama/13577.shtml
    e. http://www.nursingworld.org/MainMenuCategories/ANAMarketplace/ANAPeriodicals/OJIN/TableofContents/Volume72002/No1Jan2002.aspx

Movie Connections

    The Burning Bed (domestic violence) • *Life With Billy (domestic violence)* • *Two Story House (child abuse)* • *The Prince of Tides (domestic violence)* • *Radio Flyer (child abuse)* • *Flowers in the Attic (child abuse)* • *A Case of Rape (sexual assault)*

Premenstrual Dysphoric Disorder

● BACKGROUND ASSESSMENT DATA
Defined

Premenstrual dysphoric disorder (PMDD) is identified by a variety of physical and emotional symptoms that occur during the last week of the luteal phase of the menstrual cycle and that remit within a few days after the onset of the follicular phase. In most women, these symptoms occur in the week before, and remit within a few days after, the onset of menses. The disorder has also been reported in nonmenstruating women who have had a hysterectomy but retain ovarian function. The diagnosis is given only when the symptoms are sufficiently severe to cause marked impairment in social or occupational functioning and have occurred during a majority of menstrual cycles in the past year (American Psychiatric Association [APA], 2000).

Predisposing Factors to PMDD

1. **Physiological**
   a. ***Biochemical.*** An imbalance of the hormones estrogen and progesterone has been implicated in the predisposition to PMDD. It is postulated that excess estrogen or a high estrogen-to-progesterone ratio during the luteal phase causes water retention and that this hormonal imbalance has other effects as well, resulting in the symptoms associated with premenstrual syndrome.
   b. ***Nutritional.*** A number of nutritional alterations have been implicated in the etiology of PMDD, although the exact role is unsubstantiated. Deficiencies in the B vitamins, calcium, magnesium, manganese, vitamin E, and linolenic acid have been suggested. Glucose tolerance fluctuations, abnormal fatty acid metabolism, and sensitivity to caffeine and alcohol may also play a role in contributing to the symptoms associated with this disorder.

Symptomatology (Subjective and Objective Data)

The following symptoms have been associated with PMDD (APA, 2000; Sadock & Sadock, 2007):

1. Feelings of depression and hopelessness
2. Increased anxiety and restlessness
3. Mood swings
4. Anger and irritability
5. Decreased interest in usual activities
6. Difficulty concentrating
7. Anergia; increased fatigability
8. Appetite changes (e.g., food cravings)
9. Changes in sleep patterns (e.g., hypersomnia or insomnia)
10. Somatic complaints (e.g., breast tenderness, headaches, edema)

Other subjective symptoms that have been reported include:

11. Cramps
12. Alcohol intolerance
13. Acne
14. Cystitis
15. Oliguria
16. Altered sexual drive
17. Forgetfulness
18. Suicidal ideations or attempts

Common Nursing Diagnoses and Interventions

(Interventions are applicable to various health-care settings, such as inpatient and partial hospitalization, community outpatient clinic, home health, and private practice.)

• ACUTE PAIN

Definition: Sudden or slow onset of any intensity from mild to severe with an anticipated or predictable end and a duration of less than 6 months.

Possible Etiologies ("related to")

[Imbalance in estrogen and progesterone levels]
[Possible nutritional alterations, including the following:
    Vitamin B deficiencies
    Glucose tolerance fluctuations
    Abnormal fatty acid metabolism, which may contribute to alterations in prostaglandin synthesis

    Magnesium deficiency
    Vitamin E deficiency
    Caffeine sensitivity
    Alcohol intolerance]
[Fluid retention]

Defining Characteristics ("evidenced by")
[Subjective communication of:
    Headache
    Backache
    Joint or muscle pain
    A sensation of "bloating"
    Abdominal cramping
    Breast tenderness and swelling]
Facial mask [of pain]
Sleep disturbance
Self-focus
Changes in appetite [and eating]

Goals/Objectives
Short-term Goal
Client cooperates with efforts to manage symptoms of PMDD and minimize feelings of discomfort.

Long-term Goal
Client verbalizes relief from discomfort associated with symptoms of PMDD.

Interventions with *Selected Rationales*
1. Assess and record location, duration, and intensity of pain. ***Background assessment data are necessary to formulate an accurate plan of care for the client.***
2. Provide nursing comfort measures with a matter-of-fact approach that does not give positive reinforcement to the pain behavior (e.g., backrub, warm bath, heating pad). Give additional attention at times when client is not focusing on physical symptoms. ***These measures may serve to provide some temporary relief from pain. Absence of secondary gains in the form of positive reinforcement may discourage client's use of the pain as attention-seeking behavior.***
3. Encourage the client to get adequate rest and sleep and avoid stressful activity during the premenstrual period. ***Fatigue exaggerates symptoms associated with PMDD. Stress elicits heightened symptoms of anxiety, which may contribute to exacerbation of symptoms and altered perception of pain.***
4. Assist client with activities that distract from focus on self and pain. Demonstrate techniques such as visual or auditory

distractions, guided imagery, breathing exercises, massage, application of heat or cold, and relaxation techniques that may provide symptomatic relief. *These techniques may help to maintain anxiety at a manageable level and prevent the discomfort from becoming disabling.*

5. *In an effort to correct the possible nutritional alterations that may be contributing to PMDD,* the following guidelines may be suggested:

a. Reduce intake of fats in the diet, particularly saturated fats.

b. Limit intake of dairy products to two servings a day (excessive dairy products block the absorption of magnesium).

c. Increase intake of complex carbohydrates (vegetables, legumes, cereals, and whole grains) and *cis*-linoleic acid–containing foods (e.g., safflower oil).

d. Decrease refined and simple sugars. (Excess sugar is thought to cause nervous tension, palpitations, headache, dizziness, drowsiness, and excretion of magnesium in the urine.)

e. Decrease salt intake to 3 g per day but not less than 0.5 g per day. (Salt restriction prevents edema; too little salt stimulates norepinephrine and causes sleep disturbances.)

f. Limit intake of caffeine (coffee, tea, colas, and chocolate) and alcohol (one or two drinks a week). Caffeine increases breast tenderness and pain. Alcohol can cause reactive hypoglycemia and fluid retention.

g. Because some women crave junk food during the premenstrual period, it is important that they take a multiple vitamin or mineral tablet daily to ensure that adequate nutrients are consumed.

6. Administer medications as prescribed. Monitor client response for effectiveness of the medication, as well as for appearance of adverse side effects. *When other measures are insufficient to bring about relief,* physician may prescribe symptomatic drug therapy. Provide client with information about the medication to be administered. *Client has the right to know about the treatment she is receiving.* Some medications commonly used for symptomatic treatment of PMDD are presented in Table 18-1. Some women have experienced relief from the symptoms of PMDD through the use of herbal medications; some of these are listed in Table 18-2.

Outcome Criteria

1. Client demonstrates ability to manage premenstrual symptoms with minimal discomfort.

2. Client verbalizes relief of painful symptoms.

TABLE 18–1 Medications for Symptomatic Relief of PMDD

Medication	Indication
Fluoxetine (Sarafem), sertraline (Zoloft), paroxetine (Paxil)	These medications have been approved by the FDA for treatment of PMDD.
Hydrochlorothiazide (Ezide, HydroDiuril), furosemide (Lasix)	Diuretics may provide relief from edema when diet and sodium restriction are not sufficient.
Ibuprofen (Advil, Motrin), naproxen (Naprosyn, Aleve)	Nonsteroidal anti-inflammatory agents may provide relief from joint, muscle, and lower abdominal pain related to increased prostaglandins.
Propranolol (Inderal), verapamil (Isoptin)	β-Blockers and calcium channel blockers are often given for pro-phylactic treatment of migraine headaches.
Sumatriptan (Imitrex), naratriptan (Amerge), rizatriptan (Maxalt), zolmitriptan (Zomig), frovatriptan (Frova), almotriptan (Axert), eletriptan (Relpax)	These serotonin 5-HT$_1$ receptor agonists are highly effective in the treatment of acute migraine attack.
Bromocriptine (Parlodel)	This drug may be prescribed to relieve breast pain and other symptoms of PMDD that may be caused by elevated prolactin.

TABLE 18–2 Herbals Used for Symptoms of Premenstrual Syndrome

Herbal	Precautions/Adverse Effects	Contraindications
Black cohosh (*Cimicifuga racemosa*)	May potentiate the effects of antihypertensive medications. Some individuals may experience nausea or headache.	Pregnancy
Bugleweed (*Lycopus virginicus*)	No side effects known. Should not be taken concomitantly with thyroid preparations.	Thyroid disease
Chaste tree (*Vitex agnus-castus*)	Occasional rashes may occur. Should not be taken concomitantly with dopamine-receptor antagonists.	Pregnancy and lactation

TABLE 18–2 Herbals Used for Symptoms of Premenstrual Syndrome—cont'd

Herbal	Precautions/Adverse Effects	Contraindications
Evening primrose (*Oenothera biennis*)	May lower the seizure threshold. Should not be taken concomitantly with other drugs that lower the seizure threshold.	
Potentilla (*Potentilla anserine*)	May cause stomach irritation.	
Shepherd's purse (*Capsella bursa-pastoris*)	No side effects known.	Pregnancy
Valerian (*Valeriana officinalis*)	With long-term use: headache, restless states, sleeplessness, mydriasis, disorders of cardiac function. Should not be taken concomitantly with CNS depressants.	Pregnancy and lactation

Sources: PDR for Herbal Medicines (4th ed.). (2007). Montvale, NJ: Thomson Healthcare Inc.; and Presser, A.M. (2000). *Pharmacist's guide to medicinal herbs.* Petaluma, CA: Smart Publications.

● INEFFECTIVE COPING

Definition: Inability to form a valid appraisal of the stressors, inadequate choices of practiced responses, and/or inability to use available resources.

Possible Etiologies ("related to")

[Imbalance in estrogen and progesterone levels]
[Possible nutritional alterations, including the following:
  Vitamin B deficiencies
  Glucose tolerance fluctuations
  Abnormal fatty acid metabolism, which may contribute to alterations in prostaglandin synthesis
  Magnesium deficiency
  Vitamin E deficiency
  Caffeine sensitivity
  Alcohol intolerance]

Defining Characteristics ("evidenced by")

[Mood swings]
[Marked anger or irritability]
[Increased anxiety and restlessness]
[Feelings of depression and hopelessness]
[Decreased interest in usual activities]
[Anergia; easy fatigability]
[Difficulty concentrating; forgetfulness]
[Changes in appetite]
[Hypersomnia or insomnia]
[Altered sexual drive]
[Suicidal ideations or attempts]
Inadequate problem-solving
Inability to meet role expectations

Goals/Objectives

Short-term Goals

1. Client will seek out support person if thoughts of suicide emerge.
2. Client will verbalize ways to express anger in an appropriate manner and maintain anxiety at a manageable level.

Long-term Goals

1. Client will not harm self while experiencing symptoms associated with PMDD.
2. Client will demonstrate adaptive coping strategies to use in an effort to minimize disabling behaviors during the premenstrual and perimenstrual periods.

Interventions with *Selected Rationales*

1. Assess client's potential for suicide. Has she expressed feelings of not wanting to live? Does she have a plan? A means? *Depression is the most prevalent disorder that precedes suicide. The risk of suicide is greatly increased if the client has developed a plan and particularly if means exist for the client to execute the plan.*
2. Formulate a short-term verbal contract with the client that she will not harm herself during a specific period of time. When that contract expires, make another, and so forth. *Discussion of suicidal feelings with a trusted individual provides a degree of relief to the client. A contract gets the subject out in the open and places some of the responsibility for the client's safety with the client. An attitude of acceptance of the client as a worthwhile individual is conveyed.*
3. Secure a promise from client that she will seek out a staff member if thoughts of suicide emerge. *Suicidal clients are often very ambivalent about their feelings. Discussion of*

feelings with a trusted individual may provide assistance before the client experiences a crisis situation.

4. Encourage client to express angry feelings within appropriate limits. Provide safe method of hostility release. Help client to identify source of anger, if possible. Work on adaptive coping skills for use outside the health-care system. *Depression and suicidal behaviors are sometimes viewed as anger turned inward on the self. If this anger can be verbalized in a nonthreatening environment, the client may be able to resolve these feelings, regardless of the discomfort involved.*

5. Encourage client to discharge pent-up anger through participation in large motor activities (e.g., brisk walks, jogging, physical exercises, volleyball, punching bag, exercise bike). *Physical exercise provides a safe and effective method for discharging pent-up tension.*

6. Help client identify stressors that precipitate anxiety and irritability and develop new methods of coping with these situations (e.g., stress reduction techniques, relaxation, and visualization skills). *Knowing stress factors and ways of handling them reduces anxiety and allows client to feel a greater measure of control over the situation.*

7. Identify extent of feelings and situations when loss of control occurs. Assist with problem-solving to identify behaviors for protection of self and others (e.g., call support person, remove self from situation). *Recognition of potential for harm to self or others and development of a plan enables client to take effective actions to meet safety needs.*

8. Encourage client to reduce or shift workload and social activities during the premenstrual period as part of a total stress management program. *Stress may play a role in the exacerbation of symptoms.*

9. At each visit, evaluate symptoms. Discuss those that may be most troublesome and continue to persist well after initiation of therapy. *If traditional measures are inadequate, pharmacological intervention may be required to enhance coping abilities. For example, antidepressants may be administered for depression that remains unresolved after other symptoms have been relieved.*

10. Encourage participation in support group, psychotherapy, marital counseling, or other type of therapy as deemed necessary. *Professional assistance may be required to help the client and family members learn effective coping strategies and support lifestyle changes that may be needed.*

Outcome Criteria

1. Client participates willingly in treatment regimen and initiates necessary lifestyle changes.

2. Client demonstrates adaptive coping strategies to deal with episodes of depression and anxiety.
3. Client verbalizes that she has no suicidal thoughts or intentions.

@ INTERNET REFERENCES

a. http://www.aafp.org/afp/980700ap/daughert.html
b. http://www.drdonnica.com/display.asp?article=1086
c. http://www.obgyn.net/women/women.asp?page=/women/articles/coffee_talk/ct007
d. http://www.usdoctor.com/pms.htm
e. http://www.healthyplace.com/depression/main/premenstrual-dysphoric-disorder-pmdd/menu-id-68/
f. http://familydoctor.org/752.xml
g. http://www.obgyn.net/pmspmdd/pmspmdd.asp

HIV Disease

● BACKGROUND ASSESSMENT DATA
The Immune Response to HIV

The cells responsible for nonspecific immune reactions include neutrophils, monocytes, and macrophages. In the normal immune response, they work to destroy an invasive organism and initiate and facilitate repair to damaged tissue. If these cells are not effective in accomplishing a satisfactory healing response, specific immune mechanisms take over.

The elements of the cellular response include the T4 lymphocytes. T4 cells are also called CD4 cells. When the body is invaded by a foreign antigen, these T4 cells divide many times, producing antigen-specific T4 cells with other functions. One of these is the T4 killer cell, which serves to help destroy the antigen.

The most conspicuous immunologic abnormality associated with human immunodeficiency virus (HIV) infection is a striking depletion of T4 lymphocytes. The HIV infects the T4 lymphocyte, thereby destroying the very cell the body needs to direct an attack on the virus. An individual with a healthy immune system may present with a T4 count between 600/mm^3 and 1200/mm^3. The individual with HIV infection may experience a drop at the time of acute infection, with a subsequent increase when the acute stage subsides. Typically, the T-cell count is about 500 to 600 when the individual begins to develop **chronic persistent generalized lymphadenopathy** (PGL). Opportunistic infections are common when the T-cell count reaches 200. T4 cell counts in individuals with advanced HIV disease drop dramatically, in some cases down to zero (New Mexico AIDS Education and Training Center, 2009).

Stages and Symptoms of HIV Disease

1. **Early Stage (Category 1) HIV Disease (≥500 T4 cells/ mm^3)**
   a. *Acute (Primary) HIV Infection.* Although some people are asymptomatic at this stage, the acute HIV infection is

often identified by a characteristic syndrome of symptoms that occurs from 6 days to 6 weeks after exposure to the virus. The symptoms have an abrupt onset, are somewhat vague, and are similar to those sometimes seen in mononucleosis. Symptoms of acute HIV infection include fever, myalgia, malaise, lymphadenopathy, sore throat, anorexia, nausea and vomiting, headaches, skin rash, and diarrhea (Hare, 2006). Most symptoms resolve in 1 to 3 weeks, with the exception of fever, myalgia, lymphadenopathy, and malaise, which may continue for several months.

   b. *Seroconversion.* Seroconversion, the detectability of HIV antibodies in the blood, most often is detected between 6 and 12 weeks. Most people show positive for HIV by 3 months after infection. In some individuals it may take up to 6 months. The time between infection and seroconversion is called the *window period.*

   c. *Asymptomatic Infection.* The acute infection progresses to an asymptomatic stage. Probably the largest number of HIV-infected individuals fall within this group. Individuals may remain in this asymptomatic stage for 10 years or longer. The progression of the illness is faster in infants and children than it is in adults.

2. **Middle Stage (Category 2) Chronic HIV Disease (499 to 200 T4 cells/mm³)**

   a. *Persistent Generalized Lymphadenopathy.* Clients with HIV infection may develop a generalized lymphadenopathy, in which lymph nodes in at least two different locations in the body (usually the neck, armpit, and groin) swell and remain swollen for months, with no other signs of a related infectious disease.

   b. *Systemic Complaints.* Fever, night sweats, chronic diarrhea, fatigue, minor oral infections, headaches.

3. **Late Stage (Category 3) Clinical AIDS (<200 T4 cell/mm³)**

   a. *HIV Wasting Syndrome.* Severe weight loss, large-volume diarrhea, fever, and weakness. Involuntary weight loss of more than 10% of baseline body weight is common.

   b. *Opportunistic Infections.* Opportunistic infections are those that occur because of the altered immune state of the host. These infections, which include protozoan, fungal, viral, and bacterial infections, have long been a defining characteristic of AIDS. The most common, life-threatening opportunistic infection seen in clients with AIDS is *pneumocystis pneumonia (PCP).*

   c. *AIDS-Related Malignancies.* HIV-positive individuals are at risk for developing certain types of malignancies.

These include Kaposi's sarcoma, non-Hodgkin's lymphoma, Hodgkin's disease, squamous-cell carcinomas, malignant melanoma, testicular cancers, and primary hepatocellular carcinoma.

d. ***Altered Mental States.***

(1) The most common alterations in mental states observed in AIDS clients include delirium (fluctuating consciousness, abnormal vital signs, and psychotic phenomena) and dementia (called HIV-associated dementia [HAD]). Symptoms of HAD include cognitive, motor, and behavioral changes similar to those seen in individuals with other cognitive disorders [see Chapter 3]).

(2) Depression is the most common psychiatric disorder observed among HIV-positive clients (Sagrestano, Rogers, & Service, 2008). It can occur during any stage of the disease process. Anticipatory or actual grief is an important cause of depressive symptoms in clients with HIV disease. Transient suicidal ideation on learning of HIV positivity is quite common, although the incidence of serious suicidal behavior is low. Depression in AIDS clients may be related to receiving a new diagnosis of HIV positivity or AIDS, perceiving rejection by loved ones, experiencing multiple losses of friends to the disease, having an inadequate social and financial support system, and the presence of an early cognitive disorder.

Predisposing Factors to HIV Disease

1. **Sexual Transmission**

   a. ***Heterosexual Transmission.*** Because the virus is found in greater concentration in semen than in vaginal secretions, it is more readily transmitted from men to women than from women to men. However, female-to-male transmission is possible, as HIV has been isolated in vaginal secretions.

   b. ***Homosexual Transmission.*** The most significant risk factors for homosexual transmission of HIV are receptive anal intercourse and the number of male sexual partners. The lining of the anal canal is delicate and prone to tearing and bleeding, making anal intercourse an easy way for infections to be passed from one person to another.

2. **Bloodborne Transmission**

   a. ***Transfusion with Blood Products.*** Although laboratory tests are more than 99% sensitive, screening problems may occur when donations are received from individuals recently infected with HIV who have not yet developed antibodies or from persistently antibody-negative donors who are infected with HIV.

b. ***Transmission by Needles Infected with HIV.*** The highest number of cases occurring via this route is among IV drug users who share needles and other equipment contaminated with HIV-infected blood. Other bloodborne modes of transmission of HIV are by health-care workers who experience accidental needle sticks with contaminated needles and who may become infected from other contaminated equipment used for therapeutic purposes.

3. **Perinatal Transmission**
   a. Modes of transmission include transplacental, through exposure to maternal blood and vaginal secretions during delivery, and through breast milk. The risk of perinatal transmission has been significantly reduced in recent years with the advent of free or low-cost prenatal care, provision of access to anti-HIV medication during pregnancy, and education about the dangers of breastfeeding.

4. **Other Possible Modes of Transmission**
   a. To date, HIV has been isolated from blood, semen, vaginal secretions, saliva, tears, breast milk, cerebrospinal fluid, and amniotic fluid. However, only blood, semen, vaginal secretions, and breast milk have been epidemiologically linked to transmission of the virus.

Common Nursing Diagnoses and Interventions*

(Interventions are applicable to various health-care settings, such as inpatient and partial hospitalization, community outpatient clinic, home health, and private practice.)

● INEFFECTIVE PROTECTION

Definition: Decrease in the ability to guard self from internal or external threats such as illness or injury.

Possible Etiologies ("related to")

[Compromised immune status secondary to diagnosis of HIV disease]

Defining Characteristics ("evidenced by")

[Laboratory values indicating decreased numbers of T4 cells]
[Presence of opportunistic infections]

---

* The interventions for this care plan have been adapted from "Nursing Care Plan for the AIDS Patient," written by the nursing staff of Hospice, Inc., Wichita, KS.

[Manifestations of
    Fever, night sweats, diarrhea
    Anorexia, weight loss
    Fatigue, malaise
    Swollen lymph glands
    Cough, dyspnea
    Rash, skin lesions, white patches in mouth
    Headache
    Ataxia
    Bleeding, bruising
    Neurological defects]

Goals/Objectives

Short-term Goal

Client will exhibit no new signs or symptoms of infection.

Long-term Goal

Client safety and comfort will be maximized.

Interventions with *Selected Rationales*

1. *To prevent infection in an immunocompromised individual:*
   a. Implement Universal Precautions.
   b. Wash hands with antibacterial soap before entering and on leaving client's room.
   c. Monitor vital signs at regular intervals.
   d. Monitor complete blood counts (CBCs) for leukopenia/ neutropenia.
   e. Monitor for signs and symptoms of specific opportunistic infections.
   f. Protect client from individuals with infections.
   g. Maintain meticulous sterile technique for dressing changes and any invasive procedure.
   h. Administer antibiotics as ordered.
2. *To restore nutritional status and decrease nausea, vomiting, and diarrhea:*
   a. Provide low-residue, high-protein, high-calorie, soft, bland diet. Maintain hydration with adequate fluid intake.
   b. Obtain daily weight and record intake and output.
   c. Monitor serum electrolytes and CBCs.
   d. If client is unable to eat, provide isotonic tube feedings as tolerated. Check for gastric residual frequently.
   e. If client is unable to tolerate oral intake or tube feedings, consult physician regarding possibility of parenteral hyperalimentation. Observe hyperalimentation administration site for signs of infection.
   f. Administer antidiarrheals and antiemetics as ordered.

    g. Perform frequent oral care. Promote prevention and healing of lesions in the mouth.

    h. Have the client eat small, frequent meals with high-calorie snacks rather than three large meals per day.

3. **To promote improvement of skin and mucous membrane integrity:**

    a. Monitor skin condition for signs of redness and breakdown.

    b. Reposition client every 1 to 2 hours.

    c. Encourage ambulation and chair activity as tolerated.

    d. Use "egg crate" mattress or air mattress on bed.

    e. Wash skin daily with soap and rinse well with water.

    f. Apply lotion to skin to maintain skin softness.

    g. Provide wound care as ordered for existing pressure sores or lesions.

    h. Cleanse skin exposed to diarrhea thoroughly and protect rectal area with ointment.

    i. Apply artificial tears to eyes as appropriate.

    j. Perform frequent oral care; apply ointment to lips.

4. **To maximize oxygen consumption and minimize respiratory distress:**

    a. Assess respiratory status frequently:

       (1) Monitor depth, rate, and rhythm of respirations.

       (2) Auscultate lung fields every 2 hours and as needed.

       (3) Monitor arterial blood gases.

       (4) Check color of skin, nail beds, and sclerae.

       (5) Assess sputum for color, odor, and viscosity.

    b. Encourage coughing and deep-breathing exercises.

    c. Provide humidified oxygen as ordered.

    d. Suction as needed using sterile technique.

    e. Space nursing care to allow client adequate rest periods between procedures.

    f. Administer analgesics or sedatives judiciously to prevent respiratory depression.

    g. Administer bronchodilators and antibiotics as ordered.

5. **To minimize the potential for easy bleeding caused by HIV-induced thrombocytopenia:**

    a. Follow protocol for maintenance of skin integrity.

    b. Provide safe environment to minimize falling or bumping into objects.

    c. Provide soft toothbrush or "toothette" swabs for cleaning teeth and gums.

    d. Ensure that client does not take aspirin or other medications that increase the potential for bleeding.

    e. Clean up areas contaminated by client's blood with household bleach diluted 1:10 with water.

6. *To maintain near-normal body temperature:*
   a. Provide frequent tepid water sponge baths.
   b. Provide antipyretic as ordered by physician (avoid aspirin).
   c. Place client in cool room, with minimal clothing and bed covers.
   d. Encourage intake of cool liquids (if not contraindicated).

Outcome Criteria

1. Client does not experience respiratory distress.
2. Client maintains optimal nutrition and hydration.
3. Client has experienced no further weight loss.
4. Client maintains integrity of skin and mucous membranes.
5. Client shows no new signs or symptoms of infection.

● INTERRUPTED FAMILY PROCESSES

Definition: Change in family relationships and/or functioning.

Possible Etiologies ("related to")

[Crisis associated with having a family member diagnosed with HIV disease]

Defining Characteristics ("evidenced by")

Changes in availability for affective responsiveness and intimacy
Changes in participation in problem-solving and decision-making
Changes in communication patterns
Changes in availability for emotional support
Changes in satisfaction with family
Changes in expressions of conflict within family

Goals/Objectives

Short-term Goal

Family members will express feelings regarding loved one's diagnosis and prognosis.

Long-term Goal

Family will verbalize areas of dysfunction and demonstrate ability to cope more effectively.

Interventions with *Selected Rationales*

1. Create an environment that is comfortable, supportive, and private and promotes trust. *Basic needs of the family must be met before crisis resolution can be attempted.*
2. Encourage each individual member to express feelings regarding loved one's diagnosis and prognosis. *Each individual*

is unique and must feel that his or her private needs can be met within the family constellation.

3. If the client is homosexual, and this is the family's first awareness, help them deal with guilt and shame they may experience. Help parents to understand they are not responsible and their child is still the same individual they have always loved. *Resolving guilt and shame enables family members to respond adaptively to the crisis. Their response can affect the client's remaining future as well as the family's future.*

4. Serve as facilitator between client's family and homosexual partner. The family may have difficulty accepting the partner as a person who is as significant as a spouse. Clarify roles and responsibilities of family and partner. Do this by bringing both parties together to define and distribute the tasks involved in the client's care. *By minimizing the lack of legally defined roles and by focusing on the need for making realistic decisions about the client's care, communication and resolution of conflict are enhanced.*

5. Encourage use of stress management techniques (e.g., relaxation exercises, guided imagery, attendance at support group meetings for significant others of clients with HIV disease). *Reduction of stress and support from others who share similar experiences enable individuals to begin to think more clearly and develop new behaviors to cope with this situational crisis.*

6. Provide educational information about HIV disease and opportunity to ask questions and express concerns. *Many misconceptions about the disease abound within the public domain. Clarification may calm some of the family's fears and facilitate interaction with the client.*

7. Make family referrals to community organizations that provide supportive help or financial assistance to clients with HIV disease. *Extended care can place a financial burden on client and family members. Respite care may provide family members with occasional much-needed relief away from the stress of physical and emotional caregiving responsibilities.*

Outcome Criteria

1. Family members are able to discuss feelings regarding client's diagnosis and prognosis.
2. Family members are able to make rational decisions regarding care of their loved one and the effect on family functioning.

● DEFICIENT KNOWLEDGE (PREVENTION OF TRANSMISSION AND PROTECTION OF THE CLIENT)

Definition: Absence or deficiency of cognitive information related to a specific topic.

Possible Etiologies ("related to")

Cognitive limitation
Information misinterpretation
Lack of exposure [to accurate information]

Defining Characteristics ("evidenced by")

Verbalization of the problem
Inappropriate or exaggerated behaviors
Inaccurate follow-through of instruction
[Inaccurate statements by client and family]

Goals/Objectives

Short-term Goal

Client and family verbalize understanding about disease process, modes of transmission, and prevention of infection.

Long-term Goals

1. Client and family demonstrate ability to execute precautions for preventing transmission of HIV and infection of the client.
2. Transmission of HIV and infection of the client are prevented.

Interventions with *Selected Rationales*

1. Present the following information *in an effort to clarify misconceptions, calm fears, and support an environment of appropriate interventions for care of the client with HIV disease.* Teach that HIV cannot be contracted from:
   a. Casual or household contact with an individual with HIV infection.
   b. Shaking hands, hugging, social (dry) kissing, holding hands, or other nonsexual physical contact.
   c. Touching unsoiled linens or clothing, money, furniture, or other inanimate objects.
   d. Being near someone who has HIV disease at work, school, restaurants, or in elevators.
   e. Toilet seats, bathtubs, towels, showers, or swimming pools.

    f. Dishes, silverware, or food handled by a person with HIV disease.

    g. Animals (pets may transmit opportunistic organisms).

    h. (Very unlikely spread by) coughing, sneezing, spitting, kissing, tears, or saliva.

2. HIV dies quickly outside the body because it requires living tissue to survive. It is readily killed by soap, cleansers, hot water, and disinfectants.

3. Teach client to protect self from infections by taking the following precautions:

    a. Avoid unpasteurized milk or milk products.

    b. Cook all raw vegetables and fruits before eating. ***Raw or improperly washed foods may transmit microbes.***

    c. Cook all meals well before eating.

    d. Avoid direct contact with persons with known contagious illnesses.

    e. Consult physician before getting a pet. ***Pets require extra infection control precautions because of the opportunistic organisms carried by animals.***

    f. Avoid touching animal feces, urine, emesis, litter boxes, aquariums, or bird cages. Always wear mask and gloves when cleaning up after a pet.

    g. Avoid traveling in countries with poor sanitation.

    h. Avoid vaccines or vaccinations that contain live organisms. ***Vaccination with live organisms may be fatal to severely immunosuppressed persons.***

    i. Exercise regularly.

    j. Control stress factors. A counselor or support group may be helpful.

    k. Stop smoking. ***Smoking predisposes to respiratory infections.***

    l. Maintain good personal hygiene.

4. Teach client/significant others about prevention of transmission:

    a. Do not donate blood, plasma, body organs, tissues, or semen.

    b. Inform physician, dentist, and anyone providing care that you have HIV disease.

    c. Do not share needles or syringes.

    d. Do not share personal items, such as toothbrushes, razors, or other implements that may be contaminated with blood or body fluids.

    e. Do not eat or drink from the same dinnerware and utensils without washing them between uses.

    f. Avoid becoming pregnant if at risk for HIV infection.

    g. Engage in only "safer" sexual practices (those *not* involving exchange of body fluids).

h. Avoid sexual practices medically classified as "unsafe," such as anal or vaginal intercourse and oral sex.

i. Avoid the use of recreational drugs because of their immunosuppressive effects.

5. Teach the home caregiver(s) to protect self from HIV infection by taking the following precautions:

a. Wash hands thoroughly with liquid antibiotic soap before and after each client contact. Use moisturizing lotion afterward to prevent dry, cracking skin.

b. Wear gloves when in contact with blood or body fluids (e.g., open wounds, suctioning, feces). Gown or aprons may be worn if soiling is likely.

c. Wear a mask:
   (1) When client has a productive cough and tuberculosis has not been ruled out.
   (2) To protect client if caregiver has a cold.
   (3) During suctioning.

d. Bag disposable gloves and masks with client's trash.

e. Dispose of the following in the toilet:
   (1) Organic material on clothes or linen before laundering.
   (2) Blood or body fluids.
   (3) Soiled tissue or toilet paper.
   (4) Cleaners or disinfectants used to clean contaminated articles.
   (5) Solutions contaminated with blood or body fluids.

f. Double-bag client's trash and soiled dressings in an impenetrable, plastic bag. *Tie* the bag shut and discard with household trash.

g. Do not recap needles, syringes, and other sharp items. Use puncture-proof covered containers for disposal (e.g., coffee cans and jars are appropriate for home use).

h. Place soiled linen and clothing in a plastic bag and tie shut until washed. Launder these separately from other laundry. Use bleach or other disinfectant in hot water.

i. When house cleaning, all equipment used in care of the client, as well as bathroom and kitchen surfaces, should be cleaned with a 1:10 dilute bleach solution.

j. Mops, sponges, and other items used for cleaning should be reserved specifically for that purpose.

Outcome Criteria

1. Client, family, and significant other(s) are able to verbalize information presented regarding ways in which HIV can and cannot be transmitted, ways to protect the client from infections, and ways to prevent transmission to caregivers and others.

2. Transmission to others and infection of the client have been avoided.

INTERNET REFERENCES

- Additional information about HIV/AIDS may be located at the following websites:
  a. http://www.avert.org/
  b. http://www.aegis.com/main/
  c. http://www.HIVpositive.com/index.html
  d. http://research.med.umkc.edu/teams/cml/AIDS.html
  e. http://www.cdc.gov/hiv
  f. http://hivinsite.ucsf.edu/InSite?page=KB
  g. http://www.cdc.gov/mmwr/preview/mmwrhtml/rr5212a1.htm

 Movie Connections

Philadelphia • *Longtime Companion* • *A Mother's Prayer* • *Breaking the Surface – The Greg Louganis Story* • *And the Band Played On*

Homelessness

● BACKGROUND ASSESSMENT DATA

It is difficult to determine how many individuals are homeless in the United States. Estimates have been made at somewhere between 250,000 and 4 million.

Who are the Homeless?

1. **Age.** Studies have produced a variety of statistics related to age of the homeless: 39% are younger than 18 years; individuals between the ages of 25 and 34 comprise 25%; and 6% are ages 55 to 64.
2. **Gender.** More men than women are homeless. The National Coalition for the Homeless (NCH, 2007) reports that single men comprise 51% of the homeless population and single women comprise 17%.
3. **Families.** Families with children are among the fastest growing segments of the homeless population. Families comprise 33% of the urban homeless population, but research indicates that this number is higher in rural areas, where families, single mothers, and children make up the largest group of homeless people.
4. **Ethnicity.** The homeless population is estimated to be 42% African American, 39% white, 13% Hispanic, 4% Native American, and 2% Asian (U.S. Conference of Mayors [USCM], 2006). The ethnic makeup of homeless populations varies according to geographic location.

Mental Illness and Homelessness

The USCM (2008) survey revealed that approximately 26% of the homeless population has some form of mental illness. Schizophrenia is frequently described as the most common diagnosis. Other prevalent disorders include bipolar affective disorder, substance abuse and dependence, depression, personality disorders, and organic mental disorders.

Predisposing Factors to Homelessness Among the Mentally Ill

1. **Deinstitutionalization.** Deinstitutionalization is frequently implicated as a contributing factor to homelessness among persons with mental illness. Deinstitutionalization began out of expressed concern by mental health professionals and others who described the "deplorable conditions" under which mentally ill individuals were housed. Some individuals believed that institutionalization deprived the mentally ill of their civil rights. Not the least of the motivating factors for deinstitutionalization was the financial burden that these clients placed on state governments.

2. **Poverty.** Cuts in various government entitlement programs have depleted the allotments available for individuals with severe and persistent mental illness living in the community. The job market is prohibitive for individuals whose behavior is incomprehensible or even frightening to many. The stigma and discrimination associated with mental illness may be diminishing slowly, but it is highly visible to those who suffer from its effects.

3. **A Scarcity of Affordable Housing.** The NCH (2008b) stated:

   > A lack of affordable housing and the limited scale of housing assistance programs have contributed to the current housing crisis and to homelessness. The gap between the number of affordable housing units and the number of people needing them has created a housing crisis for poor people. Between 1970 and 1995, the gap between the number of low-income renters and the amount of affordable housing units skyrocketed from a nonexistent gap to a shortage of 4.4 million affordable housing units—the largest shortfall on record.

   In addition, the number of single-room-occupancy (SRO) hotels has diminished drastically. These SRO hotels provided a means of relatively inexpensive housing, and although some people believe that these facilities nurtured isolation, they provided adequate shelter from the elements for their occupants. So many individuals currently frequent the shelters of our cities that there is concern that the shelters are becoming mini-institutions for people with serious mental illness.

4. **Lack of Affordable Health Care.** For families barely able to scrape together enough money to pay for day-to-day living, a catastrophic illness can create the level of poverty that starts the downward spiral to homelessness.

5. **Domestic Violence.** The NCH (2008b) reports that approximately half of all women and children experiencing homelessness are fleeing domestic violence. Battered women are

often forced to choose between an abusive relationship and homelessness.

5. **Addiction Disorders.** For individuals with alcohol or drug addictions, in the absence of appropriate treatment, the chances increase for being forced into life on the street. The following have been cited as obstacles to addiction treatment for homeless persons: lack of health insurance, lack of documentation, waiting lists, scheduling difficulties, daily contact requirements, lack of transportation, ineffective treatment methods, lack of supportive services, and cultural insensitivity.

Symptomatology (Commonly Associated with Homelessness)

1. Mobility and migration (the penchant for frequent movement to various geographic locations)
2. Substance abuse
3. Nutritional deficiencies
4. Difficulty with thermoregulation
5. Increased incidence of tuberculosis
6. Increased incidence of sexually transmitted diseases
7. Increased incidence of gastrointestinal (GI) and respiratory disorders
8. Among homeless children (compared with control samples), increased incidence of:
   a. Ear infections
   b. GI and respiratory disorders
   c. Infestational ailments
   d. Developmental delays
   e. Psychological problems

Common Nursing Diagnoses and Interventions

(Interventions are applicable to various health-care settings, such as inpatient and partial hospitalization, community health clinic, "street clinic," and homeless shelters.)

• INEFFECTIVE HEALTH MAINTENANCE

Definition: Inability to identify, manage, and/or seek out help to maintain health.

Possible Etiologies ("related to")

Perceptual/cognitive impairment
Deficient communication skills

Unachieved developmental tasks
Insufficient resources (e.g., equipment, finances)
Inability to make appropriate judgments
Ineffective individual coping

Defining Characteristics ("evidenced by")

History of lack of health-seeking behavior
Impairment of personal support systems
Demonstrated lack of knowledge about basic health practices
Demonstrated lack of adaptive behaviors to environmental
 changes
Inability to take responsibility for meeting basic health practices

Goals/Objectives

Short-term Goal

Client will seek and receive assistance with current health matters.

Long-term Goals

1. Client will assume responsibility for own health-care needs
   within level of ability.
2. Client will adopt lifestyle changes that support individual
   health-care needs.

Interventions with *Selected Rationales*

1. The triage nurse in the emergency department, street clinic,
   or shelter will begin the biopsychosocial assessment of the
   homeless client. *An adequate assessment is required to ensure appropriate nursing care is provided.*
2. Assess developmental level of functioning and ability to communicate. Use language that the client can comprehend. *This
   information is essential to ensure that client achieves an accurate understanding of information presented and that the
   nurse correctly interprets what the client is attempting to
   convey.*
3. Assess client's use of substances, including use of tobacco.
   Discuss eating and sleeping habits. *These actions may be
   contributing to current health problems.*
4. Assess sexual practices, *to determine level of personal risk.*
5. Assess oral hygiene practices, *to determine specific self-care
   needs.*
6. Assess client's ability to make decisions. *Client may need assistance in determining the type of care that is required,
   how to determine the most appropriate time to seek that
   care, and where to go to receive it.*
7. It is important to ask the following basic questions of the
   homeless client:
   a. Do you understand what your problem is?
   b. How will you get your prescriptions filled?

c. Where are you going when you leave here, or where will you sleep tonight? *Answers to these questions at admission will initiate discharge planning for the client.*

8. Teach client the basics of self-care (e.g., proper hygiene; facts about nutrition). *The client must have this type of knowledge if he or she is to become more self-sufficient.*

9. Teach client about safe sex practices *in an effort to avoid sexually transmitted diseases.*

10. Identify immediate problems and assist with crisis intervention. *Emergency departments, "storefront" clinics, or shelters may be the homeless client's only resource in a crisis situation.*

11. Tend to physical needs immediately. Ensure that client has thorough physical examination. *The client cannot deal with psychosocial issues until physical problems have been addressed.*

12. Assess mental health status. *Many homeless individuals have some form of mental illness.* Ensure that appropriate psychiatric care is provided. If possible, inquire about possible long-acting medication injections for client. *The client may be less likely to discontinue the medication if he or she does not have to take pills every day.*

13. Refer client to others who can provide assistance (e.g., case manager; social worker). *If the client is to be discharged to a shelter, a case manager or social worker may be the best link between the client and the health-care system to ensure that he or she obtains appropriate follow-up care.*

Outcome Criteria

1. Client verbalizes understanding of information presented regarding optimal health maintenance.
2. Client is able to verbalize signs and symptoms that should be reported to a health-care professional.
3. Client verbalizes knowledge of available resources from which he or she may seek assistance as required.

• POWERLESSNESS

Definition: Perception that one's own action will not significantly affect an outcome; a perceived lack of control over a current situation or immediate happening.

Possible Etiologies ("related to")

Lifestyle of helplessness
[Homelessness]

Defining Characteristics ("evidenced by")

Verbal expressions of having no control (e.g., over self-care, situation, outcome)
Apathy
Inadequate coping patterns

Goals/Objectives

Short-term Goal

Client will identify areas over which he or she has control.

Long-term Goal

Client will make decisions that reflect control over present situation and future outcome.

Interventions with *Selected Rationales*

1. Provide opportunities for the client to make choices about his or her present situation. *Providing client with choices will increase his or her feeling of control.*
2. Avoid arguing or using logic with the client who feels powerless. *Client will not believe it can make a difference.*
3. Accept expressions of feelings, including anger and hopelessness. *An attitude of acceptance enhances feelings of trust and self-worth.*
4. Help client identify personal strengths and establish realistic life goals. *Unrealistic goals set the client up for failure and reinforce feelings of powerlessness.*
5. Help client identify areas of life situation that he or she can control. *Client's emotional condition interferes with his or her ability to solve problems. Assistance is required to accurately perceive the benefits and consequences of available alternatives.*
6. Help client identify areas of life situation that are not within his or her ability to control. Encourage verbalization of feelings related to this inability *in an effort to deal with unresolved issues and accept what cannot be changed.*
7. Encourage client to seek out support group or shelter resources. *Social isolation promotes feelings of powerlessness and hopelessness.*

Outcome Criteria

1. Client verbalizes choices made in a plan to maintain control over his or her life situation.
2. Client verbalizes honest feelings about life situations over which he or she has no control.
3. Client is able to verbalize system for problem-solving as required to maintain hope for the future.

INTERNET REFERENCES

a. http://www.nationalhomeless.org/
b. http://www.endhomelessness.org/
c. http://portal.hud.gov/portal/page/portal/HUD/topics/homelessness
d. http://www.hhs.gov/homeless/
e. http://www.nrchmi.samhsa.gov/Default.aspx
f. http://www.abanet.org/homeless/

 Movie Connections

The Soloist • *The Grapes of Wrath* • *Generosity* • *The Redemption*

C HAPTER 21

Psychiatric Home Nursing Care

● BACKGROUND ASSESSMENT DATA

Dramatic changes in the health care delivery system and sky-rocketing costs have created a need to find a way to provide quality, cost-effective care to psychiatric clients. Home care has become one of the fastest growing areas in the healthcare system and is now recognized by many reimbursement agencies as a preferred method of community-based service. Just what is home health care? The American Nurses Association (ANA, 2008) contributed the following definition:

> Home health nursing is nursing practice applied to patients of all ages in the patients' residences, which may include private homes, assisted living, or personal care facilities. Patients and their families and other caregivers are the focus of home health nursing practice. The goal of care is to maintain or improve the quality of life for patients and the families and other caregivers, or to support patients in their transition to end of life (p. 3).

The psychiatric home care nurse must have knowledge and skills to meet both the physical and the psychosocial needs of the homebound client. Serving health care consumers in their home environment charges the nurse with the responsibility of providing holistic care.

Predisposing Factors

An increase in psychiatric home care may be associated with the following factors:

1. Earlier hospital discharges
2. Increased demand for home care as an alternative to institutional care
3. Broader third-party payment coverage
4. Greater physician acceptance of home care
5. The increasing need to contain health-care costs and the growth of managed care

348

Psychiatric home nursing care is provided through private home health agencies; private hospitals; public hospitals; government institutions, such as the Veterans Administration; and community mental health centers. Most often, home care is viewed as follow-up care to inpatient, partial, or outpatient hospitalization.

The majority of home healthcare is paid for by Medicare. Other sources include Medicaid, private insurance, self-pay, and others. Medicare requires that the following criteria be met to qualify for psychiatric home care (Jensen & Miller, 2004):

1. The client is confined to the home.
2. The client must receive services under a plan of care established and periodically reviewed by a physician.
3. The client must be in need of skilled nursing care on an intermittent basis.
4. Services must be reasonable and necessary for treating the client's psychiatric diagnosis and/or symptoms.
5. Home health psychiatric care must be provided by a skilled psychiatric nurse.

Jensen and Miller (2004) reported:

> Care can be provided in one's own home or residence, assisted living, adult family homes, or retirement homes, but not in hospitals or skilled nursing facilities. A home health psychiatric care patient is unable to leave the home without considerable difficulty or the assistance of another person. The patient can leave home infrequently or for a short duration, for example, going to church on Sunday. The patient can also go out for medical treatment, partial hospitalization, adult day care, or chemotherapy. A patient can also be homebound for psychiatric reasons, such as depression, agoraphobia, paranoia, or panic disorder (p. 3).

Although Medicare and Medicaid are the largest reimbursement providers, a growing number of health maintenance organizations (HMOs) and preferred provider organizations (PPOs) are recognizing the cost-effectiveness of psychiatric home nursing care and are including it as part of their benefit packages. Most managed care agencies require that treatment, or even a specific number of visits, be preauthorized for psychiatric home nursing care. The plan of treatment and subsequent charting must explain why the client's psychiatric disorder keeps him or her at home and justify the need for services.

Symptomatology (Subjective and Objective Data)

Homebound psychiatric clients most often have diagnoses of depression, dementia, anxiety disorders, bipolar affective disorder, and schizophrenia. Psychiatric nurses also provide consultation for clients with primary medical disorders. Many elderly clients are homebound because of medical conditions that impair mobility and necessitate home care. Psychiatric nurses may provide the following types of home nursing care:

- To clients with primary Axis I psychiatric diagnoses, the symptoms of which are immobilizing, and the client and family require assistance with management of the symptoms
- To clients who are homebound for medical conditions but have a psychiatric condition for which they have been receiving (and continue to need ongoing) treatment
- To clients who are homebound with medical conditions and who may develop serious psychiatric symptoms in response to their medical illness

Table 21-1 identifies some of the conditions for which a psychiatric nursing home care consultation may be sought.

The following components should be included in the comprehensive assessment of the homebound client:

1. The client's perception of the problem and need for assistance
2. Information regarding the client's strengths and personal habits
3. Health history, review of systems, and vital signs
4. Any recent changes (physical, psychosocial, and environmental)
5. Availability of support systems
6. Current medication regimen (including the client's understanding about the medications and reason for taking)
7. Nutritional and elimination assessment
8. Activities of daily living (ADLs) assessment
9. Substance use assessment
10. Neurological assessment

TABLE 21 – 1 Conditions that Warrant Psychiatric Nursing Consultation

- When a client has a new psychiatric diagnosis
- When a new psychotropic medication has been added to the regimen
- When the client's mental status exacerbates or causes deterioration in his or her medical condition
- When the client is suspected of abusing alcohol or drugs
- When a client is expressing suicidal ideation
- When a client is noncompliant with psychotropic medication
- When a client develops a fundamental change in mood or a thought disorder
- When a client is immobilized by severe depression or anxiety

SOURCE: Adapted from Schroeder, 2009.

11. Mental status examination (see Appendix M)
12. Global Assessment of Functioning (GAF) scale rating (see Appendix K)

Other important assessments include information about acute or chronic medical conditions, patterns of sleep and rest, solitude and social interaction, use of leisure time, education and work history, issues related to religion or spirituality, and adequacy of the home environment.

Common Nursing Diagnoses and Interventions for Psychiatric Homebound Clients

● INEFFECTIVE SELF-HEALTH MANAGEMENT

Definition: Pattern of regulating and integrating into daily living a therapeutic regime for treatment of illness and its sequelae that is unsatisfactory for meeting specific health goals.

Possible Etiologies ("related to")

Perceived barriers
Social support deficits
Powerlessness
Perceived benefits
[Mistrust of regimen and/or health care personnel]
Knowledge deficit
Complexity of therapeutic regimen

Defining Characteristics ("evidenced by")

Makes choices in daily living ineffective for meeting health goals
Failure to include treatment regimens in daily living
Failure to take action to reduce risk factors
Verbalizes difficulty with prescribed regimens
Verbalizes desire to manage the illness

Goals/Objectives

Short-term Goals

1. Client will verbalize understanding of barriers to self-health management.
2. Client will participate in problem-solving efforts toward adequate self-health management.

Long-term Goal

Client will incorporate changes in lifestyle necessary to maintain effective self-health management.

Interventions with *Selected Rationales*

1. Assess client's knowledge of condition and treatment needs. *Client may lack full comprehension of need for treatment regimen.*
2. Identify client's perception of treatment regimen. *Client may be mistrustful of treatment regimen or of health care system in general.*
3. *Promote a trusting relationship with the client* by being honest, encouraging client to participate in decision-making, and conveying genuine positive regard.
4. Assist client in recognizing strengths and past successes. *Recognition of strengths and past successes increases self-esteem and indicates to client that he or she can be successful in managing therapeutic regimen.*
5. Provide positive reinforcement for efforts. *Positive reinforcement increases self-esteem and encourages repetition of desirable behaviors.*
6. Emphasize importance of need for treatment and/or medication. *Client must understand that the consequence of lack of follow-through is possible decompensation.*
7. *In an effort to incorporate lifestyle changes and promote wellness,* help client develop plans for managing therapeutic regimen, such as support groups, social and family systems, and financial assistance.

Outcome Criteria

1. Client verbalizes understanding of information presented regarding management of therapeutic regimen.
2. Client demonstrates desire and ability to perform strategies necessary to maintain adequate management of therapeutic regimen.
3. Client verbalizes knowledge of available resources from which he or she may seek assistance as required.

● RISK-PRONE HEALTH BEHAVIOR

Definition: Impaired ability to modify lifestyle/behaviors in a manner that improves health status.

Possible Etiologies ("related to")

Inadequate comprehension
Inadequate social support
Low self-efficacy
Low socioeconomic status
Multiple stressors

Negative attitude toward healthcare
[Intense emotional state]

Defining Characteristics ("evidenced by")

Demonstrates nonacceptance of health status change
Failure to achieve optimal sense of control
Failure to take actions that prevent health problems
Minimizes health status change

Goals/Objectives

Short-term Goals

1. Client will discuss with home health nurse the kinds of life-style changes that will occur because of the change in health status.
2. With the help of home health nurse, client will formulate a plan of action for incorporating those changes into his or her lifestyle.
3. Client will demonstrate movement toward independence, considering change in health status.

Long-term Goal

Client will demonstrate competence to function independently to his or her optimal ability, considering change in health status, by time of discharge from home health care.

Interventions with Selected Rationales

1. Encourage client to talk about lifestyle prior to the change in health status. Discuss coping mechanisms that were used at stressful times in the past. *It is important to identify the client's strengths so that they may be used to facilitate adaptation to the change or loss that has occurred.*
2. Encourage client to discuss the change or loss and particularly to express anger associated with it. *Some individuals may not realize that anger is a normal stage in the grieving process. If it is not released in an appropriate manner, it may be turned inward on the self, leading to pathological depression.*
3. Encourage client to express fears associated with the change or loss or alteration in lifestyle that the change or loss has created. *Change often creates a feeling of disequilibrium and the individual may respond with fears that are irrational or unfounded. He or she may benefit from feedback that corrects misperceptions about how life will be with the change in health status.*
4. Provide assistance with ADLs as required, but encourage independence to the limit that client's ability will allow. Give positive feedback for activities accomplished independently.

Independent accomplishments and positive feedback enhance self-esteem and encourage repetition of desired behaviors. Successes also provide hope that adaptive functioning is possible and decrease feelings of powerlessness.

5. Help client with decision-making regarding incorporation of change or loss into lifestyle. Identify problems that the change or loss is likely to create. Discuss alternative solutions, weighing potential benefits and consequences of each alternative. Support client's decision in the selection of an alternative. *The great amount of anxiety that usually accompanies a major lifestyle change often interferes with an individual's ability to solve problems and to make appropriate decisions. Client may need assistance with this process in an effort to progress toward successful adaptation.*

6. Use role-playing *to decrease anxiety* as client anticipates stressful situations that might occur in relation to the health status change. *Role-playing decreases anxiety and provides a feeling of security by arming the client with a plan of action with which to respond in an appropriate manner when a stressful situation occurs.*

7. Ensure that client and family are fully knowledgeable regarding the physiology of the change in health status and its necessity for optimal wellness. Encourage them to ask questions, and provide printed material explaining the change to which they may refer following discharge.

8. Help client identify resources within the community from which he or she may seek assistance in adapting to the change in health status. Examples include self-help or support groups, counselor, or social worker. Encourage client to keep follow-up appointments with physician or to call physician's office prior to follow-up date if problems or concerns arise.

Outcome Criteria

1. Client is able to perform ADLs independently.
2. Client is able to make independent decisions regarding lifestyle considering change in health status.
3. Client is able to express hope for the future with consideration of change in health status.

● SOCIAL ISOLATION

Definition: Aloneness experienced by the individual and perceived as imposed by others and as a negative or threatening state.

Possible Etiologies ("related to")

Alterations in mental status
Inability to engage in satisfying personal relationships
Unaccepted social values
Unaccepted social behavior
Inadequate personal resources
Immature interests
Alterations in physical appearance
Altered state of wellness

Defining Characteristics ("evidenced by")

Expresses feelings of aloneness imposed by others
Expresses feelings of rejection
Developmentally inappropriate interests
Inability to meet expectations of others
Insecurity in public
Absence of supportive significant other(s)
Projects hostility
Withdrawn; uncommunicative
Seeks to be alone
Preoccupation with own thoughts
Sad, dull affect

Goals/Objectives

Short-term Goal

Client will verbalize willingness to be involved with others.

Long-term Goal

Client will participate in interactions with others at level of ability or desire.

Interventions with *Selected Rationales*

1. Convey an accepting attitude by making regular visits. *An accepting attitude increases feelings of self-worth and facilitates trust.*
2. Show unconditional positive regard. *This conveys your belief in the client as a worthwhile human being.*
3. Be honest and keep all promises. *Honesty and dependability promote a trusting relationship.*
4. Be cautious with touch until trust has been established. *A suspicious client may perceive touch as a threatening gesture.*
5. Be with the client to offer support during activities that may be frightening or difficult for him or her. *The presence of a trusted individual provides emotional security for the client.*
6. Take walks with the client. Help him or her perform simple tasks around the house. *Increased activity enhances both physical and mental status.*

7. Assess lifelong patterns of relationships. ***Basic personality characteristics will not change. Most individuals keep the same style of relationship development that they had in the past.***
8. Help the client identify present relationships that are satisfying and activities that he or she considers interesting. ***Only the client knows what he or she truly likes, and these personal preferences will facilitate success in reversing social isolation.***
9. Consider the feasibility of a pet. ***There are many documented studies of the benefits of companion animals.***

Outcome Criteria

1. Client demonstrates willingness and desire to socialize with others.
2. Client independently pursues social activities with others.

● RISK FOR CAREGIVER ROLE STRAIN

Definition: Caregiver is vulnerable for felt difficulty in performing the family caregiver role.

Risk Factors

Caregiver not developmentally ready for caregiver role
Inadequate physical environment for providing care
Unpredictable illness course or instability in the care receiver's health
Psychological or cognitive problems in care receiver
Presence of abuse or violence
Past history of poor relationship between caregiver and care receiver
Marginal caregiver's coping patterns
Lack of respite and recreation for caregiver
Addiction or codependency
Caregiver's competing role commitments
Illness severity of the care receiver
Duration of caregiving required
Family/caregiver isolation

Goals/Objectives
Short-term Goal

Caregivers will verbalize understanding of ways to facilitate the caregiver role.

Long-term Goal

Caregivers will demonstrate effective problem-solving skills and develop adaptive coping mechanisms to regain equilibrium.

Interventions with *Selected Rationales*

1. Assess caregivers' ability to anticipate and fulfill client's unmet needs. Provide information to assist caregivers with this responsibility. Ensure that caregivers encourage client to be as independent as possible. *Caregivers may be unaware of what the client can realistically accomplish. They may be unaware of the nature of the illness.*

2. Ensure that caregivers are aware of available community support systems from which they can seek assistance when required. Examples include respite care services, day treatment centers, and adult day-care centers. *Caregivers require relief from the pressures and strain of providing 24-hour care for their loved one. Studies have shown that abuse arises out of caregiving situations that place overwhelming stress on the caregivers.*

3. Encourage caregivers to express feelings, particularly anger. *Release of these emotions can serve to prevent psychopathology, such as depression or psychophysiological disorders, from occurring.*

4. Encourage participation in support groups composed of members with similar life situations. Provide information about support groups that may be helpful:
   a. National Alliance for the Mentally Ill—(800) 950-NAMI
   b. American Association on Intellectual and Developmental Disabilities—(800) 424-3688
   c. Alzheimer's Association—(800) 272-3900

   Hearing others who are experiencing the same problems discuss ways in which they have coped may help the caregiver adopt more adaptive strategies. Individuals who are experiencing similar life situations provide empathy and support for each other.

Outcome Criteria

1. Caregivers are able to problem-solve effectively regarding care of the client.
2. Caregivers demonstrate adaptive coping strategies for dealing with stress of caregiver role.
3. Caregivers openly express feelings.
4. Caregivers express desire to join support group of other caregivers.

 INTERNET REFERENCES
   a. http://www.cms.hhs.gov/
   b. http://www.nahc.org/
   c. http://www.aahomecare.org/

CHAPTER 22

Forensic Nursing

● BACKGROUND ASSESSMENT DATA

The International Association of Forensic Nurses (IAFN) (2009) has defined *forensic nursing* as:

> The practice of nursing globally when health and legal systems intersect (p. 3).

Bellfield and Catalano (2009) have stated:

> Forensic nursing is an emerging field that forms an alliance between nursing, law enforcement, and the forensic sciences. The term **forensic** means anything belonging to, or pertaining to, the law. Forensic nurses provide a continuum of care to victims and their families beginning in the emergency room or crime scene and leading to participation in the criminal investigation and the courts of law (p. 446).

Areas of forensic nursing include:

1. Clinical forensic nursing
2. The sexual assault nurse examiner (SANE)
3. Forensic psychiatric nursing specialty
4. Correctional/institutional nursing specialty
5. Nurses in general practice

Clinical Forensic Nursing in Trauma Care

Assessment

Lynch, Roach, and Sadler (2006) have stated, "Forensic nurse specialists are specifically trained to deal with cases of sexual assault, child abuse, acute psychiatric emergencies, and death investigation" (p. 603). All traumatic injuries in which liability is suspected are considered within the scope of forensic nursing. Reports to legal agencies are required to ensure follow-up investigation; however, the protection of clients' rights remains a nursing priority.

Several areas of assessment in which the clinical forensic nurse specialist in trauma care may become involved include:

1. **Preservation of Evidence.** Evidence from both crime-related and self-inflicted traumas must be safeguarded in a

manner consistent with the investigation. Evidence such as clothing, bullets, bloodstains, hairs, fibers, and small pieces of material such as fragments of metal, glass, paint, and wood should be saved and documented in all medical accident instances that have legal implications.

2. **Investigation of Wound Characteristics.** Wounds that the nurse must be able to identify include:

    a. *Sharp-Force Injuries:* Sharp-force injuries including stab wounds and other wounds resulting from penetration with a sharp object.

    b. *Blunt-Force Injuries:* Includes cuts and bruises resulting from the impact of a blunt object against the body.

    c. *Dicing Injuries:* Multiple, minute cuts and abrasions caused by contact with shattered glass (e.g., often occur in motor vehicle accidents).

    d. *Patterned Injuries:* Specific injuries that reflect the pattern of the weapon used to inflict the injury.

    e. *Bite-Mark Injuries:* A type of patterned injury inflicted by a human or an animal.

    f. *Defense Wounds:* Injuries that reflect the victim's attempt to defend himself or herself from attack.

    g. *Hesitation Wounds:* Usually superficial, sharp-force wounds; often found perpendicular to the lower part of the body and may reflect self-inflicted wounds.

    h. *Fast-Force Injuries:* Usually gunshot wounds; may reflect various patterns of injury.

3. **Deaths in the Emergency Department.** When deaths occur in the emergency department as a result of abuse or accident, evidence must be retained, the death must be reported to legal authorities, and an investigation is conducted. It is therefore essential that the nurse carefully document the appearance, condition, and behavior of the victim upon arrival at the hospital. The information gathered from the client and family (or others accompanying the client) may serve to facilitate the postmortem investigation and may be used during criminal justice proceedings.

    The critical factor is to be able to determine if the cause of death is natural or unnatural. A death is deemed *natural* if it occurs because of a congenital anomaly or a disease process that interferes with vital organ functioning (Lynch, 2006). In the emergency department, most deaths are sudden and unexpected. Those that are considered natural most commonly involve the cardiovascular, respiratory, and central nervous systems. Deaths that are considered *unnatural* include those from trauma, from self-inflicted acts, or from injuries inflicted by another. Legal authorities must be notified of all deaths related to unnatural circumstances.

Common Nursing Diagnoses and Interventions for Forensic Nursing in Trauma Care

● POST-TRAUMA SYNDROME

Definition: Sustained maladaptive response to a traumatic, overwhelming event.

Possible Etiologies ("related to")

Physical and/or psychosocial abuse
Tragic occurrence involving multiple deaths
Sudden destruction of one's home or community
Epidemics
Disasters
Rape
Serious accidents (e.g., industrial, motor vehicle)
Witnessing mutilation, violent death, [or other horrors]
Serious threat or injury to self or loved ones

Defining Characteristics ("evidenced by")

[Physical injuries related to trauma]
Avoidance
Repression
Difficulty concentrating
Grieving; guilt
Intrusive thoughts
Neurosensory irritability
Palpitations
Anger and/or rage; aggression
Intrusive dreams; nightmares; flashbacks
Panic attacks; fear
Gastric irritability
Psychogenic amnesia
Substance abuse

Goals/Objectives

Short-term Goals

1. The client's physical wounds will heal without complication.
2. The client will begin a healthy grief resolution, initiating the process of psychological healing.

Long-term Goal

The client will demonstrate ability to deal with emotional reactions in an individually appropriate manner.

Interventions with *Selected Rationales*

1. It is important to communicate the following to the victim of sexual assault:
   a. "You are safe here."
   b. "I'm sorry that it happened."
   c. "I am very glad you survived."
   d. "It is not your fault. No one deserves to be treated this way."
   e. "You did the best that you could."
   The woman who has been sexually assaulted fears for her life and must be reassured of her safety. She may also be overwhelmed with self-doubt and self-blame, and these statements instill trust and validate self-worth.

2. Explain every assessment procedure that will be conducted and why it is being conducted. Ensure that data collection is conducted in a caring, nonjudgmental manner *to decrease fear and anxiety and increase trust.*

3. Ledray (2001) suggested the following five essential components of a forensic examination of the sexual assault survivor in the emergency department:
   a. *Treatment and documentation of injuries.* Samples of blood, semen, hair, and fingernail scrapings should be sealed in paper, not plastic, bags, *to prevent the possible growth of mildew from accumulation of moisture inside the plastic container, and the subsequent contamination of the evidence.*
   b. *Maintaining the proper chain of evidence.* Samples must be properly labeled, sealed, and refrigerated when necessary and kept under observation or properly locked until rendered to the proper legal authority *in order to ensure the proper chain of evidence and freshness of the samples.*
   c. *Treatment and evaluation of sexually transmitted diseases (STDs).* If conducted within 72 hours of the attack, several tests and interventions are available for prophylactic treatment of certain STDs.
   d. *Pregnancy risk evaluation and prevention.* Prophylactic regimens are 97% to 98% effective if started within 24 hours of the sexual attack and are generally only recommended within 72 hours (Ledray, 2001).
   e. *Crisis intervention and arrangements for follow-up counseling.* *Because a survivor is often too ashamed or fearful to seek follow-up counseling,* it may be important for the nurse to obtain the individual's permission to allow a counselor to call her to make a follow-up appointment.

4. In the case of other types of trauma (e.g., gunshot victims; automobile/pedestrian hit-and-run victims), *ensure that any*

possible evidence is not lost. Clothing that is removed from a victim should not be shaken, and each separate item of clothing should be placed carefully in a paper bag, which should be sealed, dated, timed, and signed.

5. Ensure that the client has adequate privacy for all immediate postcrisis interventions. Try to have as few people as possible providing the immediate care or collecting immediate evidence. *The post-trauma client is extremely vulnerable. Additional people in the environment may increase this feeling of vulnerability and escalate anxiety.*

6. Encourage the client to give an account of the trauma/ assault. Listen, but do not probe. *Nonjudgmental listening provides an opportunity for catharsis that the client needs to begin healing. A detailed account may be required for legal follow-up, and a caring nurse, as client advocate, may help to lessen the trauma of evidence collection.*

7. Discuss with the client whom to call for support or assistance. Provide information about referrals for aftercare. *Because of severe anxiety and fear, client may need assistance from others during this immediate postcrisis period. Provide referral information in writing for later reference (e.g., psychotherapist, mental health clinic, community advocacy group).*

8. In the event of a sudden and unexpected death in the trauma care setting, the clinical forensic nurse may be called upon to present information associated with an anatomical donation request to the survivors. *The clinical forensic nurse specialist is an expert in legal issues and has the knowledge and sensitivity to provide coordination between the medical examiner and families who are grieving the loss of loved ones.*

Outcome Criteria

1. The client is no longer experiencing panic anxiety.
2. The client demonstrates a degree of trust in the primary nurse.
3. The client has received immediate attention to physical injuries.
4. The client has initiated behaviors consistent with the grief response.
5. Necessary evidence has been collected and preserved in order to proceed appropriately within the legal system.

Forensic Psychiatric Nursing in Correctional Facilities

Assessment

It was believed that deinstitutionalization increased the freedom of mentally ill individuals in accordance with the principle of "least restrictive alternative." However, because of inadequate community-based services, many of these individuals drift into poverty and homelessness, increasing their vulnerability to criminalization. Because the bizarre behavior of mentally ill individuals living on the street is sometimes offensive to community standards, law enforcement officials have the authority to protect the welfare of the public, as well as the safety of the individual, by initiating emergency hospitalization. However, legal criteria for commitment are so stringent in most cases, that arrest becomes an easier way of getting the mentally ill person off the street if a criminal statute has been violated. According to the Bureau of Justice, more than half of all prison and jail inmates have some form of mental health problem (James & Glaze, 2006). Some of these individuals are incarcerated as a result of the increasingly popular "guilty but mentally ill" verdict. With this verdict, individuals are deemed mentally ill, yet are held criminally responsible for their actions. The individual is incarcerated and receives special treatment, if needed, but it is no different from that available for and needed by any prisoner.

Psychiatric diagnoses commonly identified at the time of incarceration include schizophrenia, bipolar disorder, major depression, personality disorders, and substance disorders, and many have dual diagnoses (Yurkovich & Smyer, 2000). Common psychiatric behaviors include hallucinations, suspiciousness, thought disorders, anger/agitation, and impulsivity. Denial of problems is a common behavior among this population. Use of substances and medication noncompliance are common obstacles to rehabilitation. Substance abuse has been shown to have a strong correlation with recidivism among the prison population. Many individuals report that they were under the influence of substances at the time of their criminal actions, and dual diagnoses are common. Detoxification frequency occurs in jails and prisons, and some inmates have died from the withdrawal syndrome because of inadequate treatment during this process.

Common Nursing Diagnoses and Interventions for Forensic Nursing in Correctional Facilities

• DEFENSIVE COPING

Definition: Repeated projection of falsely positive self-evaluation based on a self-protective pattern that defends against underlying perceived threats to positive self-regard.

Possible Etiologies ("related to")

[Low self-esteem]
[Retarded ego development]
[Underdeveloped superego]
[Negative role models]
[Lack of positive feedback]
[Absent, erratic, or inconsistent methods of discipline]
[Dysfunctional family system]

Defining Characteristics ("evidenced by")

Denial of obvious problems or weaknesses
Projection of blame or responsibility
Rationalization of failures
Hypersensitivity to criticism
Grandiosity
Superior attitude toward others
Difficulty establishing or maintaining relationships
Hostile laughter or ridicule of others
Difficulty in perception of reality testing
Lack of follow-through or participation in treatment or therapy

Goals/Objectives

Short-term Goal

Client will verbalize personal responsibility for own actions, successes, and failures.

Long-term Goal

Client will demonstrate ability to interact with others and adapt to lifestyle goals without becoming defensive, rationalizing behaviors, or expressing grandiose ideas.

Interventions with *Selected Rationales*

1. Recognize and support basic ego strengths. *Focusing on positive aspects of the personality may help to improve self-concept.*
2. Encourage client to recognize and verbalize feelings of inadequacy and need for acceptance from others, and how these feelings provoke defensive behaviors, such as blaming others for own behaviors. *Recognition of the problem is the first step in the change process toward resolution.*
3. Provide immediate, matter-of-fact, nonthreatening feedback for unacceptable behaviors. *Client may lack knowledge about how he or she is being perceived by others. Direct the behavior in a nonthreatening manner to a more acceptable behavior.*
4. Help client identify situations that provoke defensiveness and practice more appropriate responses through role-playing.

Role-playing provides confidence to deal with difficult situations when they actually occur.

5. Provide immediate positive feedback for acceptable behaviors. *Positive feedback enhances self-esteem and encourages repetition of desirable behaviors.*

6. Help client set realistic, concrete goals and determine appropriate actions to meet those goals. *Success increases self-esteem.*

7. Evaluate with client the effectiveness of the new behaviors and discuss any modifications for improvement. *Because of limited problem-solving ability, assistance may be required to reassess and develop new strategies, in the event that certain of the new coping methods prove ineffective.*

8. Use confrontation judiciously *to help client begin to identify defense mechanisms (e.g., denial and projection) that are hindering development of satisfying relationships and adaptive behaviors.*

Outcome Criteria

1. Client verbalizes and accepts responsibility for own behavior.
2. Client verbalizes correlation between feelings of inadequacy and the need to defend the ego through rationalization and grandiosity.
3. Client does not ridicule or criticize others.
4. Client interacts with others in group situations without taking a defensive stance.

• COMPLICATED GRIEVING

Definition: A disorder that occurs after the death of a significant other [or any other loss of significance to the individual], in which the experience of distress accompanying bereavement fails to follow normative expectations and manifests in functional impairment.

Possible Etiologies ("related to")
[Loss of freedom]

Defining Characteristics ("evidenced by")
[Anger]
[Internalized rage]
Depression
[Labile affect]
[Suicidal ideation]
[Difficulty expressing feelings]
[Altered activities of daily living]
[Prolonged difficulty coping]

Goals/Objectives

Short-term Goal

Client will verbalize feelings of grief related to loss of freedom.

Long-term Goal

Client will progress satisfactorily through the grieving process.

Interventions with *Selected Rationales*

1. Convey an accepting attitude—one that creates a nonthreatening environment for the client to express feelings. Be honest and keep all promises. *An accepting attitude conveys to the client that you believe he or she is a worthwhile person. Trust is enhanced.*
2. Identify the function that anger, frustration, and rage serve for the client. Allow the client to express these feelings within reason. *Verbalization of feelings in a nonthreatening environment may help the client come to terms with unresolved grief.*
3. Encourage the client to discharge pent-up anger through participation in large motor activities (e.g., physical exercises, volleyball, punching bag). *Physical exercise provides a safe and effective method for discharging pent-up tension.*
4. Anger may be displaced onto the nurse or therapist, and caution must be taken to guard against the negative effects of countertransference. These are very difficult clients who have the capacity for eliciting a whole array of negative feelings from the therapist. These feelings must be acknowledged but not allowed to interfere with the therapeutic process.
5. Explain the behaviors associated with the normal grieving process. Help the client to recognize his or her position in this process. *This knowledge about normal grieving may help facilitate the client's progression toward resolution of grief.*
6. Help the client understand appropriate ways to express anger. Give positive reinforcement for behaviors used to express anger appropriately. Act as a role model. *Positive reinforcement enhances self-esteem and encourages repetition of desirable behaviors. It is appropriate to let the client know when he or she has done something that has generated angry feelings in you. Role-modeling ways to express anger in an appropriate manner is a powerful learning tool.*
7. Set limits on acting-out behaviors and explain consequences of violation of those limits. Be supportive, yet consistent and firm in working with this client. *Client lacks sufficient self-control to limit maladaptive behaviors; therefore, assistance is required from staff. Without consistency on the part of all staff members working with the client, a positive outcome will not be achieved.*

8. Provide a safe and protective environment for the client against risk of self-directed violence. ***Depression is the emotion that most commonly precedes suicidal attempts.***

Outcome Criteria
1. Client is able to verbalize ways in which anger and acting-out behaviors are associated with maladaptive grieving.
2. Client is expresses anger and hostility outwardly in a safe and acceptable manner.
3. Client has not harmed self or others.

• RISK FOR INJURY

Definition: At risk of injury as a result of [internal or external] environmental conditions interacting with the individual's adaptive and defensive resources.

Related/Risk Factors ("related to")
[Substance use/detoxification at time of incarceration, exhibiting any of the following:
  Substance intoxication
  Substance withdrawal
  Disorientation
  Seizures
  Hallucinations
  Psychomotor agitation
  Unstable vital signs
  Delirium
  Flashbacks
  Panic level of anxiety]

Goals/Objectives
Short-term Goal
Client's condition will stabilize within 72 hours.

Long-term Goal
Client will not experience physical injury.

Interventions with *Selected Rationales*
1. Assess client's level of disorientation to determine specific requirements for safety. ***Knowledge of client's level of functioning is necessary to formulate appropriate plan of care.***
2. Obtain a drug history, if possible, to determine
   a. Type of substance(s) used.
   b. Time of last ingestion and amount consumed.

    c. Duration and frequency of consumption.

    d. Amount consumed on a daily basis.

3. Obtain urine sample for laboratory analysis of substance content. *Subjective history often is not accurate. Knowledge regarding substance ingestion is important for accurate assessment of client condition.*

4. Place client in quiet room, if possible. *Excessive stimuli increase client agitation.*

5. Institute necessary safety precautions. *Client safety is a nursing priority.*

    a. Observe client behaviors frequently; assign staff on one-to-one basis if condition warrants it; accompany and assist client when ambulating; use wheelchair for transporting long distances.

    b. Be sure that side rails are up when client is in bed.

    c. Pad headboard and side rails of bed with thick towels to protect client in case of seizure.

    d. Use mechanical restraints as necessary to protect client if excessive hyperactivity accompanies the disorientation.

6. Ensure that smoking materials and other potentially harmful objects are stored outside client's access. *Client may harm self or others in disoriented, confused state.*

7. Monitor vital signs every 15 minutes initially and less frequently as acute symptoms subside. *Vital signs provide the most reliable information regarding client condition and need for medication during acute detoxification period.*

8. Follow medication regimen, as ordered by physician. Common medical interventions for detoxification from the following substances include:

    a. **Alcohol.** Benzodiazepines are the most widely used group of drugs for substitution therapy in alcohol withdrawal. The approach to treatment is to start with relatively high doses and reduce the dosage by 20% to 25% each day until withdrawal is complete. In clients with liver disease, accumulation of the longer-acting agents, such as chlordiazepoxide (Librium), may be problematic, and the use of the shorter-acting benzodiazepine, oxazepam (Serax), is more appropriate. Some physicians may order anticonvulsant medication to be used prophylactically; however, this is not a universal intervention. Multivitamin therapy, in combination with daily thiamine (either orally or by injection), is common protocol.

    b. **Narcotics.** Narcotic antagonists, such as naloxone (Narcan), naltrexone (ReVia), or nalmefene (Revex), are administered for opioid intoxication. Withdrawal is managed with rest and nutritional therapy. Substitution therapy may be instituted to decrease withdrawal symptoms using propoxyphene (Darvon) for weaker effects or methadone

(Dolophine) for longer effects. In October 2002, the U.S. Food and Drug Administration approved two forms of the drug buprenorphine for treating opiate dependence. Buprenorphine is less powerful than methadone but is considered to be somewhat safer and causes fewer side effects, making it especially attractive for clients who are mildly or moderately addicted.

c. **Depressants.** Substitution therapy may be instituted to decrease withdrawal symptoms using a long-acting barbiturate, such as phenobarbital (Luminal). Some physicians prescribe oxazepam (Serax) as needed for objective symptoms, gradually decreasing the dosage until the drug is discontinued. Long-acting benzodiazepines are commonly used for substitution therapy when the abused substance is a nonbarbiturate central nervous system depressant.

d. **Stimulants.** Treatment of stimulant intoxication is geared toward stabilization of vital signs. Intravenous antihypertensives may be used, along with intravenous diazepam (Valium) to control seizures. Minor tranquilizers, such as chlordiazepoxide, may be administered orally for the first few days while the client is "crashing." Treatment is aimed at reducing drug craving and managing severe depression. Suicide precautions may be required. Therapy with antidepressant medication is not uncommon.

e. **Hallucinogens and Cannabinols.** Medications are normally not prescribed for withdrawal from these substances. However, in the event of overdose or the occurrence of adverse reactions (e.g., anxiety or panic), benzodiazepines (e.g., diazepam or chlordiazepoxide) may be given as needed to decrease agitation. Should psychotic reactions occur, they may be treated with antipsychotics.

Outcome Criteria

1. Client is no longer exhibiting any signs or symptoms of substance intoxication or withdrawal.
2. Client shows no evidence of physical injury obtained during substance intoxication or withdrawal.

@ INTERNET REFERENCES

Additional information related to forensic nursing may be found at the following websites:

a. http://www.forensiceducation.com/
b. http://www.iafn.org/
c. http://www.amrn.com/
d. http://nursing.advanceweb.com/common/Editorial/Editorial.aspx?CC=40302
e. http://www.forensicnursemag.com

Chapter 23

Complementary Therapies

● INTRODUCTION

The connection between mind and body, and the influence of each on the other, is well recognized by all clinicians, and particularly by psychiatrists. Traditional medicine as it is currently practiced in the United States is based on scientific methodology. Traditional medicine is also known as *allopathic* medicine and is the type historically taught in U.S. medical schools.

The term *alternative medicine* has come to be recognized as practices that differ from the usual traditional practices in the treatment of disease. "Alternative" refers to an intervention that is used *instead of* conventional treatment. "Complementary therapy" is an intervention that is different from, but used *in conjunction with*, traditional or conventional medical treatment. In the United States, approximately 38% of adults and 12% of children use some form of complementary or alternative therapy (National Institutes of Health [NIH], 2008). When prayer specifically for health reasons is included in the definition of alternative medicine, the numbers are even higher. More than $27 billion a year is spent on alternative medical therapies in the United States.

In 1991, an Office of Alternative Medicine (OAM) was established by the NIH to study nontraditional therapies and to evaluate their usefulness and their effectiveness. Since that time, the name has been changed to the National Center for Complementary Medicine and Alternative Medicine (NCCAM or CAM). The mission statement of the CAM states (NIH, 2008):

> NCCAM's mission is to explore complementary and alternative healing practices in the context of rigorous science, train CAM researchers, and disseminate authoritative information to the public and professionals.

Some health insurance companies and health maintenance organizations (HMOs) appear to be bowing to public pressure by including alternative providers in their networks of providers for treatments such as acupuncture and massage therapy. Chiropractic care has been covered by some third-party payers for many years. Individuals who seek alternative therapy, however, are often reimbursed at lower rates than are those who choose traditional practitioners.

Client education is an important part of complementary care. Positive lifestyle changes are encouraged, and practitioners serve as educators as well as treatment specialists. Complementary medicine is viewed as *holistic* health-care, which deals with not only the physical perspective but also the emotional and spiritual components of the individual. Dr. Tom Coniglione, former professor of medicine at the University of Oklahoma Health Sciences Center, has stated,

> We must look at treating the "total person" in order to be more efficient and balanced within the medical community. Even finding doctors who are well-rounded and balanced has become a criterion in the admitting process for medical students. Medicine has changed from just looking at the "scientist perspective of organ and disease" to the total perspective of lifestyle and real impact/results to the patient. This evolution is a progressive and very positive shift in the right direction (Coniglione, 1998, p. 2).

Terms such as *harmony* and *balance* are often associated with complementary care. In fact, restoring harmony and balance between body and mind is often the goal of complementary health-care approaches.

● TYPES OF COMPLEMENTARY THERAPIES

Herbal Medicine

The use of plants to heal is probably as old as humankind. Virtually every culture in the world has relied on herbs and plants to treat illness. Clay tablets from about 4000 B.C. reveal that the Sumerians had apothecaries for dispensing medicinal herbs. At the root of Chinese medicine is the *Pen Tsao*, a Chinese text written around 3000 B.C. that contained hundreds of herbal remedies. When the Pilgrims came to America in the 1600s, they brought with them a variety of herbs to be established and used for medicinal purposes. The new settlers soon discovered that the Native Americans had their own varieties of plants that they used for healing.

Many people are seeking a return to herbal remedies, because they perceive these remedies as being less potent than prescription drugs and as being free of adverse side effects. However, because the U.S. Food and Drug Administration (FDA) classifies herbal remedies as dietary supplements or food additives, their labels cannot indicate medicinal uses. They are not subject to FDA approval, and they lack uniform standards of quality control.

Several organizations have been established to attempt regulation and control of the herbal industry. They include the Council for Responsible Nutrition, the American Herbal Association, and the American Botanical Council. The Commission E of the German Federal Health Agency is the group responsible for researching and regulating the safety and efficacy of herbs and plant medicines in Germany. All of the Commission E monographs of herbal medicines have been translated into English and compiled into one text (Blumenthal, 1998).

Until more extensive testing has been completed on humans and animals, the use of herbal medicines must be approached with caution and responsibility. *The notion that something being "natural" means it is therefore completely safe is a myth.* In fact, some of the plants from which prescription drugs are derived are highly toxic in their natural state. Also, because of lack of regulation and standardization, ingredients may be adulterated. Their method of manufacture also may alter potency. For example, dried herbs lose potency rapidly because of exposure to air. In addition, it is often safer to use preparations that contain only one herb. There is a greater likelihood of unwanted side effects with combined herbal preparations.

Table 23-1 lists information about common herbal remedies, with possible implications for psychiatric/mental health nursing. Botanical names, medicinal uses, and safety profiles are included.

TABLE 23–1 Herbal Remedies

Common Name (Botanical Name)	Medicinal Uses/ Possible Action	Safety Profile
Black cohosh (*Cimicifuga racemosa*)	May provide relief of menstrual cramps; improved mood; calming effect. Extracts from the roots are thought to have action similar to estrogen.	Generally considered safe in low doses. Occasionally causes GI discomfort. Toxic in large doses, causing dizziness, nausea, headaches, stiffness, and trembling. Should not take with heart problems, concurrently with antihypertensives, or during pregnancy.
Cascara sagrada (*Rhamnus purshiana*)	Relief of constipation	Generally recognized as safe; sold as over-the-counter drug in the U.S. Should not be used during pregnancy. Contraindicated in bowel obstruction or inflammation.

TABLE 23–1 Herbal Remedies—cont'd

Common Name (Botanical Name)	Medicinal Uses/ Possible Action	Safety Profile
Chamomile (*Matricaria chamomilla*)	As a tea, is effective as a mild sedative in the relief of insomnia. May also aid digestion, relieve menstrual cramps, and settle upset stomach.	Generally recognized as safe when consumed in reasonable amounts.
Echinacea (*Echinacea angustifolia* and *Echinacea purpurea*)	Stimulates the immune system; may have value in fighting infections and easing the symptoms of colds and flu.	Considered safe in reasonable doses. Observe for side effects or allergic reaction.
Fennel (*Foeniculum vulgare* or *Foeniculum officinale*)	Used to ease stomachaches and to aid digestion. Taken in a tea or in extracts to stimulate the appetites of people with anorexia (1-2 tsp. seeds steeped in boiling water for making tea)	Generally recognized as safe when consumed in reasonable amounts.
Feverfew (*Tanacetum parthenium*)	Prophylaxis and treatment of migraine headaches. Effective in either the fresh leaf or freeze-dried forms (2-3 fresh leaves [or equivalent] per day)	A small percentage of individuals may experience the adverse effect of temporary mouth ulcers. Considered safe in reasonable doses.
Ginger (*Zingiber officinale*)	Ginger tea to ease stomachaches and to aid digestion. Two powdered ginger-root capsules have been shown to be effective in preventing motion sickness.	Generally recognized as safe in designated therapeutic doses.

Continued

TABLE 23–1 Herbal Remedies—cont'd		
Common Name (Botanical Name)	**Medicinal Uses/ Possible Action**	**Safety Profile**
Ginkgo (*Ginkgo biloba*)	Used to treat senility, short-term memory loss, and peripheral insufficiency. Has been shown to dilate blood vessels. Usual dosage is 120-240 mg/day.	Safety has been established with recommended dosages. Possible side effects include headache, GI problems, and dizziness. Contraindicated in pregnancy and lactation and in patients with bleeding disorder. Possible compound effect with concomitant use of aspirin or anticoagulants.
Ginseng (*Panax ginseng*)	The ancient Chinese saw this herb as one that increased wisdom and longevity. Current studies support a possible positive effect on the cardiovascular system. Action not known.	Generally considered safe. Side effects may include headache, insomnia, anxiety, skin rashes, diarrhea. Avoid concomitant use with anticoagulants.
Hops (*Humulus lupulus*)	Used in cases of nervousness, mild anxiety, and insomnia. Also may relieve the cramping associated with diarrhea. May be taken as a tea, in extracts, or capsules.	Generally recognized as safe when consumed in recommended dosages.
Kava-Kava (*Piper methylsticum*)	Used to reduce anxiety while promoting mental acuity. Dosage: 150-300 mg BID.	Scaly skin rash may occur when taken at high dosage for long periods. Motor reflexes and judgment when driving may be reduced while taking the herb. Concurrent use with CNS depressants may produce additive tranquilizing effects. Reports of potential for liver damage. Investigations continue. Should not be taken for longer than 3 months without a physician's supervision.

TABLE 23–1 Herbal Remedies—cont'd

Common Name (Botanical Name)	Medicinal Uses/ Possible Action	Safety Profile
Passion flower (*Passiflora incarnata*)	Used in tea, capsules, or extracts to treat nervousness and insomnia. Depresses the central nervous system to produce a mild sedative effect.	Generally recognized as safe in recommended doses.
Peppermint (*Mentha piperita*)	Used as a tea to relieve upset stomachs and headaches and as a mild sedative. Pour boiling water over 1 tbsp. dried leaves and steep to make a tea. Oil of peppermint is also used for inflammation of the mouth, pharynx, and bronchus.	Considered to be safe when consumed in designated therapeutic dosages.
Psyllium (*Plantago ovata*)	*Psyllium* seeds are a popular bulk laxative commonly used for chronic constipation. Also found to be useful in the treatment of hypercholesterolemia.	Approved as an over-the-counter drug in the U.S.
Scullcap (*Scutellaria lateriflora*)	Used as a sedative for mild anxiety and nervousness.	Considered safe in reasonable amounts.
St. John's Wort (*Hypericum perforatum*)	Used in the treatment of mild to moderate depression. May block reuptake of serotonin/norepinephrine and have a mild monoamine oxide-inhibiting effect. Effective dose: 900 mg/day. May also have antiviral, antibacterial, and anti-inflammatory properties.	Generally recognized as safe when taken at recommended dosages. Side effects include mild GI irritation that is lessened with food; photosensitivity when taken in high dosages over long periods. Should not be taken with other psychoactive medications.

Continued

TABLE 23–1 Herbal Remedies—cont'd

Common Name (Botanical Name)	Medicinal Uses/ Possible Action	Safety Profile
Valerian (*Valeriana officinals*)	Used to treat nervousness and insomnia. Produces restful sleep without morning "hangover." The root may be used to make a tea, or capsules are available in a variety of dosages. Mechanism of action is similar to benzodiazepines, but without addicting properties. Daily dosage range: 100-1000 mg.	Generally recognized as safe when taken at recommended dosages. Side effects may include mild headache or upset stomach. Taking doses higher than recommended may result in severe headache, nausea, morning grogginess, blurry vision. Should not be taken concurrently with CNS depressants.

Sources: Sadock and Sadock (2007), Trivieri and Anderson (2002), Holt and Kouzi (2002), *PDR for Herbal Medicines* (2007), and Pranthikanti (2007).

Acupressure and Acupuncture

Acupressure and acupuncture are healing techniques based on the ancient philosophies of traditional Chinese medicine dating back to 3000 B.C. The main concept behind Chinese medicine is that healing energy (*qi*) flows through the body along specific pathways called *meridians*. It is believed that these meridians of *qi* connect various parts of the body in a way similar to the way in which lines on a road map link various locations. The pathways link a conglomerate of points, called *acupoints*. Therefore, it is possible to treat a part of the body distant to another because they are linked by a meridian. Trivieri and Anderson (2002) have stated, "The proper flow of qi along energy channels (meridians) within the body is crucial to a person's health and vitality."

In acupressure, the fingers, thumbs, palms, or elbows are used to apply pressure to the acupoints. This pressure is thought to dissolve any obstructions in the flow of healing energy and to restore the body to a healthier functioning. In acupuncture, hair-thin, sterile, disposable, stainless-steel needles are inserted into acupoints to dissolve the obstructions along the meridians. The needles may be left in place for a specified length of time, they may be rotated, or a mild electric current may be applied. An occasional tingling or numbness is experienced, but little to no pain is associated with the treatment (NCCAM, 2007).

The Western medical philosophy regarding acupressure and acupuncture is that they stimulate the body's own painkilling chemicals—the morphine-like substances known as *endorphins*. The treatment has been found to be effective in the treatment of asthma, dysmenorrhea, cervical pain, insomnia, anxiety, depression, substance abuse, stroke rehabilitation, nausea of pregnancy, postoperative and chemotherapy-induced nausea and vomiting, tennis elbow, fibromyalgia, low back pain, carpal tunnel syndrome, and many other conditions (Council of Acupuncture and Oriental Medicine Associations [CAOMA], 2009; NCCAM, 2007; Sadock & Sadock, 2007). Recent studies suggest that acupuncture may aid in the treatment of cocaine dependence and chronic daily headaches (Avants et al., 2000; Coeytaux et al., 2005).

Acupuncture is gaining wide acceptance is the United States by both patients and physicians. This treatment can be administered at the same time other techniques are being used, such as conventional Western techniques, although it is essential that all health-care providers have knowledge of all treatments being received. Acupuncture should be administered by a physician or an acupuncturist who is licensed by the state in which the service is provided. Typical training for licensed acupuncturists, doctors of oriental medicine, and acupuncture physicians is a 3- or 4-year program of 2500 to 3500 hours.

Diet and Nutrition

The value of nutrition in the healing process has long been underrated. Lutz and Przytulski (2006) stated:

> Today many diseases are linked to lifestyle behaviors such as smoking, lack of adequate physical activity, and poor nutritional habits. The World Health Organization (WHO) reports that nearly one-third of early death and disability stems from nutritional or dietary causes. Healthcare providers emphasize the relationship between lifestyle and the risk of disease. Many people, at least in industrialized countries, are increasingly managing their health problems and making personal commitments to lead healthier lives. Nutrition is, in part, a preventive science. Given sufficient resources, how and what one eats is a lifestyle choice (p. 4).

Individuals select the foods they eat based on a number of factors, not the least of which is enjoyment. Eating must serve social and cultural, as well as nutritional, needs. The U.S. Department of Agriculture (USDA) and Department of Health and Human Services (USDHHS) have collaborated on a set of guidelines to help individuals understand what types of foods to eat and the healthy lifestyle they need to pursue in order to promote health and prevent disease. Following is a list of key recommendations from these guidelines (USDA/USDHHS, 2005).

1. Adequate Nutrients within Calorie Needs

a. Consume a variety of nutrient-dense foods and beverages within and among the basic food groups while choosing foods that limit the intakes of fat, cholesterol, added sugars, salt, and alcohol.

b. Meet recommended intakes within energy needs by adopting a balanced eating pattern, such as the guidelines in Table 23-2. Table 23-3 provides a summary of information about essential vitamins and minerals.

TABLE 23–2 Sample USDA Food Guide at the 2000-Calorie Level

Food Groups and Subgroups	USDA Food Guide Daily Amount	Examples/Equivalent Amounts
Fruit group	2 cups (4 servings)	½ cup equivalent is: • ½ cup fresh, frozen, or canned fruit • 1 medium fruit • ¼ cup dried fruit • ½ cup fruit juice
Vegetable group	2.5 cups (5 servings) • Dark green vegetables: 3 cups/week • Orange vegetables: 2 cups/week • Legumes (dry beans/peas): 3 cups/week • Starchy vegetables: 3 cups/week • Other vegetables: 6.5 cups/week	½ cup equivalent is: • ½ cup cut-up raw or cooked vegetable • 1 cup raw leafy vegetable • ½ cup vegetable juice
Grain group	6 ounce-equivalents • Whole grains: 3 ounce-equivalents • Other grains: 3 ounce-equivalents	1 ounce-equivalent is: • 1 slice bread • 1 cup dry cereal • ½ cup cooked rice, pasta, cereal
Meat and beans group	5.5 ounce-equivalents	1 ounce-equivalent is: • 1 oz. cooked lean meat, poultry, or fish • 1 egg • ¼ cup cooked dry beans or tofu • 1 tbsp. peanut butter • ½ oz. nuts or seeds

Complementary Therapies • 379

TABLE 23–2 Sample USDA Food Guide at the 2000-Calorie Level—cont'd

Food Groups and Subgroups	USDA Food Guide Daily Amount	Examples/ Equivalent Amounts
Milk group	3 cups	1 cup equivalent is: • 1 cup low fat/fat-free milk • 1 cup low fat/fat-free yogurt • 1½ oz low-fat or fat-free natural cheese • 2 oz. low-fat or fat-free processed cheese
Oils	24 grams (6 tsp.)	1 tsp. equivalent is: • 1 tbsp. low-fat mayo • 2 tbsp. light salad dressing • 1 tsp. vegetable oil • 1 tsp. soft margarine with zero *trans*-fat
Discretionary calorie allowance	267 calories Example of distribution: • Solid fats 18 grams (e.g., saturated & *trans* fats) • Added sugars 32 grams (8 tsp.) (e.g., sweetened cereals)	1 tbsp. added sugar equivalent is: • ½ oz. jelly beans • 8 oz. lemonade Examples of solid fats: • Fat in whole milk/ice cream • Fatty meats Essential oils (above) are not considered part of the discretionary calories

Source: *Dietary Guidelines for Americans 2005*. Washington, D.C.: USDA/USDHHS, 2005.

2. Weight Management
a. Maintain body weight in a healthy range; balance calories from foods and beverages with calories expended.
b. To prevent gradual weight gain over time, make small decreases in food and beverage calories and increase physical activity.

3. Physical Activity
a. Engage in regular physical activity and reduce sedentary activities to promote health, psychological well-being, and a healthy body weight.
b. To reduce the risk of chronic disease in adulthood, engage in at least 30 minutes of moderate-intensity physical activity, above usual activity, at work or home on most days of the week.

TABLE 23–3 Essential Vitamins and Minerals

Vitamin/Mineral	Function	New DRI (UL)*	Food Sources	Comments
Vitamin A	Prevention of night blindness; calcification of growing bones; resistance to infection	Men: 900 mcg (3000 mcg) Women: 700 mcg (3000 mcg)	Liver, butter, cheese, whole milk, egg yolk, fish, green leafy vegetables, carrots, pumpkin, sweet potatoes	May be of benefit in prevention of cancer, because of its antioxidant properties, which are associated with control of free radicals that damage DNA and cell membranes.
Vitamin D	Promotes absorption of calcium and phosphorus in the small intestine; prevention of rickets	Men and women: 5 mcg (50 mcg) (5–10 for ages 50–70 and 15 for >70)	Fortified milk and dairy products, egg yolk, fish liver oils, liver, oysters; formed in the skin by exposure to sunlight	Without vitamin D, very little dietary calcium can be absorbed.
Vitamin E	An antioxidant that prevents cell membrane destruction	Men and women: 15 mg (1000 mg)	Vegetable oils, wheat germ, whole grain or fortified cereals, green leafy vegetables, nuts	As an antioxidant, may have implications in the prevention of Alzheimer's disease, heart disease, breast cancer
Vitamin K	Synthesis of prothrombin and other clotting factors; normal blood coagulation	Men: 120 mcg (ND)*** Women: 90 mcg (ND)***	Green vegetables (collards, spinach, lettuce, kale, broccoli, brussels sprouts, cabbage), plant oils, and margarine	Individuals on anticoagulant therapy should monitor vitamin K intake.
Vitamin C	Formation of collagen in connective tissues; a powerful antioxidant; facilitates iron absorption; aids in the release of epinephrine from the adrenal glands during stress	Men: 90 mg (2000 mg) Women: 75 mg (2000 mg)	Citrus fruits, tomatoes, potatoes, green leafy vegetables, strawberries	As an antioxidant, may have implications in the prevention of cancer, cataracts, heart disease. It may stimulate the immune system to fight various types of infection.

	Function	Dosage	Sources	Comments
Vitamin B$_1$ (thiamine)	Essential for normal functioning of nervous tissue; coenzyme in carbohydrate metabolism	Men: 1.2 mg (ND)*** Women: 1.1 mg (ND)***	Whole grains, legumes, nuts, egg yolk, meat, green leafy vegetables	Large doses may improve mental performance in people with Alzheimer's disease.
Vitamin B$_2$ (riboflavin)	Coenzyme in the metabolism of protein and carbohydrate for energy	Men: 1.3 mg (ND)*** Women: 1.1 mg (ND)***	Meat, dairy products, whole or enriched grains, legumes, nuts	May help in the prevention of cataracts; high-dose therapy may be effective in migraine prophylaxis (Schoenen et al., 1998).
Vitamin B$_3$ (niacin)	Coenzyme in the metabolism of protein and carbohydrates for energy	Men: 16 mg (35 mg) Women: 14 mg (35 mg)	Milk, eggs, meats, legumes, whole grain and enriched cereals, nuts	High doses of niacin have been successful in decreasing levels of cholesterol in some individuals.
Vitamin B$_6$ (pyridoxine)	Coenzyme in the synthesis and catabolism of amino acids; essential for metabolism of tryptophan to niacin	Men and women: 1.3 mg (100 mg) After age 50: Men: 1.7 mg Women: 1.5 mg	Meat, fish, grains, legumes, bananas, nuts, white and sweet potatoes	May decrease depression in some individuals by increasing levels of serotonin; deficiencies may contribute to memory problems; also used in the treatment of migraines and premenstrual discomfort.
Vitamin B$_{12}$	Necessary in the formation of DNA and the production of red blood cells; associated with folic acid metabolism	Men and women: 2.4 mcg (ND)***	Found in animal products (e.g., meats, eggs, dairy products)	Deficiency may contribute to memory problems. Vegetarians can get this vitamin from fortified foods. Intrinsic factor must be present in the stomach for absorption of vitamin B$_{12}$.

Continued

TABLE 23 – 3 Essential Vitamins and Minerals—cont'd

Vitamin/Mineral	Function	New DRI (UL)*	Food Sources	Comments
Folic acid (folate)	Necessary in the formation of DNA and the production of red blood cells	Men and women: 400 mcg (1000 mcg) Pregnant women: 600 mcg	Meat; green leafy vegetables; beans; peas; fortified cereals, breads, rice, and pasta	Important in women of child-bearing age to prevent fetal neural tube defects; may contribute to prevention of heart disease and colon cancer.
Calcium	Necessary in the formation of bones and teeth; neuron and muscle functioning; blood clotting	Men and women: 1000 mg (2500 mg) After age 50: Men and women: 1200 mg	Dairy products, kale, broccoli, spinach, sardines, oysters, salmon	Calcium has been associated with preventing headaches, muscle cramps, osteoporosis, and pre-menstrual problems. Requires vitamin D for absorption.
Phosphorus	Necessary in the formation of bones and teeth; a component of DNA, RNA, ADP, and ATP; helps control acid-base balance in the blood	Men and women: 700 mg (4000 mg)	Milk, cheese, fish, meat, yogurt, ice cream, peas, eggs	
Magnesium	Protein synthesis and carbohydrate metabolism; muscular relaxation following contraction; bone formation	Men: 420 mg (350 mg)** Women: 320 mg (350 mg)**	Green vegetables, legumes, seafood, milk, nuts, meat	May aid in prevention of asthmatic attacks and migraine headaches. Deficiencies may contribute to insomnia, pre-menstrual problems.

	Function	Amount	Sources	Notes
Iron	Synthesis of hemoglobin and myoglobin; cellular oxidation	Men: 8 mg (45 mg); Women: (45 mg) Childbearing age: 18 mg; Over 50: 8 mg; Pregnant: 27 mg; Breastfeeding: 9 mg	Meat, fish, poultry, eggs, nuts, dark green leafy vegetables, dried fruit, enriched pasta and bread	Iron deficiencies can result in headaches and feeling chronically fatigued.
Iodine	Aids in the synthesis of T_3 and T_4	Men and women: 150 mcg (1100 mcg)	Iodized salt, seafood	Exerts strong controlling influence on overall body metabolism.
Selenium	Works with Vitamin E to protect cellular compounds from oxidation	Men and women: 55 mcg (400 mcg)	Seafood, low-fat meats, dairy products, liver	As an antioxidant combined with vitamin E, may have some anti-cancer effect. Deficiency has also been associated with depressed mood.
Zinc	Involved in synthesis of DNA and RNA; energy metabolism and protein synthesis; wound healing; increased immune functioning; necessary for normal smell and taste sensation.	Men: 11 mg (40 mg); Women: 8 mg (40 mg)	Meat, seafood, fortified cereals, poultry, eggs, milk	An important source for the prevention of infection and improvement in wound healing.

* Dietary Reference Intakes (UL), the most recent set of dietary recommendations for adults established by the Food and Nutrition Board of the Institute of Medicine, © 2004. UL is the upper limit of intake considered to be safe for use by adults (includes total intake from food, water, and supplements). In addition to the UL, DRIs are composed of the Recommended Dietary Allowance (RDA, the amount considered sufficient to meet the requirements of 97% to 98% of all healthy individuals) and the Adequate Intake (AI, the amount considered sufficient where no RDA has been established).

** UL for magnesium applies only to intakes from dietary supplements, excluding intakes from food and water.

*** ND = Not determined

Source: Adapted from National Academies of Sciences (2004).

    c. To help manage body weight and prevent gradual, unhealthy body weight gain in adulthood, engage in approximately 60 minutes of moderate- to vigorous-intensity activity on most days of the week while not exceeding caloric intake requirements.

    d. To sustain weight loss in adulthood, participate in at least 60 to 90 minutes of daily moderate-intensity physical activity while not exceeding caloric intake requirements.

    e. Achieve physical fitness by including cardiovascular conditioning, stretching exercises for flexibility, and resistance exercises or calisthenics for muscle strength and endurance.

4. **Food Groups to Encourage**

    a. **Fruits and Vegetables.** Choose a variety of fruits and vegetables each day. In particular, select from all five vegetable subgroups several times a week.

    b. **Whole Grains.** Half the daily servings of grains should come from whole grains.

    c. **Milk and Milk Products.** Daily choices of fat-free or low-fat milk or milk products are important. To help meet calcium needs, non-dairy calcium-containing alternatives may be selected by individuals with lactose intolerance or those who choose to avoid all milk products (e.g., vegans).

5. **Food Groups to Moderate**

    a. **Fats.** Keep total fat intake between 20% and 35% of calories, with most fats coming from sources of polyunsaturated and monounsaturated fatty acids, such as fish, nuts, and vegetable oils. Consume less than 10% of calories from saturated fatty acids and less than 300 mg/day of cholesterol, and keep *trans*–fatty acid consumption as low as possible.

    b. **Carbohydrates.** Carbohydrate intake should comprise 45% to 64% of total calories, with the majority coming from fiber-rich foods. Important sources of nutrients from carbohydrates include fruits, vegetables, whole grains, and milk. Added sugars, caloric sweeteners, and refined starches should be used prudently.

    c. **Sodium Chloride.** Consume less than 2300 mg (approximately 1 teaspoon of salt) of sodium per day. Choose and prepare foods with little salt. At the same time, consume potassium-rich foods, such as fruits and vegetables.

    d. **Alcoholic Beverages.** Individuals who choose to drink alcoholic beverages should do so sensibly and in moderation— defined as the consumption of up to one drink per day for women and up to two drinks per day for men. One drink should count as:

- 12 ounces of regular beer (150 calories)
- 5 ounces of wine (100 calories)
- 1.5 ounces of 80-proof distilled spirits (100 calories)

Alcohol should be avoided by individuals who are unable to restrict their intake; women who are pregnant, may become pregnant, or are breastfeeding and individuals who are taking medications that may interact with alcohol or who have specific medical conditions.

Chiropractic Medicine

Chiropractic medicine is probably the most widely used form of alternative healing in the United States. It was developed in the late 1800s by a self-taught healer named David Palmer. It was later reorganized and expanded by his son Joshua, a trained practitioner. Palmer's objective was to find a cure for disease and illness that did not use drugs but instead relied on more natural methods of healing (Trivieri & Anderson, 2002). Palmer's theory of chiropractic medicine was that energy flows from the brain to all parts of the body through the spinal cord and spinal nerves. When vertebrae of the spinal column become displaced, they may press on a nerve and interfere with the normal nerve transmission. Palmer named the displacement of these vertebrae *subluxation*, and he alleged that the way to restore normal function was to manipulate the vertebrae back into their normal positions. These manipulations are called *adjustments*.

Adjustments are usually performed by hand, although some chiropractors have special treatment tables equipped to facilitate these manipulations. Other processes used to facilitate the outcome of the spinal adjustment by providing muscle relaxation include massage tables, application of heat or cold, and ultrasound treatments.

The chiropractor takes a medical history and performs a clinical examination, which usually includes x-ray films of the spine. Today's chiropractors may practice "straight" therapy—that is, the only therapy provided is that of subluxation adjustments. *Mixer* is a term applied to a chiropractor who combines adjustments with adjunct therapies, such as exercise, heat treatments, or massage.

Individuals seek treatment from chiropractors for many types of ailments and illnesses; the most common is back pain. In addition, chiropractors treat clients with headaches, neck injuries, scoliosis, carpal tunnel syndrome, respiratory and gastrointestinal disorders, menstrual difficulties, allergies, sinusitis, and certain sports injuries (Trivieri & Anderson, 2002). Some chiropractors are employed by professional sports teams as their team physicians.

Chiropractors are licensed to practice in all 50 states and treatment costs are covered by government and most private insurance plans. They treat more than 20 million people in the United States annually (Sadock & Sadock, 2007).

Therapeutic Touch and Massage

Therapeutic Touch

The technique of therapeutic touch was developed in the 1970s by Dolores Krieger, a nurse associated with the New York University School of Nursing. This therapy is based on the philosophy that the human body projects a field of energy around it. When this field of energy becomes blocked, pain or illness occurs. Practitioners of therapeutic touch use this technique to correct the blockages, thereby relieving the discomfort and improving health.

Based on the premise that the energy field extends beyond the surface of the body, the practitioner need not actually touch the client's skin. The therapist's hands are passed over the client's body, remaining 2 to 4 inches from the skin. The goal is to repattern the energy field by performing slow, rhythmic, sweeping hand motions over the entire body. Heat should be felt where the energy is blocked. The therapist "massages" the energy field in that area, smoothing it out, and thus correcting the obstruction. Therapeutic touch is thought to reduce pain and anxiety and promote relaxation and health maintenance. It has been useful in the treatment of chronic health conditions.

Massage

Massage is the technique of manipulating the muscles and soft tissues of the body. Chinese physicians prescribed massage for the treatment of disease more than 5000 years ago. The Eastern style focuses on balancing the body's vital energy (*qi*) as it flows through pathways (meridians), as described earlier in the discussion of acupressure and acupuncture. The Western style of massage affects muscles, connective tissues (e.g., tendons and ligaments), and the cardiovascular system. Swedish massage, which is probably the best-known Western style, uses a variety of gliding and kneading strokes along with deep circular movements and vibrations to relax the muscles, improve circulation, and increase mobility (Trivieri & Anderson, 2002).

Massage has been shown to be beneficial in the following conditions: anxiety, chronic back and neck pain, arthritis, sciatica, migraine headaches, muscle spasms, insomnia, pain of labor and delivery, stress-related disorders, and whiplash. Massage is contraindicated in certain conditions, such as high blood pressure, acute infection, osteoporosis, phlebitis, skin conditions, and varicose veins. It also should not be performed over the site of a recent injury, bruise, or burn.

Massage therapists require specialized training in a program accredited by the American Massage Therapy Association and must pass the National Certification Examination for Therapeutic Massage and Bodywork.

Yoga

Yoga is thought to have developed in India some 5000 years ago and is attributed to an Indian physician and Sanskrit scholar named Patanjali. The objective of yoga is to integrate the physical, mental, and spiritual energies that enhance health and well-being (Trivieri & Anderson, 2002). Yoga has been found to be especially helpful in relieving stress and in improving overall physical and psychological wellness. Proper breathing is a major component of yoga. It is believed that yoga breathing—a deep, diaphramatic breathing—increases oxygen to the brain and body tissues, thereby easing stress and fatigue and boosting energy.

Another component of yoga is meditation. Individuals who practice the meditation and deep breathing associated with yoga find that they are able to achieve a profound feeling of relaxation.

The most familiar type of yoga practiced in Western countries is hatha yoga. Hatha yoga uses body postures, along with the meditation and breathing exercises, to achieve a balanced, disciplined workout that releases muscle tension, tones the internal organs, and energizes the mind, body, and spirit, to allow natural healing to occur. The complete routine of poses is designed to work all parts of the body—stretching and toning muscles and keeping joints flexible. Studies have shown that yoga has provided beneficial effects to some individuals with back pain, stress, migraine, insomnia, high blood pressure, rapid heart rates, and limited mobility (Sadock & Sadock, 2007; Steinberg, 2002; Trivieri & Anderson, 2002).

Pet Therapy

The therapeutic value of pets is no longer just theory. Evidence has shown that animals can directly influence a person's mental and physical well-being. Many pet-therapy programs have been established across the country and the numbers are increasing regularly.

Several studies have provided information about the positive results of human interaction with pets. Some of these include the following:

1. Petting a dog or cat has been shown to lower blood pressure. In one study, volunteers experienced a 7.1 mm Hg drop in systolic and an 8.1 mm Hg decrease in diastolic blood pressure when they talked to and petted their dogs, as opposed to reading aloud or resting quietly (Whitaker, 2000).
2. Bringing a pet into a nursing home or other institution for the elderly has been shown to enhance a client's mood and

social interaction (Godenne, 2001). Another study revealed that animal-assisted therapy with nursing home residents significantly reduced loneliness for those in the study group (Banks & Banks, 2002).

3. One study of 96 patients who had been admitted to a coronary care unit for heart attack or angina revealed that in the year following hospitalization, the mortality rate among those who did not own pets was 22% higher than that among pet owners (Whitaker, 2000).

4. Individuals with AIDS who have pets are less likely to suffer from depression than people with AIDS who do not own pets (Siegel et al., 1999).

Some researchers believe that animals may actually retard the aging process among those who live alone. Loneliness often results in premature death, and having a pet mitigates the effects of loneliness and isolation.

Whitaker (2000) has suggested:

> Though owning a pet doesn't make you immune to illness, pet owners are, on the whole, healthier than those who don't own pets. Study after study shows that people with pets have fewer minor health problems, require fewer visits to the doctor and less medication, and have fewer risk factors for heart disease, such as high blood pressure or cholesterol levels (p. 7).

It may never be known precisely why animals affect humans they way they do, but for those who have pets to love, the therapeutic benefits come as no surprise. Pets provide unconditional, nonjudgmental love and affection, which can be the perfect antidote for a depressed mood or a stressful situation. The role of animals in the human healing process requires more research, but its validity is now widely accepted in both the medical and lay communities.

● SUMMARY

Complementary therapies help the practitioner view the client in a holistic manner. Most complementary therapies consider the mind and body connection and strive to enhance the body's own natural healing powers. The OAM of the NIH has established a list of alternative therapies to be used in practice and for investigative purposes. More than $27 billion a year is spent on alternative medical therapies in the United States.

This chapter examined herbal medicine, acupressure, acupuncture, diet and nutrition, chiropractic medicine, therapeutic touch, massage, yoga, and pet therapy. Nurses must be familiar with these therapies, as more and more clients seek out the healing properties of these complementary care strategies.

INTERNET REFERENCES

a. http://www.herbalgram.org/
b. http://www.herbmed.org/
c. http://nutritiondata.self.com/
d. http://www.nutrition.gov/
e. http://www.chiropractic.org/
f. http://www.pawssf.org/
g. http://www.therapydogs.com/
h. http://www.angelonaleash.org/
i. http://www.holisticmed.com/www/acupuncture.html
j. http://www.americanyogaassociation.org/

Loss and Bereavement

● BACKGROUND ASSESSMENT DATA

Loss is the experience of separation from something of personal importance. Loss is anything that is perceived as such by the individual. The separation from loved ones or the giving up of treasured possessions, for whatever reason; the experience of failure, either real or perceived; or life events that create change in a familiar pattern of existence—all can be experienced as loss, and all can trigger behaviors associated with the grieving process. Loss and bereavement are universal events encountered by all beings who experience emotions. Following are examples of some notable forms of loss:

1. A significant other (person or pet) through death, divorce, or separation for any reason.
2. Illness or debilitating conditions. Examples include (but are not limited to) diabetes, stroke, cancer, rheumatoid arthritis, multiple sclerosis, Alzheimer's disease, hearing or vision loss, and spinal cord or head injuries. Some of these conditions not only incur a loss of physical and/or emotional wellness but may also result in the loss of personal independence.
3. Developmental/maturational changes or situations, such as menopause, andropause, infertility, "empty nest" syndrome, aging, impotence, or hysterectomy.
4. A decrease in self-esteem, if one is unable to meet self-expectations or the expectations of others (even if these expectations are only perceived by the individual as unfulfilled). This includes a loss of potential hopes and dreams.
5. Personal possessions that symbolize familiarity and security in a person's life. Separation from these familiar and personally valued external objects represents a loss of material extensions of the self.

Some texts differentiate the terms *mourning* and *grief* by describing mourning as the psychological process (or stages) through which the individual passes on the way to successful adaptation to the loss of a valued object. Grief may be viewed as the subjective states that accompany mourning, or the emotional work involved in the mourning process. For purposes of this text, grief work and the process of mourning are collectively referred to as the *grief response.*

Theoretical Perspectives on Loss and Bereavement (Symptomatology)

Stages of Grief

Behavior patterns associated with the grief response include many individual variations. However, sufficient similarities have been observed to warrant characterization of grief as a syndrome that has a predictable course with an expected resolution. Early theorists, including Kübler-Ross (1969), Bowlby (1961), and Engel (1964), described behavioral stages through which individuals advance in their progression toward resolution. A number of variables influence one's progression through the grief process. Some individuals may reach acceptance, only to revert to an earlier stage; some may never complete the sequence; and some may never progress beyond the initial stage.

A more contemporary grief specialist, J. William Worden (2009), offers a set of tasks that must be processed to complete the grief response. He suggests that it is possible for a person to accomplish some of these tasks and not others, resulting in an incomplete bereavement and thus impairing further growth and development.

ELISABETH KÜBLER-ROSS

These well-known stages of the grief process were identified by Kübler-Ross in her extensive work with dying patients. Behaviors associated with each of these stages can be observed in individuals experiencing the loss of any concept of personal value.

Stage I: Denial. The individual does not acknowledge that the loss has occurred. He or she may say, "No, it can't be true!" or "It's just not possible." This stage may protect the individual against the psychological pain of reality.

Stage II: Anger. This is the stage when reality sets in. Feelings associated with this stage include sadness, guilt, shame, helplessness, and hopelessness. Self-blame or blaming of others may lead to feelings of anger toward the self and others. The anxiety level may be elevated, and the individual may experience confusion and a decreased ability to function independently. He or she may be preoccupied with an idealized image of what has been lost. Numerous somatic complaints are common.

Stage III: Bargaining. The individual attempts to strike a bargain with God for a second chance or for more time.

The person acknowledges the loss, or impending loss, but holds out hope for additional alternatives, as evidenced by such statements as, "If only I could..." or "If only I had... ."

Stage IV: Depression. The individual mourns for that which has been or will be lost. This is a very painful stage, during which the individual must confront feelings associated with having lost someone or something of value (called *reactive* depression). An example might be the individual who is mourning a change in body image. Feelings associated with an impending loss (called *preparatory* depression) are also confronted. Examples include permanent lifestyle changes related to the altered body image or even an impending loss of life itself. Regression, withdrawal, and social isolation may be observed behaviors with this stage. Therapeutic intervention should be available, but not imposed, and with guidelines for implementation based on client readiness.

Stage V: Acceptance. The individual has worked through the behaviors associated with the other stages and either accepts or is resigned to the loss. Anxiety decreases, and methods for coping with the loss have been established. The client is less preoccupied with what has been lost and increasingly interested in other aspects of the environment. If this is an impending death of self, the individual is ready to die. The person may become very quiet and withdrawn, seemingly devoid of feelings. These behaviors are an attempt to facilitate the passage by slowly disengaging from the environment.

JOHN BOWLBY

John Bowlby hypothesized four stages in the grief process. He implied that these behaviors can be observed in all individuals who have experienced the loss of something or someone of value, even in infants as young as 6 months.

Stage I: Numbness or Protest. This stage is characterized by a feeling of shock and disbelief that the loss has occurred. Reality of the loss is not acknowledged.

Stage II: Disequilibrium. During this stage, the individual has a profound urge to recover what has been lost. Behaviors associated with this stage include a preoccupation with the loss, intense weeping and expressions of anger toward the self and others, and feelings of ambivalence and guilt associated with the loss.

Stage III: Disorganization and Despair. Feelings of despair occur in response to the realization that the loss has occurred. Activities of daily living become increasingly disorganized, and behavior is characterized by restlessness and aimlessness. Efforts to regain productive patterns of behavior are ineffective and the individual experiences fear, helplessness, and hopelessness. Somatic complaints are common. Perceptions of visualizing or being in the presence of that which has been lost may occur. Social isolation is common, and the individual may feel a great deal of loneliness.

Stage IV: Reorganization. The individual accepts or becomes resigned to the loss. New goals and patterns of organization are established. The individual begins a reinvestment in new relationships and indicates a readiness to move forward within the environment. Grief subsides and recedes into valued remembrances.

GEORGE ENGEL

Stage I: Shock and Disbelief. The initial reaction to a loss is a stunned, numb feeling and refusal by the individual to acknowledge the reality of the loss. Engel states that this stage is an attempt by the individual to protect the self "against the effects of the overwhelming stress by raising the threshold against its recognition or against the painful feelings evoked thereby."

Stage II: Developing Awareness. This stage begins within minutes to hours of the loss. Behaviors associated with this stage include excessive crying and regression to a state of helplessness and a childlike manner. Awareness of the loss creates feelings of emptiness, frustration, anguish, and despair. Anger may be directed toward the self or toward others in the environment who are held accountable for the loss.

Stage III: Restitution. The various rituals associated with loss within a culture are performed. Examples include funerals, wakes, special attire, a gathering of friends and family, and religious practices customary to the spiritual beliefs of the bereaved. Participation in these rituals is thought to assist the individual to accept the reality of the loss and to facilitate the recovery process.

Stage IV: Resolution of the Loss. This stage is characterized by a preoccupation with the loss. The concept of the loss is idealized, and the individual may even imitate admired qualities of a person who has been lost. Preoccupation with the loss gradually decreases over a year or more, and the individual eventually begins to reinvest feelings in others.

Stage V: Recovery. Obsession with the loss has ended, and the individual is able to go on with his or her life.

J. WILLIAM WORDEN

Worden views the bereaved as active and self-determining rather than passive participants in the grief process. He proposes that bereavement includes a set of tasks that must be reconciled in order to complete the grief process. Worden's four tasks of mourning include the following:

Task I: Accepting the Reality of the Loss. When something of value is lost, it is common for individuals to refuse to believe that the loss has occurred. Behaviors include misidentifying individuals in the environment for their lost loved one, retaining possessions of the lost loved one as though he or she has not died, and removing all reminders of the lost loved one so as not to have to face the reality of the loss. Worden (2009) stated:

Coming to an acceptance of the reality of the loss takes time since it involves not only an intellectual acceptance but also an emotional one. The bereaved person may be intellectually aware of the finality of the loss long before the emotions allow full acceptance of the information as true (p. 42).

Belief and denial are intermittent while grappling with this task. It is thought that traditional rituals such as the funeral help some individuals move toward acceptance of the loss.

Task II: Processing the Pain of Grief. Pain associated with a loss includes both physical pain and emotional pain. This pain must be acknowledged and worked through. To avoid or suppress it serves only to delay or prolong the grieving process. People accomplish this by refusing to allow themselves to think painful thoughts, by idealizing or avoiding reminders of what has been lost, and by using alcohol or drugs. The intensity of the pain and the manner in which it is experienced are different for all individuals. But the commonality is that it *must* be experienced. Failure to do so generally results in some form of depression that commonly requires therapy, which then focuses on working through the pain of grief that the individual failed to work through at the time of the loss. In this very difficult Task II, individuals must "allow themselves to process the pain—to feel it and to know that one day it will pass" (Worden, 2009, p. 45).

Task III: Adjusting to a World without the Lost Entity. It usually takes a number of months for a bereaved person to realize what his or her world will be like without the lost entity. In the case of a lost loved one, how the environment changes will depend on the types of roles that person fulfilled in life. In the case of a changed lifestyle, the individual will be required to make adaptations to his or her environment in terms of the changes as they are presented in daily life. In addition, those individuals who had defined their identity through the lost entity will require an adjustment to their own sense of self. Worden (2009) stated, "The coping strategy of redefining the loss in such a way that it can redound to the benefit of the survivor is often part of the successful completion of Task III" (p. 47).

If the bereaved person experiences failures in his or her attempt to adjust in an environment without the lost entity, feelings of low self-esteem may result. Regressed behaviors and feelings of helplessness and inadequacy are not uncommon. Worden (2009) stated:

[Another] area of adjustment may be to one's sense of the world. Loss through death can challenge one's fundamental life values and philosophical beliefs—beliefs that are influenced by our families, peers, education, and religion as well as life experiences. The bereaved person searches for meaning in the loss and its attendant life changes in order to make sense of it and to regain some control of his or her life (pp. 48–49).

To be successful in Task III, bereaved individuals must develop new skills to cope and adapt to their new environment without the lost entity. Successful achievement of this task determines the outcome of the mourning process—that of continued growth or a state of arrested development.

Task IV: Finding an Enduring Connection with the Lost Entity in the Midst of Embarking on a New Life. This task allows for the bereaved person to identify a special place for the lost entity. Individuals need not purge from their history or find a replacement for that which has been lost. Instead, there is a kind of continued presence of the lost entity that only becomes *relocated* in the life of the bereaved. Successful completion of Task IV involves letting go of past attachments and forming new ones. However, there is also the recognition that although the relationship between the bereaved and what has been lost is changed, it is nonetheless still a relationship. Worden (2009) suggests that one never loses memories of a significant relationship. He stated:

For many people Task IV is the most difficult one to accomplish. They get stuck at this point in their grieving and later realize that their life in some way stopped at the point the loss occurred (p. 52).

Worden (2009) relates the story of a teenaged girl who had a difficult time adjusting to the death of her father. After 2 years, when she began to finally fulfill some of the tasks associated with successful grieving, she wrote these words that express rather clearly what bereaved people in Task IV are struggling with: "There are other people to be loved, and it doesn't mean that I love Dad any less" (p. 52).

Length of the Grief Process

Stages of grief allow bereaved persons an orderly approach to the resolution of mourning. Each stage presents tasks that must be overcome through a painful experiential process. Engel (1964) stated that successful resolution of the grief response is thought to have occurred when a bereaved individual is able "to remember comfortably and realistically both the pleasures and disappointments of [what has been lost]." The duration of the grief process depends on the individual and can last for a number of years without being maladaptive. The acute phase of normal grieving usually lasts 6 to 8 weeks—longer in older adults—but complete resolution of the grief response may take much longer. Sadock and Sadock (2007) stated:

> Ample evidence suggests that the bereavement process does not end within a prescribed interval; certain aspects persist indefinitely for many otherwise high-functioning, normal individuals. Common manifestations of protracted grief occur intermittently. Most grief does not fully resolve or permanently disappear; rather grief becomes circumscribed and submerged only to reemerge in response to certain triggers (p. 64).

A number of factors influence the eventual outcome of the grief response. The grief response can be more difficult if:

- The bereaved person was strongly dependent on or perceived the lost entity as an important means of physical and/or emotional support.
- The relationship with the lost entity was highly ambivalent. A love-hate relationship may instill feelings of guilt that can interfere with the grief work.
- The individual has experienced a number of recent losses. Grief tends to be cumulative, and if previous losses have not been resolved, each succeeding grief response becomes more difficult.
- The loss is that of a young person. Grief over loss of a child is often more intense than it is over the loss of an elderly person.
- The state of the person's physical or psychological health is unstable at the time of the loss.
- The bereaved person perceives (whether real or imagined) some responsibility for the loss.

The grief response may be facilitated if:

- The individual has the support of significant others to assist him or her through the mourning process.
- The individual has the opportunity to prepare for the loss. Grief work is more intense when the loss is sudden and unexpected. The experience of anticipatory grieving is thought to facilitate the grief response that occurs at the time of the actual loss.

Worden (2009) stated:

> There is a sense in which mourning can be finished, when people regain an interest in life, feel more hopeful, experience gratification again, and adapt to new roles. There is also a sense in which mourning is never finished. [People must understand] that mourning is a long-term process, and the culmination [very likely] will not be to a pre-grief state (p. 77).

Anticipatory Grief

Anticipatory grieving is the experiencing of the feelings and emotions associated with the normal grief response before the loss actually occurs. One dissimilar aspect relates to the fact that conventional grief tends to diminish in intensity with the passage of time. Anticipatory grief can become more intense as the expected loss becomes imminent.

Although anticipatory grief is thought to facilitate the actual mourning process following the loss, there may be some problems. In the case of a dying person, difficulties can arise when the family members complete the process of anticipatory grief, and detachment from the dying person occurs prematurely. The person who is dying experiences feelings of loneliness and isolation as the psychological pain of imminent death is faced without family support. Another example of difficulty associated with premature completion of the grief response is one that can occur on the return of persons long absent and presumed dead (e.g., soldiers missing in action or prisoners of war). In this instance, resumption of the previous relationship may be difficult for the bereaved person.

Anticipatory grieving may serve as a defense for some individuals to ease the burden of loss when it actually occurs. It may prove to be less functional for others who, because of interpersonal, psychological, or sociocultural variables, are unable in advance of the actual loss to express the intense feelings that accompany the grief response.

Maladaptive Responses to Loss

When, then, is the grieving response considered to be maladaptive? Three types of pathological grief reactions have been described. These include delayed or inhibited grief, an exaggerated or distorted grief response, and chronic or prolonged grief.

Delayed or Inhibited Grief

Delayed or inhibited grief refers to the absence of evidence of grief when it ordinarily would be expected. Many times, cultural influences, such as the expectation to keep a "stiff upper lip," cause the delayed response.

Delayed or inhibited grief is potentially pathological because the person is simply not dealing with the reality of the loss.

He or she remains fixed in the denial stage of the grief process, sometimes for many years. When this occurs, the grief response may be triggered, sometimes many years later, when the individual experiences a subsequent loss. Sometimes the grief process is triggered spontaneously or in response to a seemingly insignificant event. Overreaction to another person's loss may be one manifestation of delayed grief.

The recognition of delayed grief is critical because, depending on the profoundness of the loss, the failure of the mourning process may prevent assimilation of the loss and thereby delay a return to satisfying living. Delayed grieving most commonly occurs because of ambivalent feelings toward the lost entity, outside pressure to resume normal function, or perceived lack of internal and external resources to cope with a profound loss.

Distorted (Exaggerated) Grief Response

In the distorted grief reaction, all of the symptoms associated with normal grieving are exaggerated. Feelings of sadness, helplessness, hopelessness, powerlessness, anger, and guilt, as well as numerous somatic complaints, render the individual dysfunctional in terms of management of daily living. Murray, Zentner, and Yakimo (2009) described an exaggerated grief reaction in the following way:

> An intensification of grief to the point that the person is overwhelmed, demonstrates prolonged maladaptive behavior, manifests excessive symptoms and extensive interruptions in healing, and does not progress to integration of the loss, finding meaning in the loss, and resolution of the mourning process (p. 706).

When the exaggerated reaction occurs, the individual remains fixed in the anger stage of the grief response. This anger may be directed toward others in the environment to whom the individual may be attributing the loss. However, many times the anger is turned inward on the self. When this occurs, depression is the result. Depressive mood disorder is a type of exaggerated grief reaction.

Chronic or Prolonged Grieving

Some authors have discussed a chronic or prolonged grief response as a type of maladaptive grief response. Care must be taken in making this determination because, as was stated previously, length of the grief response depends on the individual. An adaptive response may take years for some people. A prolonged process may be considered maladaptive when certain behaviors are exhibited. Prolonged grief may be a problem when behaviors such as maintaining personal possessions aimed at keeping a lost loved one alive (as though he or she will eventually reenter the life of the bereaved) or disabling behaviors that prevent the bereaved from adaptively performing activities of daily living are in evidence. Another example is of a widow who refused to participate in family gatherings following the death of her husband. For many years until her own death, she took a sandwich to the cemetery on holidays, sat on the tombstone, and ate her "holiday meal" with her husband. Other bereaved individuals have been known to set a place at the table for the deceased loved one long after the completed mourning process would have been expected.

Normal versus Maladaptive Grieving

Several authors have identified one crucial difference between normal and maladaptive grieving: the loss of self-esteem. Marked feelings of worthlessness are indicative of depression rather than uncomplicated bereavement. Corr, Nabe, and Corr (2008) have stated, "Normal grief reactions do not include the loss of self-esteem commonly found in most clinical depression" (p. 215).

Cheong, Herkov, and Goodman (2009) affirmed:

> Although both conditions may have depressed mood, loss of appetite, sleep disturbance, and decreased energy, people with depression usually experience a sense of worthlessness, guilt and/or low self-esteem that is not common in normal grief reactions.

It is thought that this major difference between normal grieving and maladaptive grieving (the feeling of worthlessness or low self-esteem) ultimately precipitates depression.

Concepts of Death—Developmental Issues

Children

Birth to Age 2. Infants are unable to recognize and understand death, but they can experience the feelings of loss and separation. Infants who are separated from their mothers may become quiet, lose weight, and sleep less. Children at this age will likely sense changes in the atmosphere of the home where a death has occurred. They often react to the emotions of adults by becoming more irritable and crying more.

Ages 3 to 5. Preschoolers and kindergartners have some understanding about death but often have difficulty distinguishing between fantasy and reality. They believe death is reversible, and their thoughts about death may include magical thinking. For example, they may believe that their thoughts or behaviors caused a person to become sick or to die.

Children of this age are capable of understanding at least some of what they see and hear from adult conversations or media reports. They become frightened if they feel a threat to themselves or to their loved ones. They are concerned with safety issues and require a great deal of personal reassurance that they will be protected. Regressive behaviors, such as loss of bladder or bowel control, thumb sucking, and temper tantrums, are not uncommon. Changes in eating and sleeping patterns may also occur.

Ages 6 to 9. Children at this age begin to understand the finality of death. They are able to understand a more detailed explanation of why or how the person died, although the concept of death is often associated with old age or with accidents. They may believe that death is contagious and avoid association with individuals who have experienced a loss by death. Death is often personified in the form of a "bogey man" or a monster—someone who takes people away or someone whom they can avoid if they try hard enough. It is difficult for them to perceive their own death. Normal grief reactions at this age include regressive and aggressive behaviors, withdrawal, school phobias, somatic symptoms, and clinging behaviors.

Ages 10 to 12. Preadolescent children are able to understand that death is final and eventually affects everyone, including themselves. They are interested in the physical aspects of dying and the final disposition of the body. They may ask questions about how the death will affect them personally. Feelings of anger, guilt, and depression are common. Peer relationships and school performance may be disrupted. There may be a preoccupation with the loss and a withdrawal into the self. They will require reassurance of their own safety and self-worth.

Adolescents

Adolescents are usually able to view death on an adult level. They understand death to be universal and inevitable; however, they have difficulty tolerating the intense feelings associated with the death of a loved one. They may or may not cry. They may withdraw into themselves or attempt to go about usual activities in an effort to avoid dealing with the pain of the loss. Some teens exhibit acting-out behaviors, such as aggression and defiance. It is often easier for adolescents to discuss their feelings with peers than with their parents or other adults. Some adolescents may show regressive behaviors whereas others react by trying to take care of their loved ones who are also grieving. In general, individuals of this age group have an attitude of immortality. Although they understand that their own death is inevitable, the concept is so far-reaching as to be imperceptible.

Adults

The adult's concept of death is influenced by cultural and religious backgrounds (Murray, Zentner, & Yakimo, 2009). Behaviors associated with grieving in the adult were discussed in the section on "Theoretical Perspectives on Loss and Bereavement."

Elderly Persons

Bateman (1999) has stated:

> For the older adult, the later years have been described by philosophers and poets as the "season of loss." Loss of one's occupational role upon retirement, loss of control and competence, loss in some life experiences, loss of material possessions, and loss of dreams, loved ones, and friends must be understood and accepted if the older adult is to adapt effectively (p. 144).

By the time individuals reach their 60s and 70s, they have experienced numerous losses, and mourning has become a lifelong process. Those who are most successful at adapting to losses earlier in life will similarly cope better with the losses and grief inherent in aging. Unfortunately, with the aging process comes a convergence of losses, the timing of which makes it impossible for the aging individual to complete the grief process in response to one loss before another occurs. Because grief is cumulative, this can result in *bereavement overload*; the person is less able to adapt and reintegrate, and mental and physical health is jeopardized (Halstead, 2005). Bereavement overload has been implicated as a predisposing factor in the development of depressive disorder in the elderly person.

Depression is a common symptom in the grief response to significant losses. It is important to understand the difference between the depression of normal grieving and the disorder of clinical depression. Some of these differences are presented in Table 24-1.

Common Nursing Diagnoses and Interventions for the Individual Who Is Grieving

• RISK FOR COMPLICATED GRIEVING

Definition: At risk for a disorder that occurs after the death of a significant other [or any other loss of significance to the individual], in which the experience of distress accompanying bereavement fails to follow normative expectations and manifests in functional impairment.

TABLE 24–1 Normal Grief Reactions versus Symptoms of Clinical Depression

Normal Grief	Clinical Depression
Self-esteem intact	Self-esteem disturbed
May openly express anger	Usually does not directly express anger
Experiences a mixture of "good and bad days"	Persistent state of dysphoria
Able to experience moments of pleasure	Anhedonia prevalent
Accepts comfort and support from others	Does not respond to social interaction and support from others
Maintains feeling of hope	Feelings of hopelessness prevail
May express guilt feelings over some aspect of the loss	Has generalized feelings of guilt
Relates feelings of depression to specific loss experienced	Does not relate feelings to a particular experience
May experience transient physical symptoms	Expresses chronic physical complaints

Sources: Cheong, Herkov, and Goodman (2009); Corr, Nabe, and Corr (2008); and Sadock and Sadock (2007).

Risk Factors ("related to")

[Actual or perceived object loss (e.g., people, pets, possessions, job, status, home, ideals, parts and process of the body)]
[Denial of loss]
[Interference with life functioning]
[Reliving of past experiences with little or no reduction (diminishment) of intensity of the grief]
Lack of social support
Emotional instability

Goals/Objectives

Short-term Goals

1. Client will acknowledge awareness of the loss.
2. Client will express feelings about the loss.
3. Client will verbalize own position in the grief process.

Long-term Goal

Client will progress through the grief process in a healthful manner toward resolution.

Interventions with *Selected Rationales*

1. Assess client's stage in the grief process. *Accurate baseline data are required to provide appropriate assistance.*

2. Develop trust. Show empathy, concern, and unconditional positive regard. *Developing trust provides the basis for a therapeutic relationship.*

3. Help the client actualize the loss by talking about it. "When did it happen? How did it happen?" and so forth. *Reviewing the events of the loss can help the client come to full awareness of the loss.*

4. Help the client identify and express feelings. *Until client can recognize and accept personal feelings regarding the loss, grief work cannot progress.* Some of the more problematic feelings include:

   a. *Anger.* The anger may be directed at the deceased, at God, displaced on others, or retroflected inward on the self. Encourage the client to examine this anger and validate the appropriateness of this feeling. *Many people will not admit to angry feelings, believing it is inappropriate and unjustified. Expression of this emotion is necessary to prevent fixation in this stage of grief.*

   b. *Guilt.* The client may feel that he or she did not do enough to prevent the loss. Help the client by reviewing the circumstances of the loss and the reality that it could not be prevented. *Feelings of guilt prolong resolution of the grief process.*

   c. *Anxiety and helplessness.* Help the client to recognize the way that life was managed before the loss. Help the client to put the feelings of helplessness into perspective by pointing out ways that he or she managed situations effectively without help from others. Role-play life events and assist with decision-making situations. *The client may have fears that he or she may not be able to carry on alone.*

5. Interpret normal behaviors associated with grieving and provide client with adequate time to grieve. *Understanding of the grief process will help prevent feelings of guilt generated by these responses. Individuals need adequate time to accommodate to the loss and all its ramifications. This involves getting past birthdays and anniversaries of which the deceased was a part.*

6. Provide continuing support. If this is not possible by the nurse, then offer referrals to support groups. Support groups of individuals going through the same experiences can be very helpful for the grieving individual. *The availability of emotional support systems facilitates the grief process.*

7. Identify pathological defenses that the client may be using (e.g., drug/alcohol use, somatic complaints, social isolation). Assist the client in understanding why these are not healthy defenses and how they delay the process of grieving. *The*

bereavement process is impaired by behaviors that mask the pain of the loss.

8. Encourage the client to make an honest review of the relationship with what has been lost. Journal keeping is a facilitative tool with this intervention. *Only when the client is able to see both positive and negative aspects related to the loss will the grieving process be complete.*

Outcome Criteria

1. Client is able to express feelings about the loss.
2. Client verbalizes stages of the grief process and behaviors associated with each stage.
3. Client acknowledges own position in the grief process and recognizes the appropriateness of the associated feelings and behaviors.

● RISK FOR SPIRITUAL DISTRESS

Definition: At risk for an impaired ability to experience and integrate meaning and purpose in life through a person's connectedness with self, others, art, music, literature, nature, and/or a power greater than oneself.

Risk Factors ("related to")

Loss [of any concept of value to the individual]
Low self-esteem
Natural disasters
Physical illness
Depression; anxiety; stress
Separated from support systems
Life change

Goals/Objectives

Short-term Goal

Client will identify meaning and purpose in life, moving forward with hope for the future.

Long-term Goal

Client will express achievement of support and personal satisfaction from spiritual practices.

Interventions with *Selected Rationales*

1. Be accepting and nonjudgmental when client expresses anger and bitterness toward God. Stay with client. *The nurse's presence and nonjudgmental attitude increase the client's feelings of self-worth and promote trust in the relationship.*

2. Encourage client to ventilate feelings related to meaning of own existence in the face of current loss. *Client may believe he or she cannot go on living without the lost entity. Catharsis can provide relief and put life back into realistic perspective.*

3. Encourage client as part of grief work to reach out to previously used religious practices for support. Encourage client to discuss these practices and how they provided support in the past. *Client may find comfort in religious rituals with which he or she is familiar.*

4. Ensure client that he or she is not alone when feeling inadequate in the search for life's answers. *Validation of client's feelings and assurance that they are shared by others offer reassurance and an affirmation of acceptability.*

5. Contact spiritual leader of client's choice, if he or she requests. *These individuals serve to provide relief from spiritual distress and often can do so when other support persons cannot.*

Outcome Criteria

1. Client verbalizes increased sense of self-concept and hope for the future.
2. Client verbalizes meaning and purpose in life that reinforces hope, peace, and contentment.
3. Client expresses personal satisfaction and support from spiritual practices.

@ INTERNET REFERENCES

- Additional references related to bereavement may be located at the following websites:
    a. http://www.journeyofhearts.org
    b. http://www.nhpco.org
    c. http://www.aarp.org/family/lifeafterloss/
    d. http://www.hospicefoundation.org
    e. http://www.bereavement.org
    f. http://www.caringinfo.org/
    g. http://www.aahpm.org/
    h. http://www.hpna.org/

PSYCHOTROPIC MEDICATIONS

C HAPTER **25**

Antianxiety Agents

● CHEMICAL CLASS: ANTIHISTAMINES
Examples

Generic Name	Trade Name	Half-life (hr)	Pregnancy Category	Available Forms (mg)
Hydroxyzine	Vistaril	3	C	Caps: 10, 25, 50, 100 Oral susp: 25/5 mL Syrup: 10/5 mL Inj: 25/mL, 50/mL

Indications
- Anxiety disorders
- Temporary relief of anxiety symptoms
- Allergic reactions producing pruritic conditions
- Antiemetic
- Reduction of narcotic requirement, alleviation of anxiety, and control of emesis in preoperative/postoperative clients (parenteral only)

Action
- Exerts central nervous system (CNS)-depressant activity at the subcortical level of the CNS
- Has anticholinergic, antihistaminic, and antiemetic properties

Contraindications and Precautions:
Contraindicated in: • Hypersensitivity • Pregnancy and lactation

Use Cautiously in: • Elderly or debilitated patients (dosage reduction recommended) • Hepatic or renal dysfunction • Concomitant use of other CNS depressants

Adverse Reactions and Side Effects
- Dry mouth
- Drowsiness
- Pain at intramuscular site

Interactions
- Additive CNS depression with other **CNS depressants** (e.g., **alcohol, other anxiolytics, opioid analgesics,** and **sedative/hypnotics**) and with **herbal depressants** (e.g., **kava, valerian**)
- Additive anticholinergic effects with other **drugs possessing anticholinergic properties** (e.g., **antihistamines, antidepressants, atropine, haloperidol, phenothiazines**) and **herbal products** such as **angel's trumpet, jimson weed,** and **scopolia**
- Can antagonize the vasopressor effects of **epinephrine**

Route and Dosage
INTRAMUSCULAR
Anxiety
Adults: 50 to 100 mg 4 times a day

Pruritis
Adults: 25 mg 3 or 4 times a day

Preoperative and Postoperative Sedative
Adults: 50 to 100 mg
Children: 0.6 mg/kg

Antiemetic/Adjunctive Therapy to Analgesia
Adults: 25 to 100 mg every 4 to 6 hours as needed
Children: 0.5 to 1 mg/kg every 4 to 6 hours as needed

ORAL
Anxiety
Adults: 50 to 100 mg 4 times a day
Children (>6 years): 50 to 100 mg/day in divided doses
Children (<6 years): 50 mg/day in divided doses

Pruritus
Adults: 25 mg 3 or 4 times a day
Children (>6 years): 50 to 100 mg/day in divided doses
Children (<6 years): 50 mg/day in divided doses

Preoperative and Postoperative Sedative

Adults: 50 to 100 mg
Children: 0.6 mg/kg

● CHEMICAL CLASS: BENZODIAZEPINES
Examples

Generic (Trade) Name	Controlled/ Pregnancy Categories	Half-life (hr)	Indications	Available Forms (mg)
Alprazolam (Xanax)	C-IV/D	6.3–26.9	• Anxiety disorders • Anxiety symptoms • Anxiety associated with depression • Panic disorder	Tabs: 0.25, 0.5, 1.0, 2.0 Tabs ER: 0.5, 1.0, 2.0, 3.0 Tabs (orally disintegrating): 0.25, 0.5, 1.0, 2.0 Oral solu: 1/mL
Chlordiazepoxide (Librium)	C-IV/D	5–30	• Anxiety disorders • Anxiety symptoms • Acute alcohol withdrawal • Preoperative sedation	Caps: 5, 10, 25
Clonazepam (Klonopin)	C-IV/C	18–50	• Petit mal, akinetic, and myoclonic seizures • Panic disorder **Unlabeled uses:** • Acute manic episodes • Neuralgias • Restless leg syndrome • Adjunct therapy in schizophrenia	Tabs: 0.5, 1.0, 2.0 Tabs (orally disintegrating): 0.125, 0.25, 0.5, 1.0, 2.0
Clorazepate (Tranxene)	C-IV/UK	40–50	• Anxiety disorders • Anxiety symptoms • Acute alcohol withdrawal • Partial seizures	Tabs: 3.75, 7.5, 15 Tabs (extended release): 11.25, 22.5
Diazepam (Valium)	C-IV/D	20–80	• Anxiety disorders • Anxiety symptoms • Skeletal muscle relaxant • Acute alcohol withdrawal • Adjunct therapy in convulsive disorders • Status epilepticus • Preoperative sedation	Tabs: 2, 5, 10 Oral solu: 5/5 mL, 5/mL Inj: 5/mL Rectal gel: 2.5, 10, 20

Generic (Trade) Name	Controlled/ Pregnancy Categories	Half-life (hr)	Indications	Available Forms (mg)
Lorazepam (Ativan)	C-IV/D	10–20	• Anxiety disorders • Anxiety symptoms • Status epilepticus • Preoperative sedation **Unlabeled uses:** • Insomnia • Chemotherapy-induced nausea and vomiting	Tabs: 0.5, 1.0, 2.0 Oral solu: 2/mL Inj: 2/mL, 4/mL
Oxazepam	C-IV/D	5–20	• Anxiety disorders • Anxiety symptoms • Acute alcohol withdrawal **Unlabeled uses:** • Management of irritable bowel syndrome	Caps: 10, 15, 30

Action
- Benzodiazepines are thought to potentiate the effects of gamma-aminobutyric acid (GABA), a powerful inhibitory neurotransmitter, thereby producing a calmative effect. The activity may involve the spinal cord, brain stem, cerebellum, limbic system, and cortical areas.

Contraindications and Precautions:
Contraindicated in: • Hypersensitivity • Psychoses • Acute narrow-angle glaucoma • Preexisting CNS depression • Pregnancy and lactation • Shock • Coma

Use Cautiously in: • Elderly or debilitated patients (reduced dosage recommended) • Patients with hepatic/renal/pulmonary impairment • History of drug abuse/dependence • Depressed/suicidal patients • Children

Adverse Reactions and Side Effects
- Drowsiness; dizziness, lethargy
- Nausea and vomiting
- Ataxia
- Dry mouth
- Blurred vision
- Rash
- Hypotension
- Tolerance
- Physical and psychological dependence
- Paradoxical excitation

Interactions

- Additive CNS depression with other **CNS depressants** (e.g., **alcohol, other anxiolytics, opioid analgesics,** and **sedative/hypnotics**) and with **herbal depressants** (e.g., **kava, valerian**)
- **Cimetidine, oral contraceptives, disulfiram, fluoxetine, isoniazid, ketoconazole, metoprolol, propoxyphene, propranolol,** or **valproic acid** may enhance effects of benzodiazepines
- Benzodiazepines may decrease the efficacy of **levodopa.**
- Sedative effects of benzodiazepines may be decreased by **theophylline.**
- **Rifampin** may decrease the efficacy of benzodiazepines.
- Serum concentration of **digoxin** may be increased (and subsequent toxicity can occur) with concurrent benzodiazepine therapy.

Route and Dosage

ALPRAZOLAM **(Xanax)**

Anxiety Disorders and Anxiety Symptoms: **PO**: 0.25 to 0.5 mg 3 times a day. Maximum daily dose 4 mg in divided doses.

In elderly or debilitated patients: 0.25 mg 2 or 3 times a day. Gradually increase if needed and tolerated.

Panic Disorder: **PO**: Initial dose: 0.5 mg 3 times a day. Increase dose at intervals of 3 to 4 days in increments of no more than 1 mg/day.

CHLORDIAZEPOXIDE **(Librium)**

Mild to Moderate Anxiety: **PO**: 5 or 10 mg 3 or 4 times a day.

Severe Anxiety: **PO**: 20 or 25 mg 3 or 4 times a day.

Elderly or Debilitated Patients: **PO:** 5 mg 2 to 4 times a day.

Preoperative Sedation: **PO:** 5 to 10 mg 3 or 4 times a day.

Acute Alcohol Withdrawal: **PO**: 50 to 100 mg; repeat as needed up to 300 mg/day.

CLONAZEPAM **(Klonopin)**

Seizures: Adults: **PO**: 0.5 mg three times a day. May increase by 0.5 to 1 mg every 3 days. Total daily maintenance dose not to exceed 20 mg.

Children (<10 years or 30 kg): **PO**: Initial daily dose 0.01 to 0.03 mg/kg/day (not to exceed 0.05 mg/kg/day) given in 2 or 3 equally divided doses; increase by no more than 0.25 to 0.5 mg every third day until a daily maintenance dose of 0.1 to 0.2 mg/kg has been reached. **Therapeutic serum concentrations of clonazepam are 20 to 80 ng/ml.**

Panic Disorder: **PO**: Initial dose: 0.25 mg 2 times a day. Increase after 3 days toward target dose of 1 mg/day. Some patients may require up to 4 mg/day, in which case the dose may be increased in increments of 0.125 to 0.25 mg twice daily every 3 days until symptoms are controlled.

Acute Manic Episode: **PO**: 1 to 6 mg/day.

Neuralgia: **PO**: 1.5 to 4 mg/day.

Restless Leg Syndrome: **PO**: 0.5 to 2 mg 30 minutes before bedtime.

Adjunct Therapy in Schizophrenia: **PO**: 0.5 to 2 mg/day.

CLORAZEPATE **(Tranxene)**

Anxiety Disorders/Anxiety Symptoms: *Adults:* **PO**: 7.5 to 15 mg 2 to 4 times a day. Adjust gradually to dose within range of 15 to 60 mg/day. May also be given in a single daily dose at bedtime. The recommended initial dose is 15 mg. Adjust subsequent dosages according to patient response.

Geriatric or debilitated patients: **PO**: 7.5 to 15 mg/day.

Acute Alcohol Withdrawal: **PO**: Day 1: 30 mg initially, followed by 15 mg 2 to 4 times a day.

Day 2: 45 to 90 mg in divided doses.

Day 3: 22.5 to 45 mg in divided doses.

Day 4: 15 to 30 mg in divided doses.

Thereafter, gradually reduce the daily dose to 7.5 to 15 mg. Discontinue drug as soon as patient's condition is stable.

Partial Seizures: *Adults:* **PO**: 7.5 mg 3 times a day. Can increase by no more than 7.5 mg/day at weekly intervals (daily dose not to exceed 90 mg).

Children (9 to 12 years): **PO**: 7.5 mg 2 times a day initially; may increase by 7.5 mg/week (not to exceed 60 mg/day).

DIAZEPAM **(Valium)**

Antianxiety/Adjunct Anticonvulsant: *Adults:* **PO**: 2 to 10 mg 2 to 4 times a day.

Children (>6 months): **PO**: 1 to 2.5 mg 3 to 4 times a day.

Moderate to severe anxiety: *Adults:* **IM** or **IV**: 2 to 10 mg. Repeat in 3 to 4 hours if necessary.

Skeletal Muscle Relaxant: *Adults:* **PO**: 2 to 10 mg 3 or 4 times a day.

Children (>6 months): **PO**: 0.12 to 0.8 mg/kg/day divided into 3 or 4 equal doses.

Geriatric or debilitated patients: **PO**: 2 to 2.5 mg 1 to 2 times daily initially. Increase gradually as needed and tolerated.

Acute Alcohol Withdrawal: **PO**: 10 mg 3 to 4 times a day in first 24 hours; decrease to 5 mg 3 or 4 times a day as needed. **IM** or **IV**: 10 mg initially, then 5 to 10 mg in 3 to 4 hours, if necessary.

Status Epilepticus/Acute Seizure Activity: Adults: **IV** (IM route may be used if IV is unavailable): 5 to 10 mg; may repeat every 10 to 15 minutes to a total of 30 mg; may repeat regimen again in 2 to 4 hours.

Children (≥5 years): **IM** or **IV**: 1 mg every 2 to 5 minutes to a maximum of 10 mg. May repeat in 2 to 4 hours if necessary.

Children (1 month to 5 years): **IM** or **IV**: 0.2 to 0.5 mg every 2 to 5 minutes to maximum of 5 mg.

Preoperative Sedation: Adults: **IM**: 10 mg.

LORAZEPAM **(Ativan)**

Anxiety Disorders/Anxiety Symptoms: **PO:** 2 to 6 mg/day (varies from 1 to 10 mg/day) given in divided doses; take the largest dose before bedtime.

Geriatric or debilitated patients: **PO:** 1 to 2 mg/day in divided doses; adjust as needed and tolerated.

Insomnia: **PO:** 2 to 4 mg at bedtime.

Geriatric or debilitated patients: **PO:** 0.25 to 1 mg at bedtime.

Preoperative Sedation: **IM:** 0.05 mg/kg (maximum 4 mg) 2 hours before surgery.

IV: Initial dose is 2 mg or 0.044 mg/kg, whichever is smaller, given 15 to 20 minutes before the procedure.

Status Epilepticus: **IV:** 4 mg given slowly (2 mg/min). May be repeated after 10 to 15 minutes if seizures continue or recur.

Antiemetic: **IV:** 2 mg 30 minutes prior to chemotherapy; may be repeated every 4 hours as needed.

OXAZEPAM

Mild to Moderate Anxiety: **PO:** 10 to 15 mg 3 or 4 times a day.

Severe Anxiety States: **PO:** 15 to 30 mg 3 or 4 times a day.

Geriatric patients: **PO:** Initial dosage: 10 mg 3 times a day. If necessary, increase cautiously to 15 mg 3 or 4 times a day.

Acute alcohol withdrawal: **PO:** 15 to 30 mg 3 or 4 times a day.

● CHEMICAL CLASS: CARBAMATE DERIVATIVE

Examples

Generic Name	Controlled/ Pregnancy Categories	Half-life (hr)	Available Forms (mg)
Meprobamate	C-IV/D	6–17	Tabs: 200, 400

Indications
- Anxiety disorders
- Temporary relief of anxiety symptoms

Action
- Depresses multiple sites in the CNS, including the thalamus and limbic system. May act by blocking the reuptake of adenosine.

Contraindications and Precautions:
Contraindicated in: • Hypersensitivity to the drug • Combination with other CNS depressants • Children under age 6 • Pregnancy and lactation • Acute intermittent porphyria
Use Cautiously in: • Elderly or debilitated clients • Patients with hepatic or renal dysfunction • Individuals with a history of drug abuse/addiction • Clients with a history of seizure disorders • Depressed/suicidal clients

Adverse Reactions and Side Effects
- Palpitations, tachycardia
- Drowsiness, dizziness, ataxia
- Nausea, vomiting, diarrhea
- Tolerance
- Physical and psychological dependence

Interactions
- Additive CNS depression with other **CNS depressants** (e.g., **alcohol, other anxiolytics, opioid analgesics,** and **sedative-hypnotics**) and with **herbal depressants** (e.g., **kava, valerian**).

Route and Dosage
Anxiety Disorders/Anxiety Symptoms: Adults and children: >12 years: **PO**: 1200 to 1600 mg/day in 3 to 4 divided doses. Maximum daily dose: 2400 mg.
Children (6 to 12 years): **PO**: 100 to 200 mg 2 or 3 times a day.

● CHEMICAL CLASS: AZASPIRODECANEDIONES
Examples

Generic Name	Trade Name	Pregnancy Category	Half-life (hr)	Available Forms (mg)
Buspirone HCl	BuSpar	B	2–3	Tabs: 5, 7.5, 10, 15, 30

INDICATIONS
- Generalized anxiety states

Unlabeled use:
- Symptomatic management of premenstrual syndrome

Actions
- Unknown
- May produce desired effects through interactions with serotonin, dopamine, and other neurotransmitter receptors
- Delayed onset (a lag time of 7 to 10 days between onset of therapy and subsiding of anxiety symptoms)
- Cannot be used on a PRN basis

Contraindications and Precautions:
Contraindicated in: • Hypersensitivity to the drug • Severe hepatic or renal impairment • Concurrent use with monoamine oxidase (MAO) inhibitors

Use Cautiously in: • Elderly or debilitated clients • Pregnancy and lactation • Children • Clients with a history of chronic benzodiazepine or other sedative/hypnotic use. Buspirone will not block the withdrawal syndrome in these clients and they should be withdrawn gradually from these medications before beginning therapy with buspirone.

Adverse Reactions and Side Effects
- Drowsiness, dizziness
- Excitement, nervousness
- Fatigue, headache
- Nausea, dry mouth
- Incoordination, numbness
- Palpitations, tachycardia

Interactions
- Increased effects of buspirone with **cimetidine, erythromycin, itraconazole, nefazodone, ketoconazole, clarithromycin, diltiazem, verapamil, fluvoxamine,** and **ritonavir**
- Decreased effects of buspirone with **rifampin, rifabutin, phenytoin, phenobarbital, carbamazepine, fluoxetine, and dexamethasone**
- Increased serum concentrations of **haloperidol** when used concomitantly with buspirone
- Use of buspirone with an **MAO inhibitor** may result in elevated blood pressure.
- Increased risk of hepatic effects when used concomitantly with **trazodone**
- Additive effects when used with certain **herbal products** (e.g., **kava, valerian**)

Route and Dosage

Anxiety: Adults: **PO**: Initial dosage 7.5 mg 2 times a day. Increase by 5 mg/day every 2 to 3 days as needed. Maximum daily dosage: 60 mg.

● NURSING DIAGNOSES RELATED TO ALL ANTIANXIETY AGENTS

1. Risk for injury related to seizures, panic anxiety, acute agitation from alcohol withdrawal (indications); abrupt withdrawal from the medication after long-term use; effects of medication intoxication or overdose
2. Anxiety (specify) related to threat to physical integrity or self-concept
3. Risk for activity intolerance related to medication side effects of sedation, confusion, lethargy
4. Disturbed sleep pattern related to situational crises, physical condition, severe level of anxiety
5. Deficient knowledge related to medication regimen
6. Risk for acute confusion related to action of the medication on the CNS

● NURSING IMPLICATIONS FOR ANTIANXIETY AGENTS

1. Instruct client not to drive or operate dangerous machinery while taking the medication.
2. Advise client receiving long-term therapy not to quit taking the drug abruptly. Abrupt withdrawal can be life-threatening (with the exception of buspirone). Symptoms include depression, insomnia, increased anxiety, abdominal and muscle cramps, tremors, vomiting, sweating, convulsions, and delirium.
3. Instruct client not to drink alcohol or take other medications that depress the CNS while taking this medication.
4. Assess mood daily. *May aggravate symptoms in depressed persons.* Take necessary precautions for potential suicide.
5. Monitor lying and standing blood pressure and pulse every shift. Instruct client to arise slowly from a lying or sitting position.
6. Withhold drug and notify the physician should paradoxical excitement occur.
7. Have client take frequent sips of water or ice chips, suck on hard candy, or chew sugarless gum to relieve dry mouth.
8. Have client take drug with food or milk to prevent nausea and vomiting.
9. Symptoms of sore throat, fever, malaise, easy bruising, or unusual bleeding should be reported to the physician immediately. They may be indications of blood dyscrasias.

10. Ensure that client taking buspirone (BuSpar) understands there is a lag time of 7 to 10 days between onset of therapy and subsiding of anxiety symptoms. Client should continue to take the medication during this time. (*Note:* This medication is not recommended for PRN administration because of this delayed therapeutic onset. There is no evidence that buspirone creates tolerance or physical dependence as do the CNS-depressant anxiolytics.)

● **CLIENT/FAMILY EDUCATION RELATED TO ALL ANTIANXIETY AGENTS**

- Do not drive or operate dangerous machinery. Drowsiness and dizziness can occur.
- Do not stop taking the drug abruptly. This can produce serious withdrawal symptoms, such as depression, insomnia, anxiety, abdominal and muscle cramps, tremors, vomiting, sweating, convulsions, and delirium.
- *(With buspirone only):* Be aware of lag time between start of therapy and subsiding of symptoms. Relief is usually evident within 7 to 10 days. Take the medication regularly, as ordered, so that it has sufficient time to take effect.
- Do not consume other CNS depressants (including alcohol).
- Do not take nonprescription medication without approval from physician.
- Rise slowly from the sitting or lying position to prevent a sudden drop in blood pressure.
- Report to physician immediately symptoms of sore throat, fever, malaise, easy bruising, unusual bleeding, or motor restlessness.
- Be aware of risks of taking these drugs during pregnancy. (Congenital malformations have been associated with use during the first trimester.) If pregnancy is suspected or planned, the client should notify the physician of the desirability to discontinue the drug.
- Be aware of possible side effects. Refer to written materials furnished by health-care providers regarding the correct method of self-administration.
- Carry a card or piece of paper at all times stating the names of medications being taken.

@ **INTERNET REFERENCES**

a. http://www.mentalhealth.com/
b. http://www.nimh.nih.gov/health/publications/mental-health-medications/complete-index.shtml
c. http://www.fadavis.com/townsend
d. http://www.nlm.nih.gov/medlineplus/druginformation.html

Antidepressants

● **CHEMICAL CLASS: TRICYCLICS AND RELATED (Nonselective Reuptake Inhibitors)**

Examples

Generic (Trade) Name	Pregnancy Categories/ Half-life (hr)	Indications	Therapeutic Plasma Level Range (ng/ml)	Available Forms (mg)
TRICYCLICS				
Amitriptyline	D/31–46	• Depression **Unlabeled uses:** • Migraine prevention • Fibromyalgia • Postherpetic neuralgia	110–250 (including metabolite)	Tabs: 10, 25, 50, 75, 100, 150
Clomipramine (Anafranil)	C/19–37	• Obsessive-compulsive disorder (OCD) **Unlabeled uses:** • Premenstrual symptoms • Panic disorder	80–100	Caps: 25, 50, 75
Desipramine (Norpramin)	C/12–24	Depression **Unlabeled uses:** • Alcoholism • Attention-deficit/ hyperactivity disorder (ADHD) • Bulimia nervosa • Diabetic neuropathy • Postherpetic neuralgia	125–300	Tabs: 10, 25, 50, 75, 100, 150

Continued

417

Generic (Trade) Name	Pregnancy Categories/ Half-life (hr)	Indications	Therapeutic Plasma Level Range (ng/ml)	Available Forms (mg)
Doxepin (Sinequan)	C/8–24	• Depression or anxiety • Depression or anxiety associated with alcoholism • Depression or anxiety associated with organic disease • Psychotic depressive disorders with anxiety **Unlabeled uses:** • Migraine prevention	100–200 (including metabolite)	Caps: 10, 25, 50, 75, 100, 150 Oral conc: 10/mL
Imipramine (Tofranil)	D/11–25	• Depression • Childhood enuresis **Unlabeled uses:** • Alcoholism • ADHD • Bulimia nervosa • Migraine prevention • Urinary incontinence	200–350 (including metabolite)	HCl tabs: 10, 25, 50 Pamoate caps: 75, 100, 125, 150
Nortriptyline (Aventyl; Pamelor)	D/18–44	• Depression **Unlabeled uses:** • ADHD • Postherpetic neuralgia	50–150	Caps: 10, 25, 50, 75 Oral Solution: 10/5 mL
Protriptyline (Vivactil)	C/67–89	• Depression **Unlabeled uses:** • Migraine prevention	100–200	Tabs: 5, 10
Trimipramine (Surmontil)	C/7–30	• Depression	180 (includes active metabolite)	Caps: 25, 50, 100
DIBENZOXAZEPINE				
Amoxapine	C/8	• Depression • Depression with anxiety	200–500	Tabs: 25, 50, 100, 150
TETRACYCLIC				
Maprotiline	B/21–25	• Depression • Depression with anxiety **Unlabeled uses:** • Postherpetic neuralgia	200–300 (including metabolite)	Tabs: 25, 50, 75

Action
• Inhibit reuptake of norepinephrine or serotonin at the pre-synaptic neuron

Contraindications and Precautions:
Contraindicated in: • Hypersensitivity to any tricyclic or related drug • Concomitant use with monoamine oxidase

inhibitors (MAOIs) ● Acute recovery period following myocardial infarction ● Narrow angle glaucoma ● Pregnancy and lactation (safety not established) ● Known or suspected seizure disorder (maprotiline)

Use Cautiously in: ● Patients with history of seizures (maprotiline contraindicated) ● Patients with tendency to have urinary retention ● Benign prostatic hypertrophy ● Cardiovascular disorders ● Hepatic or renal insufficiency ● Psychotic patients ● Elderly or debilitated patients

Adverse Reactions and Side Effects

- Drowsiness; fatigue
- Dry mouth
- Blurred vision
- Orthostatic hypotension
- Tachycardia; arrhythmias
- Constipation
- Urinary retention
- Blood dyscrasias
- Nausea and vomiting
- Photosensitivity
- Increased risk of suicidality in children and adolescents (black box warning)

Interactions

- Increased effects of tricyclic antidepressants with **bupropion, cimetidine, haloperidol, selective serotonin reuptake inhibitors (SSRIs),** and **valproic acid**
- Decreased effects of tricyclic antidepressants with **carbamazepine, barbiturates,** and **rifamycins**
- Hyperpyretic crisis, convulsions, and death can occur with **MAOIs.**
- Coadministration with **clonidine** may produce hypertensive crisis.
- Decreased effects of **levodopa** and **guanethidine** with tricyclic antidepressants
- Potentiation of pressor response with direct-acting **sympathomimetics**
- Increased anticoagulation effects with **dicumarol**
- Increased serum levels of **carbamazepine** occur with concomitant use of tricyclics.
- Increased risk of seizures with concomitant use of maprotiline and **phenothiazines**
- Potential for cardiovascular toxicity of maprotiline when given concomitantly with **thyroid hormones** (e.g., **levothyroxine**)

Route and Dosage

AMITRIPTYLINE

***Depression:* PO**: 75 mg/day in divided doses. May gradually increase to 150 mg/day.

Alternative dosing: May initiate at 50 to 100 mg at bedtime; increase by 25 to 50 mg as necessary, to a total of 150 mg/day.

Hospitalized patients: may require up to 300 mg/day.

Adolescent and elderly patients: 10 mg 3 times a day and 20 mg at bedtime.

***Migraine Prevention:* PO:** Common dosage: 50 to 100 mg/day in divided doses. Range: 10 to 300 mg/day.

***Fibromyalgia:* PO:** 10 to 50 mg at bedtime

***Postherpetic Neuralgia:* PO:** 65 to 100 mg/day for at least 3 weeks.

CLOMIPRAMINE **(Anafranil)**

***Obsessive-Compulsive Disorder:* PO**: *Adults*: 25 mg/day. Gradually increase to 100 mg/day during first 2 weeks, given in divided doses. May increase gradually over several weeks to maximum of 250 mg/day.

Children and adolescents: 25 mg/day. Gradually increase during first 2 weeks to daily dose of 3 mg/kg or 100 mg, whichever is smaller. Maximum daily dose: 3 mg/kg or 200 mg, whichever is smaller.

***Premenstrual Symptoms:* PO:** 25 to 75 mg/day for irritability and dysphoria

***Panic Disorder:* PO:** Initial dose: 10 mg. Increase to a maximum dose of 150 mg given as multiple daily doses.

DESIPRAMINE **(Norpramin)**

***Depression:* PO**: 100 to 200 mg/day in divided doses or as a single daily dose. May increase to maximum dose of 300 mg/day.

Elderly and adolescents: 25 to 100 mg/day in divided doses or as a single daily dose. Maximum dose: 150 mg/day.

***Alcoholism:* PO:** 200 to 275 mg/day.

***Attention-deficit/Hyperactivity Disorder (ADHD):* PO:** 100 to 200 mg/day

***Bulimia Nervosa:* PO:** Initial dose: 25 mg 3 times a day. Titrate dosage up to 200 to 300 mg/day, depending on response and adverse effects.

***Diabetic Neuropathy:* PO:** 50 to 250 mg/day.

***Postherpetic Neuralgia:* PO:** 94 to 167 mg/day for at least 6 weeks.

DOXEPIN **(Sinequan)**

***Depression and/or Anxiety:* PO**: (Mild to moderate illness): 75 mg/day. May increase to maximum dose of 150 mg/day.

(Mild symptoms associated with organic illness): 25 to 50 mg/day.
(Severe symptoms): 50 mg 3 times a day; may gradually increase
to 300 mg/day.

Migraine Prevention: PO: 75 to 150 mg/day. Occasionally
dosages up to 300 mg/day may be required.

IMIPRAMINE **(Tofranil)**

Depression: PO: 75 mg/day. May increase to maximum of
200 mg/day. Hospitalized patients may require up to 300 mg/
day.

Adolescent and geriatric patients: 30 to 40 mg/day. May
increase to maximum of 100 mg/day.

Childhood Enuresis (children ≥6 years of age): PO:
25 mg/day 1 hour before bedtime. May increase after 1 week to
50 mg/night if <12 years of age; up to 75 mg/night if > 12 years
of age. Maximum dose 2.5 mg/kg/day

Alcoholism: PO: 50 mg/day titrated by 50 mg every 3 to 5 days
to a maximum daily dose of 300 mg.

ADHD: PO: 1 mg/kg/day titrated to a maximum dose of 4 mg/
kg/day or 200 mg/day, whichever is smaller.

Bulimia Nervosa: PO: 50 mg/day titrated to 100 mg 2 times
a day.

Migraine Prevention: PO: 10 to 25 mg 3 times a day.

Urinary Incontinence: PO: 25 mg 2 to 3 times a day.

NORTRIPTYLINE **(Aventyl; Pamelor)**

Depression: PO: 25 mg 3 or 4 times a day. The total daily dose
may be given at bedtime.

Elderly and adolescent patients: 30 to 50 mg daily in divided doses
or total daily dose may be given once a day.

ADHD: PO: *Adults:* 25 mg 3 to 4 times a day. *Children and
adolescents:* 0.5 mg/kg/day, titrated to a maximum dose of
2 mg/kg/day or 100 mg, whichever is less.

Postherpetic Neuralgia: PO: Dosage range: 58 to 89 mg/day
for at least 5 weeks.

PROTRIPTYLINE **(Vivactil)**

Depression: PO: 15 to 40 mg/day divided into 3 or 4 doses.
Maximum daily dose: 60 mg.

Adolescent and elderly patients: 5 mg 3 times a day.

TRIMIPRAMINE **(Surmontil)**

Depression: PO: 75 mg/day. Increase gradually to 150 to
200 mg/day. Adult hospitalized patients may require up to
300 mg/day.

Adolescent and elderly patients: Initially, 50 mg/day, with gradual
increments up to 100 mg/day.

AMOXAPINE

Depression and Depression with Anxiety: **PO**: 50 mg 2 or
  3 times a day. May increase to 100 mg 2 or 3 times a day by
  end of first week.
Elderly patients: 25 mg 2 or 3 times a day. May increase to 50 mg
  2 or 3 times a day by end of first week.

MAPROTILINE

Depression/Depression with Anxiety: **PO**: *Adults*—Initial
  dose: 75 mg/day. After 2 weeks, may increase gradually in
  25 mg increments. Maximum daily dose: 150 to 225 mg.
Elderly patients: Initiate dosage at 25 mg/day. 50 to 75 mg/day
  may be sufficient for maintenance therapy in elderly patients.
Postherpetic Neuralgia: **PO**: 100 mg/day for 5 weeks.

● **CHEMICAL CLASS: SELECTIVE SEROTONIN
  REUPTAKE INHIBITORS (SSRIs)**
Examples

Generic (Trade) Name	Pregnancy Categories/ Half-life	Indications	Therapeutic Plasma Level Ranges	Available Forms (mg)
Citalopram (Celexa)	C/~35	• Treatment of depression **Unlabeled uses:** • Generalized anxiety disorder (GAD) • Obsessive-compulsive disorder (OCD) • Panic disorder • Premenstrual dysphoric disorder (PMDD) • Posttraumatic stress disorder (PTSD)	Not well established	Tabs: 10, 20, 40 Oral Solution: 10/5 mL
Escitalopram (Lexapro)	C/27–32 hr	• Major depressive disorder • GAD **Unlabeled uses:** • Post traumatic stress disorder	Not well established	Tabs: 5, 10, 20 Oral Solution: 1/mL

Generic (Trade) Name	Pregnancy Categories/ Half-life	Indications	Therapeutic Plasma Level Ranges	Available Forms (mg)
Fluoxetine (Prozac; Sarafem)	C/1 to 16 days (including metabolite)	• Depression • OCD • Bulimia nervosa • Panic disorder • PMDD **Unlabeled uses:** • Alcoholism • Borderline personality disorder • Fibromyalgia • Hot flashes • PTSD • Migraine prevention • Raynaud phenomenon	Not well established	Tabs: 10, 15, 20 Caps: 10, 20, 40 Caps, delayed-release: 90 Oral solution: 20/5 mL
Fluvoxamine (Luvox)	C/13.6–15.6 hr	• OCD • Social anxiety disorder **Unlabeled uses:** • Panic disorder • PTSD • Migraine prevention	Not well established	Tabs: 25, 50, 100 Caps (ER): 100, 150
Paroxetine (Paxil)	C/21 hr (CR: 15–20 hr)	• Major depressive disorder • Panic disorder • OCD • Social anxiety disorder • GAD • PTSD • PMDD **Unlabeled uses:** • Hot flashes • Diabetic neuropathy	Not well established	Tabs: 10, 20, 30, 40 Oral Suspension: 10/5 mL Tabs (CR): 12.5, 25, 37.5
Sertraline (Zoloft)	C/26–104 hr (including metabolite)	• Major depressive disorder • OCD • Panic disorder • PTSD • PMDD • Social anxiety disorder	Not well established	Tabs: 25, 50, 100 Oral concentrate: 20/mL

Action
- Selectively inhibit the central nervous system neuronal uptake of serotonin (5-HT)

Contraindications and Precautions
Contraindicated in: • Hypersensitivity to SSRIs • Concomitant use with, or within 14 days' use of, MAOIs • *Fluoxetine:* concomitant use with thioridazine (or within 5 weeks after discontinuation of fluoxetine) • *Fluvoxamine:* concomitant use with cisapride, thioridazine, or pimozide • *Paroxetine:* concomitant use with thioridazine • *Sertraline:* concomitant use with pimozide • *Sertraline:* coadministration of oral concentrate with disulfiram

Use Cautiously in: • Patients with history of seizures • Underweight or anorexic patients • Patients with hepatic or renal insufficiency • Elderly or debilitated patients • Suicidal patients • Pregnancy and lactation

Adverse Reactions and Side Effects
- Headache
- Insomnia
- Nausea
- Anorexia
- Diarrhea
- Constipation
- Sexual dysfunction
- Somnolence
- Dry mouth
- Increased risk of suicidality in children and adolescents (black box warning)
- Serotonin syndrome. Can occur if taken concurrently with other medications that increase levels of serotonin (e.g., MAOIs, tryptophan, amphetamines, other antidepressants, buspirone, lithium, dopamine agonists, or serotonin 5-HT$_1$ receptor agonists [agents for migraine]). Symptoms of serotonin syndrome include diarrhea, cramping, tachycardia, labile blood pressure, diaphoresis, fever, tremor, shivering, restlessness, confusion, disorientation, mania, myoclonus, hyperreflexia, ataxia, seizures, cardiovascular shock, and death.

Interactions
- Toxic, sometimes fatal, reactions have occurred with concomitant use of **MAOIs**.
- Increased effects of SSRIs with **cimetidine, L-tryptophan, lithium, linezolid**, and **St. John's wort**.
- Serotonin syndrome may occur with concomitant use of SSRIs and **metoclopramide, sibutramine, tramadol, serotonin**

5-HT₁ receptor agonists (agents for migraine), or any drug that increases levels of serotonin.
- Concomitant use of SSRIs may increase effects of **hydantoins, tricyclic antidepressants, cyclosporine, benzodiazepines, beta blockers, methadone, carbamazepine, clozapine, olanzapine, pimozide, haloperidol, phenothiazines, St. John's wort, sumatriptan, sympathomimetics, tacrine, theophylline,** and **warfarin.**
- Concomitant use of SSRIs may decrease effects of **buspirone** and **digoxin.**
- **Lithium** levels may be increased or decreased by concomitant use of SSRIs.
- Decreased effects of SSRIs with concomitant use of **carbamazepine** or **cyproheptadine**

Route and Dosage

CITALOPRAM **(Celexa)**

Depression: **PO:** Initial dosage: 20 mg/day as a single daily dose. May increase in increments of 20 mg at intervals of no less than 1 week. Recommended maximum dose: 40 mg/day.
Elderly clients: 20 mg/day.

OCD: **PO:** Initial dosage: 20 mg/day. Titrate to a target dosage of 40 to 60 mg/day. Maximum dosage: 80 mg.

ESCITALOPRAM **(Lexapro)**

Depression and GAD: **PO:** Initial dosage: 10 mg/day as a single daily dose. May increase to 20 mg/day after 1 week.
Elderly clients: **PO:** 10 mg/day.

PTSD: **PO:** Initial dose: 10 mg/day. Increase to 20 mg/day after 4 weeks.

FLUOXETINE **(Prozac; Sarafem)**

Depression and OCD: **PO:** *Adults:* Initial dosage: 20 mg/day in the morning. May increase dosage after several weeks if clinical improvement is not observed. Maximum dose: 80 mg/day. *Children and adolescents:* 10 to 20 mg/day.

Bulimia Nervosa: **PO:** 60 mg/day administered in the morning. May need to titrate up to this target dose in some clients.

Panic Disorder: **PO:** Initial dose: 10 mg/day. After 1 week, increase dose to 20 mg/day. If no improvement is seen after several weeks, may consider dose increases up to 60 mg/day.

PMDD (Sarafem): **PO:** Initial dose: 20 mg/day. Maximum: 80 mg/day. May be given continuously throughout the cycle or intermittently (only during the 14 days prior to anticipated onset of menses).

Alcoholism: **PO:** Initial dosage: 20 mg/day. Titrate to 40 mg/day after 2 weeks, if needed.

Borderline Personality Disorder: **PO:** 20 to 80 mg/day.

Fibromyalgia: **PO:** 20 mg/day (in the morning) for up to 6 weeks.

Hot Flashes: **PO:** 20 mg/day.

PTSD: **PO:** *Adults:* 10 to 80 mg/day. *Children:* 10 to 20 mg/day.

Migraine Prevention: **PO:** 10 to 40 mg/day.

Raynaud Phenomenon: **PO:** 20 to 60 mg/day.

FLUVOXAMINE **(Luvox)**

OCD: **PO:** *Adults:* Initial dose: 50 mg at bedtime. May increase dose in 50 mg increments every 4 to 7 days. Maximum dose: 300 mg. Administer daily doses >100 mg in 2 divided doses. If unequal, give larger dose at bedtime.

Children 8 to 17 years: Initial dose: 25 mg single dose at bedtime. May increase the dose in 25 mg increments every 4 to 7 days to a maximum dose of 200 mg/day for children up to 11 years of age. Maximum dose for adolescents: 300 mg/day. Divide daily doses >50 mg into 2 doses. If unequal, give larger dose at bedtime.

Social Anxiety Disorder: **PO** (*extended release capsules*): Initial dose: 100 mg/day as a single daily dose at bedtime. Increase in 50 mg increments every week, as tolerated, until maximum therapeutic benefit is achieved. Maximum dose: 300 mg/day.

Panic Disorder: **PO:** Initial dosage: 50 mg/day. Gradually increase after several days to 150 mg/day. For clients who fail to respond after several weeks of treatment, further increases up to 300 mg/day may be considered.

PTSD: **PO:** *Adults:* Initial dosage: 50 mg/day. Increase gradually to target dose of 100 to 250 mg/day in adults, and 100 mg/day in older adults. Maximum recommended dosage: 300 mg/day. *Children and adolescents:* Target dose: 50 mg/day.

Migraine Prevention: **PO:** 50 mg at bedtime for 12 weeks.

PAROXETINE **(Paxil)**

Depression: **PO:** *Immediate release:* Initial dose: 20 mg/day in the morning. May increase dose in 10 mg increments at intervals of at least 1 week to a maximum of 50 mg/day.

Controlled release: Initial dose: 25 mg/day in the morning. May increase dose in 12.5 mg increments at intervals of at least 1 week to a maximum of 62.5 mg/day.

Panic Disorder: **PO:** *Immediate release:* Initial dose: 10 mg/day in the morning. May increase dose in 10 mg increments at intervals of at least 1 week to a target dose of 40 mg/day. Maximum dose: 60 mg/day. *Controlled release:* Initial dose: 12.5 mg/day. May increase dose in 12.5 mg/day increments at intervals of at least 1 week to a maximum dose of 75 mg/day.

OCD: **PO**: *Immediate release*: 20 mg/day. May increase dose in 10 mg/day increments at intervals of at least 1 week. Recommended dose: 40 mg/day. Maximum dose: 60 mg/day.

Social Anxiety Disorder: **PO**: *Immediate release*: 20 mg/day. Usual range is 20 to 60 mg/day.

Controlled release: 12.5 mg/day. May increase dosage at intervals of at least 1 week, in increments of 12.5 mg/day to a maximum of 37.5 mg/day.

GAD and PTSD: **PO**: *Immediate release*: 20 mg/day. Usual range is 20 to 50 mg/day. Change doses in increments of 10 mg/day at intervals of at least 1 week.

PMDD: **PO**: *Controlled release:* Initial dose: 12.5 mg/day. Usual range: 12.5 to 25 mg/day. Change doses at intervals of at least 1 week. May be administered daily throughout the menstrual cycle or limited to luteal phase of menstrual cycle.

Hot Flashes: **PO**: *Immediate release:* 20 mg/day.
Controlled release: 12.5 to 25 mg/day

Diabetic Neuropathy: **PO:** Initial dose: 10 mg/day. Titrate to 20 to 60 mg/day.

Elderly or Debilitated Patients: **PO**: *Immediate release:* Initial dose: 10 mg/day. Maximum dose: 40 mg/day.
Controlled release: Initial dose: 12.5 mg/day. Maximum dose: 50 mg/day.

SERTRALINE **(Zoloft)**

Depression and OCD: **PO**: 50 mg/day (either morning or evening). May increase dosage at 1 week intervals to a maximum of 200 mg/day.

Panic Disorder and PTSD: **PO**: Initial dose: 25 mg/day. After 1 week, increase dose to 50 mg/day. For patients not responding, may increase dosage at 1 week intervals to a maximum of 200 mg/day.

PMDD: **PO:** 50 mg/day given on each day of the menstrual cycle or only during each day of the luteal phase of the menstrual cycle. For patients not responding, may increase dosage in 50 mg increments per menstrual cycle up to 150 mg/day when dosing throughout the cycle or 100 mg/day when dosing only during the luteal phase. If 100 mg/day has been established with luteal phase dosing, titrate at 50 mg/day for first 3 days of each luteal phase dosing period.

Social Anxiety Disorder: **PO:** Initial dose: 25 mg/day. After 1 week, increase dose to 50 mg/day. May increase gradually to maximum dose of 200 mg/day.

● CHEMICAL CLASS: NOREPINEPHRINE-DOPAMINE REUPTAKE INHIBITORS (NDRIs)

Examples

Generic (Trade) Name	Pregnancy Categories/ Half-life (hr)	Indications	Therapeutic Plasma Level Range	Available Forms (mg)
Bupropion (Wellbutrin; Zyban)	C/8–24	• Depression (Wellbutrin) • Seasonal affective disorder (Wellbutrin XL) • Smoking cessation (Zyban) **Unlabeled uses:** • ADHD (Wellbutrin)	Not well established	Tabs: 75, 100 Tabs (SR): 100, 150, 200 Tabs (XL): 150, 300

SR = 12-hour tablets; XL = 24-hour tablets.

Action

• Action is unclear. Thought to inhibit the reuptake of norepinephrine and dopamine into presynaptic neurons.

Contraindications and Precautions

Contraindicated in: • Hypersensitivity to the drug • Concomitant use with, or within 2 weeks use of, MAOIs • Known or suspected seizure disorder • Alcohol or benzodiazepine (or other sedatives) withdrawal • Current or prior diagnosis of bulimia or anorexia nervosa • Concomitant use of Wellbutrin (for depression or ADHD) and Zyban (for smoking cessation) • Lactation

Use Cautiously in: • Patients with urinary retention • Patients with hepatic or renal function impairment • Patients with suicidal ideation • Patients with recent history of myocardial infarction or unstable heart disease • Pregnancy (safety not established) • Elderly and debilitated patients

Adverse Reactions and Side Effects

• Dry mouth
• Blurred vision
• Agitation
• Insomnia
• Tremor
• Sedation; dizziness
• Tachycardia

- Excessive sweating
- Headache
- Nausea/vomiting
- Anorexia; weight loss
- Seizures
- Constipation
- Increased risk of suicidality in children and adolescents (black box warning)

Interactions

- Increased effects of bupropion with **amantadine, levodopa, clopidogrel, CYP2B6 inhibitors** (e.g., **cimetidine**), **guanfacine, linezolid,** and **ticlopidine**
- Increased risk of acute toxicity with **MAOIs.** Coadministration is contraindicated.
- Coadministration with a **nicotine replacement agent** may cause hypertension.
- Concomitant use with **alcohol** may produce adverse neuropsychiatric events (alcohol tolerance is reduced).
- Decreased effects of bupropion with **carbamazepine** and **rifampin**
- Increased anticoagulant effect of **warfarin** with bupropion
- Increased effects of drugs metabolized by CYP2D6 isoenzyme (e.g., **nortriptyline, imipramine, desipramine, paroxetine, fluoxetine, sertraline, haloperidol, risperidone, thioridazine, metoprolol, propafenone,** and **flecainide**)

Route and Dosage

BUPROPION **(Wellbutrin; Zyban)**

Depression (Wellbutrin): **PO**: *Adults (immediate release tabs):* 100 mg 2 times a day. May increase after 3 days to 100 mg given 3 times a day. For patients who do not show improvement after several weeks of dosing at 300 mg/day, an increase in dosage up to 450 mg/day may be considered. No single dose of bupropion should exceed 150 mg. To prevent the risk of seizures, administer with an interval of 4 to 6 hours between doses.

Sustained release tabs: Give as a single 150 mg dose in the morning. May increase to twice a day (total 300 mg), with 8 hours between doses.

Extended release tabs: Begin dosing at 150 mg/day, given as a single daily dose in the morning. May increase after 3 days to 300 mg/day, given as a single daily dose in the morning.

Seasonal Affective Disorder (Wellbutrin XL): **PO:** 150 mg administered each morning beginning in the autumn prior to the onset of depressive symptoms. Dose may be uptitrated to the target dose of 300 mg/day after 1 week. Therapy should continue through the winter season before being tapered to 150 mg/day for 2 weeks prior to discontinuation in early spring.

Smoking Cessation (Zyban): PO: Begin dosing at 150 mg given once a day in the morning for 3 days. If tolerated well, increase to target dose of 300 mg/day given in doses of 150 mg 2 times a day with an interval of 8 hours between doses. Continue treatment for 7 to 12 weeks. Some patients may need treatment for as long as 6 months.

ADHD: PO: *Children:* 3 mg/kg/day. *Adults:* 150 to 450 mg/day. No single dose of bupropion should exceed 150 mg. To prevent the risk of seizures, administer with an interval of 4 to 6 hours between doses.

● **CHEMICAL CLASS: SEROTONIN-NOREPINEPHRINE REUPTAKE INHIBITORS (SNRIs)**

Examples

Generic (Trade) Name	Pregnancy Category/ Half-life (hr)	Indications	Therapeutic Plasma Level Ranges	Available Forms (mg)
Desvenlafaxine (Pristiq)	C/11	• Depression	Not well established	Tabs ER: 50, 100
Duloxetine (Cymbalta)	C/8–17	• Depression • Diabetic peripheral neuropathic pain • Fibromyalgia • Generalized anxiety disorder (GAD) **Unlabeled uses:** • Stress urinary incontinence	Not well established	Caps: 20, 30, 60
Venlafaxine (Effexor)	C/5–11 (incl. metabolite)	• Depression • GAD (extended release [ER] only) • Social anxiety disorder (ER) • Panic disorder (ER) **Unlabeled uses:** • Hot flashes • PMDD • PTSD	Not well established	Tabs: 25, 37.5, 50, 75, 100 Caps XR: 37.5, 75, 150

Action

- SNRIs are potent inhibitors of neuronal serotonin and norepinephrine reuptake; weak inhibitors of dopamine reuptake.

Contraindications and Precautions

Contraindicated in: • Hypersensitivity to the drug • Children (safety not established) • Concomitant (or within 14 days) use with MAOIs • Severe renal or hepatic impairment • Pregnancy and lactation (safety not established) • Uncontrolled narrow-angle glaucoma

Use Cautiously in: • Patients with hepatic and renal insufficiency • Elderly and debilitated patients • Patients with history of drug abuse • Patients with suicidal ideation • Patients with history of or existing cardiovascular disease • Patients with history of mania • Patients with history of seizures • Children

Adverse Reactions and Side Effects

- Headache
- Dry mouth
- Nausea
- Somnolence
- Dizziness
- Insomnia
- Asthenia
- Constipation
- Diarrhea
- Mydriasis (venlafaxine)
- Increased risk of suicidality in children and adolescents (black box warning)
- Discontinuation syndrome. Abrupt withdrawal may result in symptoms such as nausea, vomiting, nervousness, dizziness, headache, insomnia, nightmares, paresthesias, and a return of symptoms for which the medication was prescribed. A gradual reduction in dosage is recommended.

Interactions

- Concomitant use with **MAOIs** results in serious, sometimes fatal, effects resembling neuroleptic malignant syndrome. Coadministration is contraindicated.
- Serotonin syndrome may occur when SNRIs are used concomitantly with **St. John's wort, sumatriptan, sibutramine, trazodone,** or other drugs that increase levels of serotonin.
- Increased effects of **haloperidol, clozapine,** and **desipramine** when used concomitantly with venlafaxine
- Increased effects of venlafaxine with **cimetidine** and **azole antifungals**

- Decreased effects of venlafaxine with **cyproheptadine**
- Decreased effects of **indinavir** and **metoprolol** with venlafaxine
- Increased effects of **warfarin** with SNRIs
- Increased effects of duloxetine with CYP1A2 inhibitors (e.g., fluvoxamine, quinolone antibiotics) and CYP2D6 inhibitors (e.g., fluoxetine, quinidine, paroxetine)
- Increased risk of liver injury with concomitant use of **alcohol** and duloxteine
- Increased risk of toxicity or adverse effects from drugs extensively metabolized by CYP2D6 (e.g., **flecainide, phenothiazines, propafenone, tricyclic antidepressants, thioridazine**) when used concomitantly with duloxetine
- Increased effects of **desipramine** with desvenlafaxine
- Decreased effects of **midazolam** with desvenlafaxine

Route and Dosage

DESVENLAFAXINE **(Pristiq)**

***Depression:* PO:** 50 mg once daily, with or without food. (In clinical studies, doses of 50 to 400 mg/day were shown to be effective, although no additional benefit was demonstrated at doses greater than 50 mg/day and adverse events and discontinuations were more frequent at higher doses.)

DULOXETINE **(Cymbalta)**

***Depression:* PO:** 40 mg/day (given as 20 mg twice a day) to 60 mg/day (given either once a day or as 30 mg 2 times a day) without regard to meals.

***Diabetic Peripheral Neuropathic Pain:* PO:** 60 mg/day given once daily without regard to meals.

***Fibromyalgia:* PO:** 30 mg once daily for 1 week and then increase to 60 mg once daily, if needed.

***GAD:* PO:** 60 mg once daily. For some patients, it may be desirable to start at 30 mg once daily for 1 week to allow the patient to adjust to the medication before increasing to 60 mg once daily.

VENLAFAXINE **(Effexor)**

***Depression:* PO**: *Immediate-release tabs:* Initial dosage: 75 mg/day in 2 or 3 divided doses, taken with food. May increase in increments up to 75 mg/day at intervals of at least 4 days. Maximum dosage: 225 mg/day.

***Depression, GAD, and Social Anxiety Disorder:* PO**: *Extended-release caps:* Initial dosage: 75 mg/day, administered in a single dose. May increase dose in increments of up to 75 mg/day at intervals of at least 4 days to a maximum of 225 mg/day.

Panic Disorder: **PO**: *Extended-release caps:* Initial dosage: 37.5 mg/day for 7 days. After 7 days, increase dosage to 75 mg/day. May increase dose in increments of up to 75 mg/day at intervals of at least 7 days to a maximum of 225 mg/day.

● **CHEMICAL CLASS: SEROTONIN-2 ANTAGONISTS/REUPTAKE INHIBITORS (SARIs)**

Examples

Generic Name	Pregnancy Categories/ Half-life (hr)	Indications	Therapeutic-Plasma Level Ranges (ng/ml)	Available Forms (mg)
Nefazodone*	C/2–4	• Depression	Not well established	Tabs: 50, 100, 150, 200, 250
Trazodone	C/4–9	• Depression **Unlabeled uses:** • Aggressive behavior • Panic disorder and agoraphobia with panic attacks • Insomnia • Migraine prevention	800–1600	Tabs: 50, 100, 150, 300

* Bristol-Myers Squibb voluntarily removed their brand of nefazodone (Serzone) from the market in 2004. The generic equivalent is currently available through various other manufacturers.

Action

• Trazodone inhibits neuronal reuptake of serotonin; nefazodone inhibits neuronal reuptake of serotonin and norepinephrine and acts as an antagonist at central 5-HT$_2$ receptors.

Contraindications and Precautions

Contraindicated in: • Hypersensitivity • Coadministration with terfenadine, astemizole, cisapride, pimozide, carbamazepine, or triazolam (nefazodone) • Patients who were withdrawn because of liver injury (nefazodone) • Concomitant use with, or within 2 weeks of use of, MAOIs • Acute phase of myocardial infarction

Use Cautiously in: • Pregnancy and lactation (safety not established) • Children (safety not established) • Patients with suicidal ideation • Patients with hepatic, renal, or cardiovascular disease • Elderly and debilitated patients

Adverse Reactions and Side Effects

- Drowsiness; dizziness
- Fatigue
- Orthostatic hypotension
- Headache
- Nervousness; insomnia
- Dry mouth
- Nausea
- Somnolence
- Constipation
- Priapism
- Increased risk of suicidality in children and adolescents (black box warning)
- Risk of hepatic failure (*nefazodone*) (black box warning)

Interactions

- Increased effects of **CNS depressants, carbamazepine, digoxin,** and **phenytoin** with trazodone
- Increased effects of trazodone with **phenothiazines, azole antifungals,** and **protease inhibitors**
- Risk of serotonin syndrome with concomitant use of trazodone and **SSRIs** or **SNRIs**
- Decreased effects of trazodone with **carbamazepine**
- Increases or decreases in prothrombin time with concurrent use of trazodone and **warfarin**
- Symptoms of serotonin syndrome and those resembling neuroleptic malignant syndrome may occur with concomitant use of **MAOIs** and **SARIs.**
- Risk of serotonin syndrome with concomitant use of nefazodone and **sibutramine** or **sumatriptan**
- Increased effects of both drugs with concomitant use of **buspirone** and nefazodone
- Increased effects of **benzodiazepines, carbamazepine, cisapride, cyclosporine, digoxin,** and **St. John's Wort** with nefazodone
- Decreased effects of nefazodone with **carbamazepine**
- Risk of rhabdomyolysis with concomitant use of nefazodone and **HMG-CoA reductase inhibitors** (e.g., **simvastatin, atorvastatin, lovastatin**)

Route and Dosage

NEFAZODONE

Depression: PO: *Adults:* Initial dosage: 200 mg/day, in 2 divided doses. Dose may be increased in increments of 100 to 200 mg/day (on a 2 times a day schedule) at intervals of at least 1 week. Maximum dose: 600 mg/day.

Elderly and debilitated patients: **PO:** 100 mg/day, in 2 divided doses. Increases should be titrated slowly and based on careful assessment of the patient's clinical response.

TRAZODONE

Depression: **PO:** *Adults:* Initial dosage: 150 mg/day in divided doses. May be increased by 50 mg/day every 3 to 4 days to maximum dose of 400 mg/day. Inpatients or severely depressed patients may be given up to a maximum of 600 mg/day. Drowsiness may require that largest dose of the medication be taken at bedtime.

Aggressive Behavior: **PO:** 50 mg 2 times a day (along with tryptophan 500 mg 2 times a day).

Panic Disorder or Agoraphobia with Panic Attacks: **PO:** 300 mg/day.

Insomnia: **PO:** 50 to 100 mg at bedtime.

Migraine Prevention: **PO:** 100 mg/day.

● **CHEMICAL CLASS: ALPHA-2 RECEPTOR ANTAGONIST**
Examples

Generic (Trade) Name	Pregnancy Category/ Half-life (hr)	Indications	Therapeutic Plasma Level Range	Available Forms (mg)
Mirtazapine (Remeron)	C/20–40	● Depression	Not well established	Tabs: 7.5, 15, 30, 45 Tabs (orally disintegrating): 15, 30, 45

Action

- Potent antagonist of $5\text{-}HT_2$ and $5\text{-}HT_3$ receptors. Acts as antagonist at central presynaptic α_2-adrenergic inhibitory autoreceptors and heteroreceptors, resulting in an increase in central noradrenergic and serotonergic activity. It is also a potent antagonist of histamine (H_1) receptors.

Contraindications and Precautions

Contraindicated in: ● Patients with hypersensitivity to the drug ● Patients with suicidal ideation ● Concurrent use with, or within 14 days of therapy with, MAOIs

Use Cautiously in: ● History of seizures ● History of mania or hypomania ● Elderly or debilitated patients ● Patients with hepatic, renal, or cardiovascular disease ● Pregnancy and lactation (safety not established) ● Children (safety not established)

Adverse Reactions and Side Effects

- Somnolence
- Dizziness
- Dry mouth
- Constipation
- Increased appetite
- Weight gain
- Agranulocytosis
- Increases in cholesterol and triglyceride levels

Interactions

- Additive impairment in cognitive and motor skills with **CNS depressants** (e.g., **benzodiazepines, alcohol**)
- Life-threatening symptoms similar to neuroleptic malignant syndrome with concurrent use, or within 14 days of use of, **MAOIs**
- Possible interaction with drugs that are metabolized by or inhibit cytochrome P450 enzymes CYP2D6, CYP1A2, and CYP3A4
- Increased effects of mirtazapine with concomitant use of **SSRIs** (e.g., **fluoxetine, fluvoxamine**)

Route and Dosage

MIRTAZAPINE **(Remeron)**

Depression: **PO:** Initial dosage: 15 mg/day, administered in a single dose, preferably at bedtime. Dose may be increased at intervals of 1 to 2 weeks, up to a maximum dose of 45 mg/day.

When switching to or from an MAOI: At least 14 days should elapse between discontinuation of an MAOI and initiation of therapy with mirtazapine. In addition, allow at least 14 days after stopping mirtazapine before starting an MAOI.

● CHEMICAL CLASS: MONOAMINE OXIDASE INHIBITORS

Examples

Generic (Trade) Name	Pregnancy Category/ Half-life (hr)	Indications	Therapeutic Plasma Level Range	Available Forms (mg)
Isocarboxazid (Marplan)	C/Not Established	• Depression	Not well established	Tabs: 10
Phenelzine (Nardil)	C/2–3	• Depression **Unlabeled uses:** • PTSD • Migraine prevention	Not well established	Tabs: 15

Generic (Trade) Name	Pregnancy Category/ Half-life (hr)	Indications	Therapeutic Plasma Level Range	Available Forms (mg)
Tranylcypromine (Parnate)	C/2.4–2.8	• Depression **Unlabeled uses:** • Migraine prevention • Social anxiety disorder • Panic disorder	Not well established	Tabs: 10
Selegiline transdermal system (Emsam)	C/18–25 (including metabolites)	• Depression	Not well established	Transdermal patches: 6, 9, 12

Action

• Inhibition of the enzyme monoamine oxidase, which is responsible for the decomposition of the biogenic amines, epinephrine, norepinephrine, dopamine, and serotonin. This action results in an increase in the concentration of these endogenous amines.

Contraindications and Precautions

Contraindicated in: • Hypersensitivity • Pheochromocytoma • Hepatic or renal insufficiency • History of or existing cardiovascular disease • Hypertension • History of severe or frequent headaches • Concomitant use with other MAOIs, tricyclic antidepressants, carbamazepine, cyclobenzaprine, bupropion, SSRIs, SARIs, buspirone, sympathomimetics, meperidine, dextromethorphan, anesthetic agents, CNS depressants, antihypertensives, caffeine, and food with high tyramine content • Children younger than 16 years • Pregnancy and lactation (safety not established)

Use Cautiously in: • Patients with a history of seizures • Patients with diabetes mellitus • Patients with suicidal ideation • Agitated or hypomanic patients • Patients with a history of angina pectoris or hyperthyroidism

Adverse Reactions and Side Effects

• Dizziness
• Headache
• Orthostatic hypotension
• Constipation
• Nausea
• Disturbances in cardiac rate and rhythm
• Blurred vision

- Dry mouth
- Weight gain
- Hypomania
- Site reactions (itching, irritation) (with selegiline transdermal system)
- Increased risk of suicidality in children and adolescents (black box warning)

Interactions

- Serious, potentially fatal adverse reactions may occur with concurrent use of other **antidepressants, carbamazepine, cyclobenzaprine, bupropion, SSRIs, SARIs, buspirone, sympathomimetics, tryptophan, dextromethorphan, anesthetic agents, CNS depressants,** and **amphetamines.** Avoid using within 2 weeks of each other (5 weeks after therapy with **fluoxetine**).
- Hypertensive crisis may occur with **amphetamines, methyldopa, levodopa, dopamine, epinephrine, norepinephrine, guanethidine, methylphenidate, guanadrel, reserpine,** or **vasoconstrictors.**
- Hypertension or hypotension, coma, convulsions, and death may occur with **opioids** (avoid use of **meperidine** within 14 to 21 days of MAOI therapy).
- Additive hypotension may occur with **antihypertensives, thiazide diuretics,** or **spinal anesthesia.**
- Additive hypoglycemia may occur with **insulins** or **oral hypoglycemic agents.**
- **Doxapram** may increase pressor response.
- Serotonin syndrome may occur with concomitant use of **St. John's wort.**
- Hypertensive crisis may occur with ingestion of foods or other products containing high concentrations of **tyramine** (see Nursing Implications).
- Consumption of foods or beverages with high **caffeine** content increases the risk of hypertension and arrhythmias.
- Bradycardia may occur with concurrent use of MAOIs and **beta blockers.**

Route and Dosage

ISOCARBOXAZID **(Marplan)**

Depression: **PO**: Initial dose: 10 mg 2 times a day. May increase dosage by 10 mg every 2 to 4 days to 40 mg by end of first week. If needed, may continue to increase dosage by increments of up to 20 mg/week. Maximum dosage: 60 mg/day divided into 2 to 4 doses. Gradually reduce to smallest effective dose.

PHENELZINE **(Nardil)**

Depression: **PO**: Initial dose: 15 mg 3 times a day. Increase to 60 to 90 mg/day in divided doses until therapeutic response is achieved. Then gradually reduce to smallest effective dose (15 mg/day or every other day).

TRANYLCYPROMINE **(Parnate)**

Depression: **PO**: 30 mg/day in divided doses. After 2 weeks, may increase by 10 mg/day, at 1- to 3-week intervals, up to 60 mg/day.

SELEGILINE TRANSDERMAL SYSTEM **(Emsam)**

Depression: *Transdermal patch:* Initial dose: 6 mg/24 hr. If necessary, dosage may be increased in increments of 3 mg/24 hr at intervals of no less than 2 weeks up to a maximum dose of 12 mg/24 hr.

Elderly clients: The recommended dosage is 6 mg/24 hr.

● **PSYCHOTHERAPEUTIC COMBINATIONS**
Examples

Generic (Trade) Name	Indications	Available Forms (mg)
Olanzapine/fluoxetine (Symbyax)	• For the acute treatment of depressive episodes associated with bipolar I disorder in adults • For the acute treatment of treatment-resistant depression	Caps: olanzapine 3/fluoxetine 25; olanzapine 6/fluoxetine 25; olanzapine 6/fluoxetine 50; olanzapine 12/fluoxetine 25; olanzapine 12/fluoxetine 50
Chlordiazepoxide/ amitriptyline (Limbitrol)	• For the treatment of moderate to severe depression associated with moderate to severe anxiety	Tabs: chlordiazepoxide 5/ amitriptyline 12.5; chlordiazepoxide 10/ amitriptyline 25
Perphenazine/ amitriptyline HCl (Etrafon)	• For the treatment of moderate to severe anxiety or agitation and depressed mood • For the treatment of patients with schizophrenia who have associated symptoms of depression	Tabs: perphenazine 2/amitriptyline 10; perphenazine 2/amitriptyline 25; perphenazine 4/amitriptyline 10; perphenazine 4/amitriptyline 25; perphenazine 4/amitriptyline 50

* These medications are presented for general information only. For detailed information, the reader is directed to the chapters that deal with each of the specific drugs that make up these combinations.

Route and Dosage

OLANZAPINE/FLUOXETINE **(Symbyax)**

Depression Associated with Bipolar I Disorder and Treatment-resistant Depression: **PO:** Initial dosage: olanzapine 6 mg/fluoxetine 25 mg once daily in the evening. Dosage adjustments, if indicated, can be made according to efficacy and tolerability.

CHLORDIAZEPOXIDE/AMITRIPTYLINE **(Limbitrol)**

Moderate to Severe Depression Associated with Moderate to Severe Anxiety: **PO:** Initial dose: chlordiazepoxide 10/amitriptyline 25 given 3 or 4 times a day in divided doses. May increase to 6 times a day, as required. Some patients respond to smaller doses and can be maintained on 2 tablets daily.

PERPHENAZINE/AMITRIPTYLINE HCL **(Etrafon)**

Anxiety/Agitation/Depression: **PO:** Initial dose: perphenazine 2 to 4 mg/amitriptyline 10 to 50 mg, 3 or 4 times/day. Once a satisfactory response is achieved, reduce to smallest amount necessary to obtain relief.

● NURSING DIAGNOSES RELATED TO ALL ANTIDEPRESSANTS

1. Risk for suicide related to depressed mood.
2. Risk for injury related to side effects of sedation, lowered seizure threshold, orthostatic hypotension, priapism, photo-sensitivity, arrhythmias, and hypertensive crisis.
3. Social isolation related to depressed mood.
4. Risk for constipation related to side effects of the medication.

● NURSING IMPLICATIONS FOR ANTIDEPRESSANTS

The plan of care should include monitoring for the following side effects from antidepressant medications. Nursing implications are designated by an asterisk (*).

1. **May occur with all chemical classes:**
   a. **Dry mouth**
      * Offer the client sugarless candy, ice, frequent sips of water
      * Strict oral hygiene is very important.
   b. **Sedation**
      * Request an order from the physician for the drug to be given at bedtime.
      * Request that the physician decrease the dosage or perhaps order a less sedating drug.
      * Instruct the client not to drive or use dangerous equipment while experiencing sedation.

c. **Nausea**
  * Medication may be taken with food to minimize GI distress.
d. **Discontinuation syndrome**
  * All classes of antidepressants have varying potentials to cause discontinuation syndromes. Abrupt withdrawal following long-term therapy with SSRIs and SNRIs may result in dizziness, lethargy, headache, and nausea. Fluoxetine is less likely to result in withdrawal symptoms because of its long half-life. Abrupt withdrawal from tricyclics may produce hypomania, akathisia, cardiac arrhythmias, and panic attacks. The discontinuation syndrome associated with MAOIs includes confusion, hypomania, and worsening of depressive symptoms. All antidepressant medication should be tapered gradually to prevent withdrawal symptoms.

2. **Most commonly occur with tricyclics and others, such as the SARIs, bupropion, maprotiline, and mirtazapine:**
  a. **Blurred vision**
    * Offer reassurance that this symptom should subside after a few weeks
    * Instruct the client not to drive until vision is clear.
    * Clear small items from routine pathway to prevent falls.
  b. **Constipation**
    * Order foods high in fiber; increase fluid intake if not contraindicated; and encourage the client to increase physical exercise, if possible.
  c. **Urinary retention**
    * Instruct the client to report hesitancy or inability to urinate.
    * Monitor intake and output.
    * Try various methods to stimulate urination, such as running water in the bathroom or pouring water over the perineal area.
  d. **Orthostatic hypotension**
    * Instruct the client to rise slowly from a lying or sitting position.
    * Monitor blood pressure (lying and standing) frequently, and document and report significant changes.
    * Instruct the client to avoid long hot showers or tub baths.
  e. **Reduction of seizure threshold**
    * Observe clients with history of seizures closely.
    * Institute seizure precautions as specified in hospital procedure manual.
    * Bupropion (Wellbutrin) should be administered in doses of no more than 150 mg and should be given at

least 4 hours apart. Bupropion has been associated with a relatively high incidence of seizure activity in anorexic and cachectic clients.

f. **Tachycardia; arrhythmias**
   * Carefully monitor blood pressure and pulse rate and rhythm, and report any significant change to the physician.

g. **Photosensitivity**
   * Ensure that client wears sunblock lotion, protective clothing, and sunglasses while outdoors.

h. **Weight gain**
   * Provide instructions for reduced-calorie diet.
   * Encourage increased level of activity, if appropriate.

3. **Most commonly occur with SSRIs:**
   a. **Insomnia; agitation**
      * Administer or instruct client to take dose early in the day.
      * Instruct client to avoid caffeinated food and drinks.
      * Teach relaxation techniques to use before bedtime.

   b. **Headache**
      * Administer analgesics, as prescribed.
      * If relief is not achieved, physician may order another antidepressant.

   c. **Weight loss** (may occur early in therapy)
      * Ensure that client is provided with caloric intake sufficient to maintain desired weight.
      * Caution should be taken in prescribing these drugs for anorexic clients.
      * Weigh client daily or every other day, at the same time and on the same scale if possible.
      * After prolonged use, some clients may gain weight on SSRIs.

   d. **Sexual dysfunction**
      * Men may report abnormal ejaculation or impotence.
      * Women may experience delay or loss of orgasm.
      * If side effect becomes intolerable, a switch to another antidepressant may be necessary.

   e. **Serotonin syndrome** (may occur when two drugs that potentiate serotonergic neurotransmission are used concurrently [see "Interactions"]).
      * Most frequent symptoms include changes in mental status, restlessness, myoclonus, hyperreflexia, tachycardia, labile blood pressure, diaphoresis, shivering, and tremors.
      * Discontinue offending agent immediately.
      * The physician will prescribe medications to block serotonin receptors, relieve hyperthermia and muscle

rigidity, and prevent seizures. In severe cases, artificial ventilation may be required. The histamine-1 receptor antagonist cyproheptadine is commonly used to treat the symptoms of serotonin syndrome.

* Supportive nursing measures include monitoring vital signs, providing safety measures to prevent injury when muscle rigidity and changes in mental status are present, cooling blankets and tepid baths to assist with temperature regulation, and monitoring intake and output (Prator, 2006).

* The condition will usually resolve on its own once the offending medication has been discontinued. However, if the medication is not discontinued, the condition may progress to life-threatening complications such as seizures, coma, hypotension, ventricular arrhythmias, disseminated intravascular coagulation, rhabdomyolysis, metabolic acidosis, and renal failure (Prator, 2006).

4. **Most commonly occur with MAOIs:**
   a. **Hypertensive crisis**
      * Hypertensive crisis occurs if the individual consumes foods or other substances containing tyramine while receiving MAOI therapy. Foods that should be avoided include aged cheeses, raisins, fava beans, red wines, smoked and processed meats, caviar, pickled herring, soy sauce, monosodium glutamate (MSG), beer, chocolate, yogurt, and bananas. Drugs that should be avoided include other antidepressants, sympathomimetics (including over-the-counter cough and cold preparations), stimulants (including over-the-counter diet drugs), antihypertensives, meperidine and other opioid narcotics, and antiparkinsonian agents, such as levodopa.
      * Symptoms of hypertensive crisis include severe occipital headache, palpitations, nausea and vomiting, nuchal rigidity, fever, sweating, marked increase in blood pressure, chest pain, and coma.
      * Treatment of hypertensive crisis: Discontinue drug immediately; monitor vital signs; administer short-acting antihypertensive medication, as ordered by physician; use external cooling measures to control hyperpyrexia.
   b. **Application site reactions** (with selegiline transdermal system [Emsam])
      * The most common reactions include rash, itching, erythema, redness, irritation, swelling, or urticarial lesions. Most reactions resolve spontaneously, requiring no treatment. However, if reaction becomes problematic, it should be reported to the physician. Topical corticosteroids have been used in treatment.

5. **Miscellaneous side effects:**
   a. **Priapism (with trazodone)**
      * Priapism is a rare side effect, but it has occurred in some men taking trazodone.
      * If the client complains of prolonged or inappropriate penile erection, withhold medication dosage and notify the physician immediately.
      * Priapism can become very problematic, requiring surgical intervention, and, if not treated successfully, can result in impotence.
   b. **Hepatic failure (with nefazodone)**
      * Cases of life-threatening hepatic failure have been reported in clients treated with nefazodone.
      * Advise clients to be alert for signs or symptoms suggestive of liver dysfunction (e.g., jaundice, anorexia, GI complaints, or malaise) and to report them to physician immediately.

● **CLIENT/FAMILY EDUCATION RELATED TO ALL ANTIDEPRESSANTS**

- Continue to take the medication even though the symptoms have not subsided. The therapeutic effect may not be seen for as long as 4 weeks. If after this length of time no improvement is noted, the physician may prescribe a different medication.
- Use caution when driving or operating dangerous machinery. Drowsiness and dizziness can occur. If these side effects become persistent or interfere with activities of daily living, the client should report them to the physician. Dosage adjustment may be necessary.
- Do not stop taking the drug abruptly. To do so might produce withdrawal symptoms, such as nausea, vertigo, insomnia, headache, malaise, nightmares, and a return of the symptoms for which the medication was prescribed.
- Use sunblock lotion and wear protective clothing when spending time outdoors. The skin may be sensitive to sunburn.
- Report occurrence of any of the following symptoms to the physician immediately: sore throat, fever, malaise, yellowish skin, unusual bleeding, easy bruising, persistent nausea and vomiting, severe headache, rapid heart rate, difficulty urinating, anorexia or weight loss, seizure activity, stiff or sore neck, and chest pain.
- Rise slowly from a sitting or lying position to prevent a sudden drop in blood pressure.
- Take frequent sips of water, chew sugarless gum, or suck on hard candy if dry mouth is a problem. Good oral care (frequent brushing, flossing) is very important.

- Do not consume the following foods or medications while taking MAOIs: aged cheese, wine (especially Chianti), beer, chocolate, colas, coffee, tea, sour cream, smoked and processed meats, chicken or beef liver, soy sauce, pickled herring, yogurt, raisins, caviar, broad beans, cold remedies, or diet pills. To do so could cause a life-threatening hypertensive crisis.
- Follow the correct procedure for applying the selegiline transdermal patch:
  - Apply to dry, intact skin on upper torso, upper thigh, or outer surface of upper arm.
  - Apply approximately same time each day to new spot on skin, after removing and discarding old patch.
  - Wash hands thoroughly after applying the patch.
  - Avoid exposing application site to direct heat (e.g., heating pads, electric blankets, heat lamps, hot tub, or prolonged direct sunlight).
  - If patch falls off, apply new patch to a new site and resume previous schedule.
- Avoid smoking while receiving tricyclic therapy. Smoking increases the metabolism of tricyclics, requiring an adjustment in dosage to achieve the therapeutic effect.
- Do not drink alcohol while taking antidepressant therapy. These drugs potentiate the effects of each other.
- Do not consume other medications (including over-the-counter medications) without the physician's approval while receiving antidepressant therapy. Many medications contain substances that, in combination with antidepressant medication, could precipitate a life-threatening hypertensive crisis.
- Notify physician immediately if inappropriate or prolonged penile erections occur while taking trazodone. If the erection persists longer than 1 hour, seek emergency department treatment. This condition is rare but has occurred in some men who have taken trazodone. If measures are not instituted immediately, impotence can result.
- Do not "double up" on medication if a dose of bupropion (Wellbutrin) is missed, unless advised to do so by the physician. Taking bupropion in divided doses will decrease the risk of seizures and other adverse effects.
- Be aware of possible risks of taking antidepressants during pregnancy. Safe use during pregnancy and lactation has not been fully established. These drugs are believed to readily cross the placental barrier; if so, the fetus could experience adverse effects of the drug. Inform the physician immediately if pregnancy occurs, is suspected, or is planned.

- Be aware of the side effects of antidepressants. Refer to written materials furnished by health care providers for safe self-administration.
- Carry a card or other identification at all times describing the medications being taken.

 INTERNET REFERENCES

a. http://www.mentalhealth.com/
b. http://www.nimh.nih.gov/publicat/medicate.cfm
c. http://www.fadavis.com/townsend
d. http://www.nlm.nih.gov/medlineplus/druginformation .html

Mood-Stabilizing Drugs

● CHEMICAL CLASS: ANTIMANIC
Examples

Generic (Trade) Name	Pregnancy Category/ Half-life (hrs)	Indications	Therapeutic Plasma Level Range mEq/L	Available Forms (mg)
Lithium carbonate (Eskalith; Lithobid) Lithium citrate	D/20–27	• Manic episodes associated with bipolar disorder • Maintenance therapy to prevent or diminish intensity of subsequent manic episodes **Unlabeled uses:** • Borderline personality disorder • Neutropenia • Cluster headaches (prophylaxis) • Alcohol dependence • Bulimia • Postpartum affective psychosis • Corticosteroid-induced psychosis	Acute mania: 1.0–1.5 Maintenance: 0.6–1.2	Caps: 150, 300, 600 Tabs: 300 Tabs (ER): 300, 450 Syrup: 8 mEq (as citrate equivalent to 300 mg lithium carbonate)/ 5 mL

Action
• Not fully understood, but lithium may have an influence on the reuptake of norepinephrine and serotonin. Effects on other neurotransmitters have also been noted. Lithium also alters sodium transport in nerve and muscle cells.

Contraindications and Precautions:
Contraindicated in: • Hypersensitivity • Severe cardiovascular or renal disease • Dehydrated or debilitated patients • Sodium depletion • Pregnancy and lactation

Use Cautiously in: • Elderly patients • Any degree of cardiac, renal, or thyroid disease • Diabetes mellitus • Urinary retention • Children younger than 12 years (*safety not established*)

Adverse Reactions and Side Effects

- Drowsiness, dizziness, headache
- Seizures
- Dry mouth, thirst
- Indigestion, nausea, anorexia
- Fine hand tremors
- Hypotension, arrhythmias, electrocardiogram (ECG) changes
- Polyuria, glycosuria
- Weight gain
- Hypothyroidism
- Dehydration
- Leukocytosis

Interactions

- The effects of lithium (and potential for toxicity) are increased with concurrent use of **carbamazepine, fluoxetine, haloperidol, loop diuretics, methyldopa, nonsteroidal anti-inflammatory drugs (NSAIDs),** and **thiazide diuretics.**
- The effects of lithium are decreased with concurrent use of **acetazolamide, osmotic diuretics, theophylline,** and **urinary alkalinizers.**
- Increased effects of **neuromuscular blocking agents** and **tricyclic antidepressants** are seen with concurrent use of lithium.
- Decreased pressor sensitivity of **sympathomimetics** with lithium
- Neurotoxicity may occur with concurrent use of lithium and **high-potency antipsychotics** or **calcium channel blockers.**

Route and Dosage

Acute Mania: **PO:** 600 mg three times a day or 900 mg twice daily for the slow release form. Serum levels should be taken twice weekly at the initiation of therapy and until therapeutic level has been achieved.

Long-Term (Maintenance) Use: **PO:** 300 mg three to four times a day. Serum levels should be monitored in uncomplicated cases during maintenance therapy every 1 to 2 months.

Borderline Personality Disorder: **PO:** 900 to 2400 mg/day in 3 to 4 divided doses (or 900 to 1800 mg/day [ER tabs] in 2 divided doses). Titrate dosage to maintain serum levels of 0.8 to 1 mEq/L.

● CHEMICAL CLASS: ANTICONVULSANTS
Examples

Generic (Trade) Name	Pregnancy Categories/ Half-life (hr)	Indications	Therapeutic Plasma Level Range	Available Forms (mg)
Carbamazepine* (Tegretol, Epitol, Carbatrol, Equetro, Teril, Tegretol-XR)	D/25–65 (initial) 12–17 (repeated doses)	• Epilepsy • Trigeminal neuralgia **Unlabeled uses:** • Bipolar disorder (FDA approved: *Equetro* only) • Borderline personality disorder • Management of alcohol withdrawal • Restless legs syndrome • Postherpetic neuralgia	4–12 mcg/mL	Tabs: 100, 200 Tabs XR: 100, 200, 400 Caps XR: 100, 200, 300 Oral suspension: 100/5 mL
Clonazepam (C-IV) (Klonopin)	C/18–60	• Petit mal, akinetic, and myoclonic seizures • Panic disorder **Unlabeled uses:** • Acute manic episodes • Restless leg syndrome • Neuralgias	20–80 ng/mL	Tabs: 0.5, 1, 2
Valproic acid* (Depakene, Depakote, Stavzor, Depacon)	D/5–20	• Epilepsy **Unlabeled uses:** • Manic episodes (FDA approved: *Stavzor* only) • Migraine prophylaxis (FDA approved: *Stavzor* only) • Borderline personality disorder	50–150 mcg/mL	Caps: 250 Caps (DR): 125, 250, 500 Syrup: 250/5 mL Tabs (DR): 125, 250, 500 Tabs (ER): 250, 500 Caps (sprinkle): 125 Injection: 100/mL in 5 mL vial

Continued

Generic (Trade) Name	Pregnancy Categories/ Half-life (hr)	Indications	Therapeutic Plasma Level Range	Available Forms (mg)
Lamotrigine* (Lamictal)	C/-33	• Epilepsy • Bipolar disorder	Not established	Tabs: 25, 100, 150, 200 Tabs (chewable): 2, 5, 25
Gabapentin* (Neurontin; Gabarone)	C/5–7	• Epilepsy • Postherpetic neuralgia **Unlabeled uses:** • Bipolar disorder • Migraine prophylaxis • Neuropathic pain • Tremors associated with multiple sclerosis	Not established	Caps: 100, 300, 400 Tabs: 100, 300, 400, 600, 800 Oral Solution: 250/5 mL
Topiramate* (Topamax)	C/21	• Epilepsy • Migraine prophylaxis **Unlabeled uses:** • Bipolar disorder • Cluster headaches • Bulimia • Weight loss in obesity	Not established	Tabs: 25, 50, 100, 200 Caps (sprinkle): 15, 25
Oxcarbazepine* (Trileptal)	C/2 (metabolite 9)	• Epilepsy **Unlabeled uses:** • Alcohol withdrawal • Bipolar disorder • Diabetic neuropathy	Not established	Tabs: 150, 300, 600 Oral Susp: 60/mL

* The FDA has issued a warning indicating reports of suicidal behavior or ideation associated with the use of these drugs (and other antiepileptic medications). The FDA now requires that all manufacturers of drugs in this class include a warning in their labeling to this effect. Results of a study published in the December 2009 issue of *Archives of General Psychiatry* indicate that antiepileptic medications "do not increase risk of suicide attempts in patients with bipolar disorder" (Gibbons et al., 2009).

Action
• Action in the treatment of bipolar disorder is unclear.

Contraindications and Precautions

Carbamazepine
• **Contraindicated in** hypersensitivity, with monoamine oxidase inhibitors (MAOIs), lactation, history of previous bone marrow depression.
• **Use cautiously in** elderly, liver/renal/cardiac disease, pregnancy.

Clonazepam
• **Contraindicated in** hypersensitivity, acute narrow-angle glaucoma, liver disease, lactation.
• **Use cautiously in** elderly, liver/renal disease, pregnancy.

Valproic Acid
• **Contraindicated in** hypersensitivity, liver disease.
• **Use cautiously in** elderly, renal/cardiac diseases, pregnancy, lactation.

Lamotrigine
• **Contraindicated in** hypersensitivity.
• **Use cautiously in** renal/hepatic/cardiac insufficiency, pregnancy, lactation.

Gabapentin
• **Contraindicated in** hypersensitivity, children <3 years of age.
• **Use cautiously in** renal insufficiency, pregnancy, lactation, children, elderly.

Topiramate
• **Contraindicated in** hypersensitivity.
• **Use cautiously in** renal and hepatic impairment, pregnancy, lactation, children, elderly.

Oxcarbazepine
• **Contraindicated in** hypersensitivity (cross-sensitivity with carbamazepine may occur), lactation.
• **Use cautiously in** renal impairment, pregnancy, children <4 years old.

Adverse Reactions and Side Effects

Carbamazepine
• Drowsiness, ataxia
• Nausea, vomiting
• Blood dyscrasias

Clonazepam
• Drowsiness, ataxia
• Dependence, tolerance
• Blood dyscrasias

Valproic Acid
- Drowsiness, dizziness
- Nausea, vomiting
- Prolonged bleeding time
- Tremor

Gabapentin
- Drowsiness, dizziness, ataxia
- Nystagmus
- Tremor

Lamotrigine
- Ataxia, dizziness, headache
- Nausea, vomiting
- Risk of severe rash
- Photosensitivity

Topiramate
- Drowsiness, dizziness, fatigue, ataxia
- Impaired concentration, nervousness
- Vision changes
- Nausea, weight loss
- Decreased efficacy with oral contraceptives

Oxcarbazepine
- Dizziness, drowsiness
- Headache
- Nausea and vomiting
- Abnormal vision, diplopia, nystagmus
- Ataxia
- Tremor

Interactions

The effects of:	Are increased by:	Are decreased by:	Concurrent use may result in:
Carbamazepine	Verapamil, diltiazem, propoxyphene, erythromycin, clarithromycin, SSRIs, tricyclic antidepressants, cimetidine, isoniazid, danazol, lamotrigine, niacin, acetazolamide, dalfopristin, valproate, nefazodone	Cisplatin, doxorubicin, felbamate, rifampin, barbiturates, hydantoins, primidone, theophylline	Decreased levels of **corticosteroids, doxycycline, felbamate, quinidine, warfarin, estrogen-containing contraceptives, cyclosporine, benzodiazepines, theophylline, lamotrigine, valproic acid, bupropion, haloperidol, olanzapine, tiagabine, topiramate, voriconazole, ziprasidone. felbamate, levothyroxine, antidepressants** Increased levels of **lithium** Life-threatening hypertensive reaction with **MAOIs**

The effects of:	Are increased by:	Are decreased by:	Concurrent use may result in:
Clonazepam	CNS depressants, cimetidine, hormonal contraceptives, disulfiram, fluoxetine, isoniazid, ketoconazole, metoprolol, propoxyphene, propranol, valproic acid, probenecid	Rifampin, theophylline (↓ sedative effects), phenytoin	Increased **phenytoin** levels; decreased efficacy of **levodopa**
Valproic acid	Chlorpromazine, cimetidine, erythromycin, felbamate, salicylates	Rifampin, carbamazepine, cholestyramine, lamotrigine, phenobarbital, ethosuximide, hydantoins	Increased effects of **tricyclic antidepressants, carbamazepine, CNS depressants, ethosuximide, lamotrigine, phenobarbital, hydantoins, warfarin, zidovudine, hydantoins**
Gabapentin	Cimetidine, hydrocodone, morphine, naproxin	Antacids	Decreased effects of **hydrocodone**
Lamotrigine	Valproic acid	Primidone, phenobarbital, phenytoin, rifamycin, succinimides, oral contraceptives, oxcarbazepine, carbamazepine, acetaminophen	Decreased levels of **valproic acid;** Increased levels of **carbamazepine** and **topiramate**
Topiramate	Metformin; hydrochlorothiazide	Phenytoin, carbamazepine, valproic acid, lamotrigine	Increased risk of CNS depression with **alcohol** or other **CNS depressants.** Increased risk of kidney stones with **carbonic anhydrase inhibitors.** Increased effects of **phenytoin, metformin, amitriptyline.** Decreased effects of **oral contraceptives, digoxin, lithium, riseridone,** and **valproic acid.**
Oxcarbazepine		Carbamazepine, phenobarbital, phenytoin, valproic acid, verapamil	Increased concentrations of **phenobarbital** and **phenytoin;** decreased effects of **oral contraceptives, felodipine,** and **lamotrigine**

Route and Dosage

CARBAMAZEPINE **(Tegretol)**

Seizure Disorders: *Adults and children > 12 years:* **PO**: Initial dosage: Either 200 mg 2 times a day for tablets and extended-release (ER) tablets/capsules, or 5 mL (100 mg) 4 times a day for suspension. Increase by 200 mg/day every 7 days until therapeutic levels are achieved. Maximum dose: 1000 mg/day in children 12 to 15 years; 1200 mg/day in patients >15 years.

Children 6 to 12 years: **PO**: 100 mg 2 times a day (50 mg 4 times a day of suspension). Increase by 100 mg weekly until therapeutic levels are obtained. (Usual range: 400 to 800 mg/day.) Maximum daily dose: 1000 mg.

Children <6 years: **PO**: 10 to 20 mg/kg/day in 2 to 3 divided doses. May increase weekly to achieve optimal clinical response administered 3 or 4 times a day. Maximum daily dose: 35 mg/kg/day.

***Trigeminal Neuralgia:* PO**: Initial dose 100 mg 2 times a day. May increase by up to 200 mg/day using 100 mg increments every 12 hours. Maximum daily dose: 1200 mg.

Bipolar Disorder, Mania: (Equetro only) **PO**: Initial dose: 200 mg 2 times a day. Dosage may be adjusted in 200 mg daily increments to achieve optimal clinical response. Doses higher than 1600 mg/day have not been studied.

***Borderline Personality Disorder:* PO**: 400 mg/day in 2 divided doses. May increase dose in increments of 200 mg/day depending on response, tolerability, and plasma concentrations. Maximum dosage: 1600 mg/day.

***Management of Alcohol Withdrawal:* PO**: Dosage on day 1: 600 to 1200 mg. Dosage is then tapered over 5 to 10 days to 0 mg.

***Restless Leg Syndrome:* PO**: 100 to 600 mg daily for up to 5 weeks.

***Postherpetic Neuralgia:* PO**: 100 to 200 mg/day, slowly increased to a maximum of 1200 mg/day.

CLONAZEPAM **(Klonopin)**

Seizures: *Adults:* **PO**: 0.5 mg 3 times a day; may increase by 0.5 to 1 mg every third day. Maximum daily dose 20 mg.

Children <10 years or 30 kg: **PO**: Initial daily dose 0.01 to 0.03 mg/kg/day (not to exceed 0.05 mg/kg/day) given in 2 to 3 divided doses; increase by no more than 0.25 to 0.5 mg every third day until a daily maintenance dose of 0.1 to 0.2 mg/kg has been reached, unless seizures are controlled or side effects preclude further increase.

***Panic Disorder:* PO**: Initial dose: 0.25 mg 2 times a day. Increase after 3 days toward target dose of 1 mg/day. Some patients may require up to 4 mg/day, in which case the dose may be increased in increments of 0.125 to 0.25 mg twice daily every 3 days until symptoms are controlled.

Bipolar Disorder, Mania: **PO**: 1 to 6 mg/day.

Restless Leg Syndrome: **PO**: 0.5 to 2 mg/night.

Neuralgias: **PO**: 1.5 to 4 mg/day.

VALPROIC ACID **(Depakene; Depakote)**

Epilepsy: **PO**: *Adults and children ≥10 years old:* Initial dose: 5 to 15 mg/kg/day. Increase by 5 to 10 mg/kg/week until therapeutic levels are reached. Maximum recommended dosage: 60 mg/kg/day. When daily dosage exceeds 250 mg, give in 2 divided doses.

Manic Episodes: **PO** (Stavzor only): Initial dose: 750 mg/day in divided doses. Titrate rapidly to desired clinical effect or trough plasma levels of 50 to 125 mcg/mL. Maximum recommended dose: 60/mg/kg/day.

Migraine Prophylaxis: **PO** (Stavzor only): 250 mg twice daily. Some patients may require up to 1000 mg/day. No evidence that higher doses lead to greater efficacy.

Borderline Personality Disorder: **PO**: 750 mg/day in divided doses. Titrate to maintain a therapeutic plasma level of 50 to 100 mcg/mL.

LAMOTRIGINE **(Lamictal)**

Epilepsy *Adults and children >12 years: Adjunctive therapy with carbamazepine, phenobarbital, phenytoin, or primidone:* **PO**: 50 mg as a single daily dose for 2 weeks, then 50 mg twice daily for next 2 weeks; then increase by 100 mg/day on a weekly basis to maintenance dose of 300 to 500 mg/day in 2 doses. If valproic acid is also being taken, the initial dose should be 25 mg every other day for 2 weeks, then 25 mg once daily for next 2 weeks; then increase by 25 to 50 mg/day every 1 to 2 weeks to maintenance dose of 50 to 200 mg twice a day.

Children 2 to 12 years: Refer to manufacturer's dosing recommendations.

Bipolar Disorder: *Escalation regimen: For patients not taking carbamazepine, valproic acid, or other enzyme-inducing drugs:* **PO**: Weeks 1 and 2: 25 mg/day; weeks 3 and 4: 50 mg/day; week 5: 100 mg/day; then 200 mg/day.

For patients taking valproic acid: **PO**: Weeks 1 and 2: 25 mg every other day; weeks 3 and 4: 25 mg/day; week 5: 50 mg/day; then 100 mg/day.

For patients taking carbamazepine or other enzyme-inducing drugs, but not valproic acid: **PO**: Weeks 1 and 2: 50 mg/day; weeks 3 and 4: 100 mg/day in divided doses; week 5: 200 mg/day in divided doses; week 6: 300 mg/day in divided doses; then up to 400 mg/day in divided doses.

GABAPENTIN **(Neurontin)**

Epilepsy: *Adults and children >12 years*: **PO**: Initial dose: 300 mg 3 times a day. Titration may be continued until desired results have been achieved (range is 900 to 1800 mg/day in 3 divided doses). Doses should not be more than 12 hours apart. Doses of 2400 to 3600 mg have been well tolerated.

Children 5 to 12 years: **PO:** Initial dose: 10 to 15 mg/kg/day in 3 divided doses. Titrate dosage over a period of 3 days to 25 to 35 mg/kg/day in 3 divided doses. Dosage interval should not exceed 12 hours. Dosages up to 50 mg/kg/day have been used.

Children 3 to 4 years: **PO:** Initial dose: 10 to 15 mg/kg/day in 3 divided doses. Titrate dosage over a period of 3 days to 40 mg/kg/day in 3 divided doses. Dosage interval should not exceed 12 hours. Dosages up to 50 mg/kg/day have been used.

Bipolar Disorder: **PO**: 900 to 2400 mg/day in 2 or 3 divided doses.

Postherpetic Neuralgia: **PO:** *Adults:* 300 mg once daily on first day; 300 mg twice daily on second day; then 300 mg three times a day on day 3. May then be titrated upward as needed up to 600 mg three times a day.

Migraine Prophylaxis: **PO:** *Adults:* 1200 to 2400 mg/day.

Tremors in Multiple Sclerosis: **PO:** 1200 to 1800 mg/day.

TOPIRAMATE **(Topamax)**

Epilepsy: *Adults and children ≥17 years (adjunctive therapy):* **PO**: Initial dose: 25 to 50 mg/day. Gradually increase by 25 to 50 mg weekly up to 200 to 400 mg/day in 2 divided doses (200 to 400 mg/day in 2 divided doses for partial seizures and 400 mg/day in 2 divided doses for primary generalized tonic/clonic seizures).

Children 2 to 17 years (adjunctive therapy): **PO**: 5 to 9 mg/kg/day in 2 divided doses; initiate with 25 mg (or less, based on 1 to 3 mg/kg) nightly for 7 days, then increase at 1- to 2-week intervals in increments of 1 to 3 mg/kg/day in 2 divided doses. Titration should be based on clinical outcome.

Adults and children ≥10 years (monotherapy): **PO:** 50 mg/day initially in 2 divided doses. Gradually increase over 6 weeks to 400 mg/day in 2 divided doses.

Migraine Prophylaxis: **PO:** Target dose of 100 mg/day in 2 divided doses, titrated weekly according to the following schedule: *Week 1:* 25 mg in the evening; *Week 2:* 25 mg in the morning and 25 mg in the evening; *Week 3:* 25 mg in the morning and 50 mg in the evening; *Week 4:* 50 mg in the morning and 50 mg in the evening.

***Bipolar Disorder:* PO:** Initial dose: 25 to 50 mg/day. Increase to target range of 100 to 200 mg/day in divided doses. Maximum dosage: 400 mg/day.

OXCARBAZEPINE **(Trileptal)**

***Epilepsy:* PO:** *Adults: (adjunctive therapy):* 300 mg twice daily, may be increased by up to 600 mg/day at weekly intervals up to 1200 mg/day (up to 2400 mg/day may be needed). *Conversion to monotherapy:* 300 mg twice daily; may be increased by 600 mg/day at weekly intervals, whereas other antiepileptic drugs are tapered over 3 to 6 weeks; dose of oxcarbazepine should be increased up to 2400 mg/day over a period of 2 to 4 weeks. *Initiation of monotherapy:* 300 mg twice daily, increase by 300 mg/day every third day, up to 1200 mg/day. Maximum maintenance dose should be achieved over 2 to 4 weeks.

Children 2 to 16 years: (adjunctive therapy): 4 to 5 mg/kg twice daily (up to 600 mg/day), increased over 2 weeks to achieve 900 mg/day in patients 20 to 29 kg, 1200 mg/day in patients 29.1 to 39 kg, and 1800 mg/day in patients >39 kg (range 6 to 51 mg/kg/day). In patients <20 kg, initial dose of 16 to 20 mg/kg/day may be used, not to exceed 60 mg/kg/day. *Conversion to monotherapy:* 8 to 10 mg/kg/day given twice daily; may be increased by 10 mg/kg/day at weekly intervals, whereas other antiepileptic drugs are tapered over 3 to 6 weeks; dose of oxcarbazepine should be increased up to 600 to 900 mg/day in patient ≤20 kg, 900 to 1200 mg/day in patients 25 to 30 kg, 900 to 1500 mg/day in patients 35 to 40 kg, 1200 to 1500 mg/day in patients 45 kg, 1200 to 1800 mg/day in patients 50 to 55 kg, 1200 to 2100 mg/day in patients 60 to 65 kg, and 1500 to 2100 mg/day in patients 70 kg. Maximum maintenance dose should be achieved over 2 to 4 weeks.

***Alcohol Withdrawal:* PO:** 600 to 1800 mg in divided doses for 6 weeks to 6 months.

***Bipolar Disorder:* PO:** *Adults:* Initial dose: 300 mg/day. Titrate to a maximum dose of 900 to 2400 mg/day.

***Diabetic Neuropathy:* PO:** Initial dose: 150 to 300 mg/day. Titrate to recommended dose of 900 to 1200 mg/day. Maximum dose: 1800 mg/day.

● CHEMICAL CLASS: CALCIUM CHANNEL BLOCKERS

Examples

Generic (Trade) Name	Pregnancy Categories/ Half-life (hr)	Indications	Therapeutic Plasma Level Range	Available Forms (mg)
Verapamil (Calan; Isoptin)	C/3–7 (initially) 4.5–12 (repeated dosing) ~12 (SR) 2–5 (IV)	• Angina • Arrhythmias • Hypertension **Unlabeled uses:** • Bipolar mania • Migraine headache prophylaxis	80–300 ng/ml	Tabs: 40, 80, 120 Tabs (XR; SR): 120, 180, 240 Caps XR: 100, 120, 180, 200, 240, 300, 360 Injection: 2.5/mL

Action
• Action in the treatment of bipolar disorder is unclear.

Contraindications and Precautions
Contraindicated in: • Hypersensitivity • Severe left ventricular dysfunction • Heart block • Hypotension • Cardiogenic shock • Congestive heart failure • Patients with atrial flutter or atrial fibrillation and an accessory bypass tract

Use Cautiously in: • Liver or renal disease • Cardiomyopathy • Intracranial pressure • Elderly patients • Pregnancy and lactation (*safety not established*)

Adverse Reactions and Side Effects
• Drowsiness
• Dizziness
• Headache
• Hypotension
• Bradycardia
• Nausea
• Constipation

Interactions
• Effects of verapamil are increased with concomitant use of **amiodarone, beta-blockers, cimetidine, ranitidine,** and **grapefruit juice.**
• Effects of verapamil are decreased with concomitant use of **barbiturates, calcium salts, hydantoins, rifampin,** and **antineoplastics.**
• Effects of the following drugs are increased with concomitant use of verapamil: **beta-blockers, disopyramide, flecainide, doxorubicin, benzodiazepines, buspirone, carbamazepine, digoxin, dofetilide, ethanol, imipramine,**

nondepolarizing muscle relaxants, prazosin, quinidine, siro-limus, tacrolimus, theophylline, and **HMG-CoA reductase inhibitors.**
* Serum **lithium** levels may be altered when administered concurrently with verapamil.

Route and Dosage
Angina: **PO**: 80 to 120 mg 3 times a day.
Arrhythmias: **PO**: 240 to 320 mg/day in 3 or 4 divided doses
Hypertension: **PO**: 40 to 80 mg 3 times a day. Maximum recommended daily dose: 360 mg.
Bipolar Mania: **PO**: 80 to 320 mg/day in divided doses.
Migraine Prophylaxis: **PO**: 160 to 320 mg/day in 3 to 4 divided doses.

● CHEMICAL CLASS: ANTIPSYCHOTICS
Examples

Generic (Trade) Name	Pregnancy Categories/ Half-life (hr)	Indications	Available Forms (mg)
Olanzapine (Zyprexa)	C/21–54	• Schizophrenia • Bipolar disorder • Agitation associated with schizophrenia and mania (IM)	Tabs: 2.5, 5, 7.5, 10, 15, 20 Tabs (Orally disintegrating): 5, 10, 15, 20 Powder for injection: 10 mg/vial
Olanzapine and fluoxetine (Symbyax)†		• For the treatment of depressive episodes associated with bipolar disorder • Treatment-resistant depression	Caps: 3 olanzapine/25 fluoxetine; 6 olanzapine/25 fluoxetine; 6 olanzapine/50 fluoxetine; 12 olanzapine/25 fluoxetine; 12 olanzapine/50 fluoxetine
Aripiprazole (Abilify)	C/75–94 (including metabolite)	• Bipolar mania • Schizophrenia • Major depressive disorder (adjunctive treatment)	Tabs: 2, 5, 10, 15, 20, 30 Tabs (orally disintegrating): 10, 15 Oral solution: 1/mL Injection: 7.5/mL
Chlorpromazine	C/24	• Bipolar mania • Schizophrenia • Emesis/hiccoughs • Acute intermittent porphyria • Hyperexcitable, combative behavior in children • Preoperative apprehension **Unlabeled uses:** • Migraine headaches	Tabs: 10, 25, 50, 100, 200 Injection: 25/mL

Continued

Generic (Trade) Name	Pregnancy Categories/ Half-life (hr)	Indications	Available Forms (mg)
Quetiapine (Seroquel	C/6	• Schizophrenia • Acute manic episodes	Tabs: 25, 50, 100, 200, 300, 400 Tabs (XR): 200, 300, 400
Risperidone (Risperdal)	C/3–21 (including metabolite)	• Bipolar mania • Schizophrenia • Behavioral problems associated with autism **Unlabeled uses:** • Severe behavioral problems in children • Obsessive-compulsive disorder	Tabs: 0.25, 0.5, 1, 2, 3, 4 Tabs (orally disintegrating): 0.5, 1, 2, 3, 4 Oral solution: 1/mL Powder for injection: 12.5/vial, 25/vial, 37.5/vial, 50/vial
Ziprasidone (Geodon)	C/7 (oral); 2–5 (IM)	• Bipolar mania • Schizophrenia • Acute agitation in schizophrenia (IM)	Caps: 20, 40, 60, 80 Powder for injection: 20/vial
Asenapine (Saphris)	C/24	• Schizophrenia • Bipolar disorder	Tabs (Sublingual): 5, 10

[1] For information related to action, contraindications/precautions, adverse reactions and side effects, and interactions, refer to the monographs for olanzapine (see Chapters 27 and 28) and fluoxetine (see Chapter 26).

Action

• Efficacy in schizophrenia is achieved through a combination of dopamine and serotonin type 2 (5-HT$_2$) antagonism.
• Mechanism of action in the treatment of acute manic episodes is unknown.

Contraindications and Precautions
Olanzapine
• **Contraindicated in** hypersensitivity; lactation. *Orally disintegrating tablets only:* Phenylketonuria (orally disintegrating tablets contain aspartame).
• **Use cautiously in** hepatic insufficiency, elderly clients (reduce dosage), pregnancy and children (*safety not established*), cardiovascular or cerebrovascular disease, history of glaucoma, history of seizures, history of attempted suicide, prostatic hypertrophy, diabetes or risk factors for diabetes, narrow-angle glaucoma, history of paralytic ileus; patients with preexisting low white blood cell count and/or history of drug-induced leukopenia/neutropenia; elderly patients with dementia-related psychosis (**black box warning**).

Aripiprazole
- **Contraindicated in** hypersensitivity; lactation.
- **Use cautiously in** cardiovascular or cerebrovascular disease; conditions that cause hypotension (dehydration, treatment with antihypertensives or diuretics); elderly patients; pregnancy, children, and adolescents (*safety not established*); elderly patients with dementia-related psychosis (**black box warning**).

Chlorpromazine
- **Contraindicated in** hypersensitivity (cross-sensitivity with other phenothiazines may occur); narrow-angle glaucoma; bone marrow depression; severe liver or cardiovascular disease; concurrent pimozide use.
- **Use cautiously in** elderly and debilitated patients; children with acute illnesses, infections, gastroenteritis, or dehydration (increased risk of extrapyramidal reactions); diabetes; respiratory disease; prostatic hypertrophy; central nervous system (CNS) tumors; epilepsy; intestinal obstruction; pregnancy or lactation (*safety not established*); elderly patients with dementia-related psychosis (**black box warning**).

Quetiapine
- **Contraindicated in** hypersensitivity; lactation.
- **Use cautiously in** cardiovascular or cerebrovascular disease; dehydration or hypovolemia (increased risk of hypotension); elderly patients; hepatic impairment; hypothyroidism; history of suicide attempt; pregnancy or children (*safety not established*); elderly patients with dementia-related psychosis (**black box warning**).

Risperidone
- **Contraindicated in** hypersensitivity; lactation.
- **Use cautiously in** elderly or debilitated patients; renal or hepatic impairment; cardiovascular disease; history of seizures; history of suicide attempt or drug abuse; diabetes or risk factors for diabetes; pregnancy or children (*safety not established*); elderly patients with dementia-related psychosis (**black box warning**).

Ziprasidone
- **Contraindicated in** hypersensitivity; history of QT prolongation, arrhythmias, recent myocardial infarction (MI), or uncompensated heart failure; concurrent use of other drugs known to prolong QT interval; hypokalemia or hypomagnesemia; lactation.
- **Use cautiously in** concurrent diuretic therapy or diarrhea (may increase the risk of hypotension, hypokalemia, or hypomagnesemia); hepatic impairment; cardiovascular or cerebrovascular disease; hypotension, concurrent antihypertensive

therapy, dehydration, or hypovolemia (may increase risk of orthostatic hypotension); elderly patients; patients at risk for aspiration pneumonia; history of suicide attempt; pregnancy and children (*safety not established*); patients with preexisting low white blood cell count and/or history of drug-induced leukopenia/neutropenia; elderly patients with dementia-related psychosis (**black box warning**).

Asenapine
- **Contraindicated in** hypersensitivity; lactation; history of QT prolongation or arrhythmias; concurrent use of other drugs known to prolong QT interval.
- **Use cautiously in** patients with hepatic, renal, or cardio-vascular insufficiency; diabetes or risk factors for diabetes; patients with preexisting low white blood cell count and/or history of drug-induced leukopenia/neutropenia; history of seizures; history of suicide attempt; patients at risk for aspiration pneumonia; elderly patients; pregnancy and children (*safety not established*); elderly patients with dementia-related psychosis (**black box warning**).

Adverse Reactions and Side Effects
Olanzapine
- Drowsiness, dizziness, weakness
- Dry mouth, constipation, increased appetite
- Nausea
- Weight gain or loss
- Orthostatic hypotension, tachycardia
- Restlessness
- Rhinitis
- Tremor
- Headache

Aripiprazole
- Drowsiness, lightheadedness
- Headache
- Insomnia, restlessness
- Constipation
- Nausea
- Weight gain

Chlorpromazine
- Sedation
- Blurred vision
- Hypotension
- Constipation
- Dry mouth
- Photosensitivity
- Extrapyramidal symptoms

- Weight gain
- Urinary retention

Quetiapine
- Drowsiness, dizziness
- Hypotension, tachycardia
- Headache
- Constipation
- Dry mouth
- Nausea
- Weight gain

Risperidone
- Agitation, anxiety
- Drowsiness, dizziness
- Extrapyramidal symptoms
- Headache
- Insomnia
- Constipation
- Nausea/vomiting
- Weight gain
- Rhinitis
- Sexual dysfunction
- Diarrhea
- Dry mouth

Ziprasidone
- Drowsiness, dizziness
- Restlessness
- Headache
- Constipation
- Diarrhea
- Dry mouth
- Nausea
- Weight gain
- Prolonged QT interval

Asenapine
- Constipation
- Dry mouth
- Nausea and vomiting
- Weight gain
- Restlessness
- Extrapyramidal symptoms
- Drowsiness, dizziness
- Insomnia
- Headache

Interactions

The effects of:	Are increased by:	Are decreased by:	Concurrent use may result in:
Olanzapine	Fluvoxamine and other CYP-1A2 inhibitors, fluoxetine	Carbamazepine and other CYP-1A2 inducers, omeprazole, rifampin	Decreased effects of levodopa and dopamine agonists. Increased hypotension with antihypertensives. Increased CNS depression with alcohol or other CNS depressants.
Aripiprazole	Ketoconazole and other CYP-3A4 inhibitors; quinidine, fluoxetine, paroxetine, or other potential CYP-2D6 inhibitors	Carbamazepine, famotidine, valproate	Increased CNS depression with alcohol or other CNS depressants. Increased hypotension with antihypertensives.
Chlorproma-zine	Beta-blockers, paroxetine	Centrally acting anticholinergics	Increased effects of beta-blockers; excessive sedation and hypotension with meperidine; decreased hypotensive effect of guanethidine; decreased effect of oral anticoagulants; decreased or increased phenytoin levels; increased orthostatic hypotension with thiazide diuretics; Increased CNS depression with alcohol or other CNS depressants. Increased hypotension with antihypertensives. Increased anticholinergic effects with anticholinergic agents.
Quetiapine	Cimetidine; keto-conazole, itracon-azole, fluconazole, erythromycin, or other CYP-3A4 inhibitors	Phenytoin, thioridazine	Decreased effects of levodopa and dopamine agonists. Increased CNS depression with alcohol or other CNS depressants. Increased hypotension with antihypertensives.
Risperidone	Clozapine, fluoxetine, paroxetine, or ritonavir	Carbamazepine	Decreased effects of levodopa and dopamine agonists. Increased effects of clozapine and valproate. Increased CNS depression with alcohol or other CNS depressants. Increased hypotension with antihypertensives.

The effects of:	Are increased by:	Are decreased by:	Concurrent use may result in:
Ziprasidone	Ketoconazole and other CYP-3A4 inhibitors	Carbamazepine	Life-threatening prolongation of QT interval with quinidine, dofetilide, other class Ia and III antiarrhythmics, pimozide, sotalol, thioridazine, chlorpromazine, floquine, pentamidine, arsenic trioxide, mefloquine, dolasetron, tacrolimus, droperidol, gatifloxacin, or moxifloxacin. Decreased effects of levodopa and dopamine agonists. Increased CNS depression with alcohol or other CNS depressants. Increased hypotension with antihypertensives.
Asenapine	Fluvoxamine, imipramine, valproate	Carbamazepine, cimetidine, paroxetine	Increased effects of paroxetine and dextromethorphan; Increased CNS depression with alcohol or other CNS depressants. Increased hypotension with antihypertensives; Additive effects on QT interval prolongation with quinidine, dofetilide, other Class Ia and III antiarrhythmics, pimozide, sotalol, thioridazine, chlorpromazine, floquine, pentamadine, arsenic trioxide, mefloquine, dolasetron, tacrolimus, droperidol, gatifloxacin, or moxifloxacin.

Route and Dosage

OLANZAPINE (Zyprexa)

Bipolar Disorder: Adults: **PO:** 10 to 15 mg/day initially; may increase every 24 hours by 5 mg/day (not to exceed 20 mg/day).

Schizophrenia: Adults: **PO:** 5 to 10 mg/day initially; may increase at weekly intervals by 5 mg/day (not to exceed 20 mg/day).

Agitation Associated with Schizophrenia or Mania: Adults: **IM:** 2.5 to 10 mg, administered slowly, deep into muscle mass. May repeat in 2 hours and again 4 hours later, if needed.

OLANZAPINE AND FLUOXETINE **(Symbyax)**

Depressive Episodes Associated with Bipolar Disorder:
Adults: **PO:** Initial dosage: 6/25 given once daily in the evening. Adjust dosage according to efficacy and tolerability to within a range of 6 to 12 olanzapine/25 to 50 fluoxetine.

ARIPIPRAZOLE **(Abilify)**

Bipolar Mania: *Adults:* **PO:** Usual starting dose: 15 mg/day. Dosage may be increased to 30 mg/day based on clinical response. The safety of dosages higher than 30 mg have not been evaluated.

Major Depressive Disorder (adjunctive treatment): *Adults:* **PO:** Initial dosage: 2 to 5 mg/day for patients already taking another antidepressant. May increase dosage by up to 5 mg/day at intervals of at least a week. Maintenance dosage range: 2 to 15 mg/day.

Schizophrenia: *Adults:* **PO:** Initial dosage: 10 or 15 mg/day as a single dose. Doses up to 30 mg have been used. Dosage increases should not be made before 2 weeks, the time required to achieve steady state.

CHLORPROMAZINE **(Thorazine)**

Psychotic Disorders: *Adults*: **PO**: 10 mg 3 or 4 times a day or 25 mg 2 or 3 times a day. Increase by 20 to 50 mg every 3 to 4 days until effective dose is reached, usually 200 to 400 mg/day. **IM**: Initial dose: 25 mg. May give additional 25 to 50 mg in 1 hour. Increase gradually over several days (up to 400 mg every 4 to 6 hours in severe cases).

Pediatric Behavioral Disorders: *Children >6 months*: **PO**: 0.5 mg/kg every 4 to 6 hours as needed. **IM**: 0.5 mg/kg every 6 to 8 hours (not to exceed 40 mg/day in children 6 months to 5 years or 75 mg/day in children 6 to 12 years).

Nausea and Vomiting: *Adults*: **PO**: 10 to 25 mg every 4 to 6 hours. **IM**: 25 mg initially, may repeat 25-50 mg every 3 to 4 hours.
Children >6 months: **PO**: 0.55 mg/kg every 4 to 6 hours. **IM:** 0.55 mg/kg every 6 to 8 hours (not to exceed 40 mg/day in children up to 5 years or 75 mg/day in children 5 to 12 years).

Intractable Hiccoughs: *Adults:* **PO**: 25 to 50 mg 3 or 4 times daily. If symptoms persist for 2 or 3 days, give 25 to 50 mg **IM**.

Preoperative Sedation: *Adults*: **PO**: 25 to 50 mg 2 or 3 hours before surgery, or **IM**: 12.5 to 25 mg 1 to 2 hours before surgery.
Children: **PO**: 0.5 mg/kg 2 or 3 hours before surgery, or **IM**: 0.5 mg/kg 1 to 2 hours before surgery.

Acute Intermittent Porphyria: Adults: **PO**: 25 to 50 mg 3 or 4 times a day, or **IM**: 25 mg 3 or 4 times a day until patient can take **PO**.

QUETIAPINE **(Seroquel)**

Schizophrenia: Adults: **PO**: 25 mg twice daily initially, increased by 25 to 50 mg 2 or 3 times daily over 3 days, up to 300 to 400 mg/day in 2 or 3 divided doses by the fourth day (not to exceed 800 mg/day).

Bipolar Mania: Adults: **PO**: 100 mg/day in 2 divided doses on day 1; increase dose by 100 mg/day up to 400 mg/day by day 4 given in twice daily divided doses. May increase in 200 mg/day increments up to 800 mg/day by day 6 if required.

RISPERIDONE **(Risperdal)**

Bipolar mania: Adults: **PO**: 2 or 3 mg/day as a single daily dose; dose may be increased at 24-hour intervals by 1 mg (range 1 to 6 mg/day).

Schizophrenia: Adults: **PO**: Initial dosage: 2 mg/day administered as a single dose or in two divided doses. May increase dose at 24-hour intervals in increments of 1 to 2 mg/day to a recommended dose of 4 to 8 mg/day.

IM: Adults: 25 mg every 2 weeks; some patients may require larger dose of 37.5 or 50 mg every 2 weeks.

Adolescents (13 to 17 years): **PO**: 0.5 mg once daily, increased by 0.5 to 1.0 mg no more frequently than every 24 hours to 3 mg daily. May administer half the daily dose twice daily if drowsiness persists.

Behavioral Problems Associated with Autistic Disorder: Children and adolescents 5 to 16 years weighing <20 kg: **PO**: 0.25 mg/day initially. After at least 4 days of therapy, may increase to 0.5 mg/day. Dose increases in increments of 0.25 mg/day may be considered at 2-week or longer intervals. May be given as a single dose or in divided doses.

Children and adolescents 5 to 16 years weighing >20 kg: **PO**: 0.5 mg/day initially. After at least 4 days of therapy, may increase to 1.0 mg/day. Dose increases in increments of 0.5 mg/day may be considered at 2-week or longer intervals. May be given as a single dose or in divided doses.

ZIPRASIDONE **(Geodon)**

Bipolar Mania: Adults: **PO:** 40 mg twice daily with food. Increase dose to 60 or 80 mg twice/day on the second day of treatment. Adjust dose on the basis of toleration and efficacy within the range of 40 to 80 mg twice/day.

Schizophrenia: Adults: **PO:** Initial dose: 20 mg twice daily with food. Dose increments may be made at 2-day intervals up to 80 mg twice daily.

Acute Agitation in Schizophrenia: Adults: **IM:** 10 to 20 mg as needed up to 40 mg/day. May be given as 10 mg every 2 hours or 20 mg every 4 hours. Maximum dosage: 40 mg/day.

ASENAPINE **(Saphris)**

Schizophrenia: Adults: **PO:** Usual starting and target dose: 5 mg twice daily. The safety of doses above 10 mg twice daily has not been evaluated in clinical trials.

Bipolar Disorder: Adults: **PO:** Recommended initial dose: 10 mg twice daily. The dose can be decreased to 5 mg twice daily if there are adverse effects. The safety of doses above 10 mg twice daily has not been evaluated in clinical trials.

● **NURSING DIAGNOSES RELATED TO ALL MOOD-STABILIZING DRUGS**

1. Risk for injury related to manic hyperactivity.
2. Risk for self-directed or other-directed violence related to unresolved anger turned inward on the self or outward on the environment.
3. Risk for injury related to lithium toxicity.
4. Risk for injury related to adverse effects of mood-stabilizing drugs.
5. Risk for activity intolerance related to side effects of drowsiness and dizziness.

● **NURSING IMPLICATIONS FOR MOOD-STABILIZING DRUGS**

The plan of care should include monitoring for the following side effects from mood-stabilizing drugs. Nursing implications are designated by an asterisk (*).

1. **May occur with lithium:**
   a. **Drowsiness, dizziness, headache**
      * Ensure that client does not participate in activities that require alertness, or operate dangerous machinery.
   b. **Dry mouth; thirst**
      * Provide sugarless candy, ice, frequent sips of water. Ensure that strict oral hygiene is maintained.
   c. **GI upset; nausea/vomiting**
      * Administer medications with meals to minimize GI upset.
   d. **Fine hand tremors**
      * Report to physician, who may decrease dosage. Some physicians prescribe a small dose of beta-blocker propranolol to counteract this effect.

  e. **Hypotension; arrhythmias; pulse irregularities**
    * Monitor vital signs two or three times a day. Physician may decrease dose of medication.
  f. **Polyuria; dehydration**
    * May subside after initial week or two. Monitor daily intake and output and weight. Monitor skin turgor daily.
  g. **Weight gain**
    * Provide instructions for reduced calorie diet. Emphasize importance of maintaining adequate intake of sodium.
2. **May occur with anticonvulsants:**
  a. **Nausea/vomiting**
    * May give with food or milk to minimize GI upset.
  b. **Drowsiness; dizziness**
    * Ensure that client does not operate dangerous machinery or participate in activities that require alertness.
  c. **Blood dyscrasias**
    * Ensure that client understands the importance of regular blood tests while receiving anticonvulsant therapy.
  d. **Prolonged bleeding time (with valproic acid)**
    * Ensure that platelet counts and bleed time are determined before initiation of therapy with valproic acid. Monitor for spontaneous bleeding or bruising.
  e. **Risk of severe rash (with lamotrigine)**
    * Ensure that client is informed that he or she must report evidence of skin rash to physician immediately.
  f. **Decreased efficacy of oral contraceptives (with topiramate)**
    * Ensure that client is aware of decreased efficacy of oral contraceptives with concomitant use.
  g. **Risk of suicide with all antiepileptic drugs** (warning by FDA, December 2008)
    * Monitor for worsening of depression, suicidal thoughts or behavior, or any unusual changes in mood or behavior.
3. **May occur with calcium channel blockers:**
  a. **Drowsiness; dizziness**
    * Ensure that client does not operate dangerous machinery or participate in activities that require alertness.
  b. **Hypotension; bradycardia**
    * Take vital signs just before initiation of therapy and before daily administration of the medication. Physician will provide acceptable parameters for administration. Report marked changes immediately.
  c. **Nausea**
    * May give with food to minimize GI upset.

 d. **Constipation**
  * Encourage increased fluid (if not contraindicated) and fiber in the diet.
4. **May occur with antipsychotics:**
 a. **Drowsiness; dizziness**
  * Ensure that client does not operate dangerous machinery or participate in activities that require alertness.
 b. **Dry mouth; constipation**
  * Provide sugarless candy or gum, ice, and frequent sips of water. Provide foods high in fiber; encourage physical activity and fluid if not contraindicated.
 c. **Increased appetite; weight gain**
  * Provide calorie-controlled diet. Provide opportunity for physical exercise. Provide diet and exercise instruction.
 d. **ECG changes**
  * Monitor vital signs. Observe for symptoms of dizziness, palpitations, syncope, or weakness.
 e. **Extrapyramidal symptoms**
  * Monitor for symptoms. Administer prn medication at first sign.
 f. **Hyperglycemia and diabetes**
  * Monitor blood glucose regularly. Observe for the appearance of symptoms of polydipsia, polyuria, polyphagia, and weakness at any time during therapy.

● CLIENT/FAMILY EDUCATION RELATED TO MOOD-STABILIZING DRUGS

* Do not drive or operate dangerous machinery. Drowsiness or dizziness can occur.
* Do not stop taking the drug abruptly. Can produce serious withdrawal symptoms. The physician will administer orders for tapering the drug when therapy is to be discontinued.
* Report the following symptoms to the physician immediately:
 * *Client taking anticonvulsant:* unusual bleeding, spontaneous bruising, sore throat, fever, malaise, skin rash, dark urine, and yellow skin or eyes.
 * *Client taking calcium channel blocker:* irregular heartbeat, shortness of breath, swelling of the hands and feet, pronounced dizziness, chest pain, profound mood swings, severe and persistent headache.
 * *Client taking lithium:* ataxia, blurred vision, severe diarrhea, persistent nausea and vomiting, tinnitus, excessive urine output, increasing tremors, or mental confusion.
 * *Client taking antipsychotic:* sore throat, fever, malaise, unusual bleeding, easy bruising, persistent nausea and vomiting, severe headache, rapid heart rate, difficulty urinating,

muscle twitching, tremors, dark urine, excessive urination, excessive thirst, excessive hunger, weakness, pale stools, yellow skin or eyes, muscular incoordination, or skin rash.

- For the client on lithium: ensure that the diet contains adequate sodium. Drink 6 to 8 glasses of water each day. Avoid drinks that contain caffeine (that have a diuretic effect). Have serum lithium level checked every 1 to 2 months, or as advised by physician.
- For the client on asenapine: Place the tablet *under* the tongue and allow to dissolve completely. Do not chew or swallow tablet. Do not eat or drink for 10 minutes.
- Avoid consuming alcoholic beverages and nonprescription medications without approval from physician.
- Carry card at all times identifying the name of medications being taken.

 INTERNET REFERENCES

  a. http://www.rxlist.com
  b. http://www.nimh.nih.gov/publicat/medicate.cfm
  c. http://www.fadavis.com/townsend
  d. http://www.mentalhealth.com/
  e. http://www.nlm.nih.gov/medlineplus/druginformation .html

Chapter 28

Antipsychotic Agents

● **CHEMICAL CLASS: PHENOTHIAZINES**
Examples

Generic (Trade) Name	Pregnancy Categories/ Half-life	Indications	Available Forms (mg)
Chlorpromazine	C/24 hr	• Bipolar mania • Schizophrenia • Emesis/hiccoughs • Acute intermittent porphyria • Hyperexcitable, combative behavior in children • Preoperative apprehension **Unlabeled uses:** • Migraine headaches	Tabs: 10, 25, 50, 100, 200 Injection: 25/mL
Fluphenazine	C/HCl: 18 hr Decanoate: 6.8–9.6 days	• Psychotic disorders	Tabs: 1, 2.5, 5, 10 Elixir: 2.5/5 mL Conc: 5/mL Inj: 2.5/mL Inj (Decanoate): 25/mL
Perphenazine	C/9–12 hr	• Psychotic disorders • Nausea and vomiting	Tabs: 2, 4, 8, 16 Conc: 16/5 mL
Prochlorperazine	C/3–5 hr (oral) 6.9 hr (IV)	• Schizophrenia • Nonpsychotic anxiety • Nausea and vomiting **Unlabeled uses:** • Migraine headache	Tabs: 5, 10 Supp: 25 Inj: 5/mL
Thioridazine	C/24 hr	• Management of schizophrenia in patients who do not have an acceptable response to other antipsychotic therapy	Tabs: 10, 15, 25, 50, 100, 150, 200
Trifluoperazine	C/18 hr	• Schizophrenia • Nonpsychotic anxiety	Tabs: 1, 2, 5, 10

Action
- These drugs are thought to work by blocking postsynaptic dopamine receptors in the basal ganglia, hypothalamus, limbic system, brainstem, and medulla.
- They also demonstrate varying affinity for cholinergic, alpha$_1$-adrenergic, and histaminic receptors.
- Antipsychotic effects may also be related to inhibition of dopamine-mediated transmission of neural impulses at the synapses.

Contraindications and Precautions
Contraindicated in: • Hypersensitivity (cross-sensitivity may exist among phenothiazines) • In comatose or severely central nervous system (CNS)-depressed clients • Poorly controlled seizure disorders • Clients with blood dyscrasias • Narrow angle glaucoma • Clients with liver, renal, or cardiac insufficiency • Bone marrow depression • Concurrent **pemozide** use • Co-administration with other drugs that prolong QT interval, or in patients with long-QT syndrome or history of cardiac arrhythmias

Use Cautiously in: • Elderly and debilitated patients • Children with acute illnesses, infections, gastroenteritis, or dehydration (increased risk of extrapyramidal reactions) • Diabetes • Respiratory disease • Prostatic hypertrophy • CNS tumors • Epilepsy • Intestinal obstruction • Pregnancy or lactation (*safety not established*) • Elderly patients with dementia-related psychosis (**black box warning**)

Adverse Reactions and Side Effects
- Dry mouth
- Blurred vision
- Constipation
- Urinary retention
- Nausea
- Skin rash
- Sedation
- Orthostatic hypotension
- Photosensitivity
- Decreased libido
- Amenorrhea
- Retrograde ejaculation
- Gynecomastia
- Weight gain
- Reduction of seizure threshold
- Agranulocytosis
- Extrapyramidal symptoms

- Tardive dyskinesia
- Neuroleptic malignant syndrome
- Prolongation of QT interval (**thioridazine**)

Interactions

- Coadministration of phenothiazines and **beta-blockers** may increase effects from either or both drugs.
- Increased effects of phenothiazines with **paroxetine**
- Concurrent administration with **meperidine** may produce excessive sedation and hypotension.
- Therapeutic effects of phenothiazines may be decreased by **centrally acting anticholinergics.** Anticholinergic effects are increased.
- Concurrent use may result in decreased hypotensive effect of **guanethidine.**
- Phenothiazines may reduce effectiveness of **oral anticoagulants.**
- Concurrent use with phenothiazines may increase or decrease **phenytoin** levels.
- Increased orthostatic hypotension with **thiazide diuretics**
- Increased CNS depression with **alcohol** or other **CNS depressants**
- Increased hypotension with **antihypertensives**
- Concurrent use with **epinephrine** or **dopamine** may result in severe hypotension.

Route and Dosage

CHLORPROMAZINE

Psychotic Disorders: *Adults*: **PO**: 10 mg 3 or 4 times a day or 25 mg 2 or 3 times a day. Increase by 20 to 50 mg every 3 to 4 days until effective dose is reached, usually 200 to 400 mg/day. **IM**: Initial dose: 25 mg. May give additional 25 to 50 mg in 1 hour. Increase gradually over several days (up to 400 mg every 4 to 6 hours in severe cases).

Pediatric Behavioral Disorders: *Children >6 months*: **PO**: 0.5 mg/kg every 4 to 6 hours as needed. **IM**: 0.5 mg/kg every 6 to 8 hours (not to exceed 40 mg/day in children 6 months to 5 years or 75 mg/day in children 6 to 12 years).

Nausea and Vomiting: *Adults*: **PO**: 10 to 25 mg every 4 to 6 hours. **IM**: 25 mg initially, may repeat 25 to 50 mg every 3 to 4 hours.
Children >6 months: **PO**: 0.55 mg/kg every 4 to 6 hours. **IM**: 0.55 mg/kg every 6 to 8 hours (not to exceed 40 mg/day in children up to 5 years or 75 mg/day in children 5 to 12 years).

Intractable Hiccoughs: *Adults:* **PO**: 25 to 50 mg 3 or 4 times daily. If symptoms persist for 2 to 3 days, give 25 to 50 mg **IM**.

Preoperative Sedation: *Adults:* **PO**: 25 to 50 mg 2 to 3 hours before surgery, or **IM**: 12.5 to 25 mg 1 to 2 hours before surgery.
Children: **PO**: 0.5 mg/kg 2 to 3 hours before surgery or **IM**: 0.5 mg/kg 1 to 2 hours before surgery.

Acute Intermittent Porphyria: *Adults:* **PO**: 25 to 50 mg 3 or 4 times a day or **IM**: 25 mg 3 or 4 times a day until patient can take **PO**.

FLUPHENAZINE

Psychotic Disorders: *Adults:* **PO**: Initial dose: 2.5 to 10 mg/day in divided doses every 6 to 8 hours. Maintenance dose: 1 to 5 mg/day. **IM**: 1.25 to 2.5 mg every 6 to 8 hours.
Elderly or debilitated patients: **PO:** 1 to 2.5 mg/day initially. Adjust dosage according to response.

Decanoate Formulation: *Adults:* **IM, SC:** Initial dose: 12.5 to 25 mg. May be repeated every 3 to 4 weeks. Dosage may be slowly increased in 12.5 mg increments as needed (not to exceed 100 mg/dose).

PERPHENAZINE

Psychotic Disorders: *Adults:* **PO**: *Outpatients*: 4 to 8 mg 3 times a day initially. Reduce as soon as possible to minimum effective dose.
Hospitalized patients with schizophrenia: 8 to 16 mg 2 to 4 times a day, not to exceed 64 mg/day.

Nausea and Vomiting: *Adults:* **PO**: 8 to 16 mg daily in divided doses, up to 24 mg, if necessary.

PROCHLORPERAZINE

Schizophrenia: *Adults (mild conditions):* **PO**: 5 to 10 mg 3 or 4 times a day. *(Moderate conditions):* 10 mg 3 or 4 times a day. Gradually increase dosage by small increments over 2 or 3 days to 50 to 75 mg/day. *(Severe conditions):* 100 to 150 mg/day. **IM**: 10 to 20 mg every 2 to 4 hours for up to 4 doses, then 10 to 20 mg every 4 to 6 hours, if needed. When control is achieved, switch to oral dosage.
Children ≥12 years: **PO:** 5 to 10 mg 3 to 4 times a day.
Children 2 to 12 years: **PO:** 2.5 mg 2 to 3 times a day.

Nonpsychotic Anxiety: *Adults:* **PO**: 5 mg 3 to 4 times a day, not to exceed 20 mg/day or longer than 12 weeks.

Nausea and Vomiting: *Adults:* **PO**: 5 to 10 mg 3 or 4 times a day. **SR caps:** 15 mg once daily or 10 mg 2 times a day. **Rectal**: 25 mg 2 times a day. **IM**: 5 to 10 mg. May repeat every 3 or 4 hours, not to exceed 40 mg/day.
Children 20 to 29 lb: **PO/Rectal:** 2.5 mg 1 or 2 times a day, not to exceed 7.5 mg/day.

Children 30 to *39 lb:* **PO/Rectal:** 2.5 mg 2 or 3 times a day, not to exceed 10 mg/day.

Children 40 to *85 lb:* **PO/Rectal:** 2.5 mg 3 times a day or 5 mg 2 times a day, not to exceed 15 mg/day.

Children >20 lb or 2 years of age: **IM:** 0.132 mg/kg. Usually only 1 dose is required.

THIORIDAZINE

Schizophrenia (Intractable to Other Antipsychotics): *Adults:* **PO:** Initial dose: 50 to 100 mg 3 times a day. May increase gradually to maximum dosage of 800 mg/day. Once effective response has been achieved, may reduce gradually to determine the minimum maintenance dose. Usual daily dosage range: 200 to 800 mg, divided into 2 to 4 doses.

Children: **PO:** Initial dose: 0.5 mg/kg/day given in divided doses. Increase gradually until therapeutic effect has been achieved or maximum dose of 3 mg/kg/day has been reached.

TRIFLUOPERAZINE

Schizophrenia: *Adults:* **PO:** 2 to 5 mg 2 times a day. Usual optimum dosage range: 15 to 20 mg/day, although a few may require 40 mg/day or more.

Children 6 to 12 years: **PO:** Initial dose: 1 mg once or 2 times a day. May increase dose gradually to a maximum of 15 mg/day.

Nonpsychotic Anxiety: *Adults:* **PO:** 1 or 2 mg 2 times a day. Do not administer more than 6 mg/day or for longer than 12 weeks.

● CHEMICAL CLASS: THIOXANTHENES
Examples

Generic (Trade) Name	Pregnancy Categories/ Half-life (hr)	Indications	Available Forms (mg)
Thiothixene (Navane)	C/34	● Schizophrenia	Caps: 1, 2, 5, 10, 20

Action

- Blocks postsynaptic dopamine receptors in the basal ganglia, hypothalamus, limbic system, brainstem, and medulla
- Demonstrates varying affinity for cholinergic, alpha$_1$-adrenergic, and histaminic receptors

Contraindications and Precautions
Contraindicated in: ● Hypersensitivity ● Comatose or severely CNS-depressed patients ● Bone marrow depression or

blood dyscrasias • Parkinson's disease • Severe hypotension or hypertension • Circulatory collapse • Children <12 years old • Pregnancy and lactation (*safety not established*)

Use Cautiously in: • Patients with history of seizures • Respiratory, renal, hepatic, thyroid, or cardiovascular disorders • Elderly or debilitated patients • Patients exposed to extreme environmental heat • Patients taking atropine or atropine-like drugs • Elderly patients with dementia-related psychosis (**black box warning**)

Adverse Reactions and Side Effects
• Refer to this section under Phenothiazines.

Interactions
• Additive CNS depression with **alcohol** and other **CNS depressants**
• Additive anticholinergic effects with other drugs that have anticholinergic properties
• Possible additive hypotension with **antihypertensive agents**
• Concurrent use with **epinephrine** or **dopamine** may result in severe hypotension.

Route and Dosage
Schizophrenia: Adults and children ≥12 years: **PO**: *(Mild conditions):* Initial dosage: 2 mg three times a day. May increase to 15 mg/day. *(Severe conditions):* Initial dosage: 5 mg 2 times a day. Optimal dose is 20 to 30 mg/day. If needed, may increase gradually, not to exceed 60 mg/day.

● CHEMICAL CLASS: PHENYLBUTYLPIPERADINES
Examples

Generic (Trade) Name	Pregnancy Categories/ Half-life	Indications	Available Forms (mg)
Haloperidol (Haldol)	C/~18 hr (oral); ~3 wk (IM decanoate)	• Psychotic disorders • Tourette's disorder • Pediatric behavior problems and hyperactivity **Unlabeled uses:** • Intractable hiccoughs • Nausea and vomiting	Tabs: 0.5, 1, 2, 5, 10, 20 Conc: 2/mL Inj (lactate): 5/mL Inj (decanoate): 50/mL; 100/mL

Continued

Generic (Trade) Name	Pregnancy Categories/ Half-life	Indications	Available Forms (mg)
Pimozide (Orap)	C/~55 hr	• Tourette's disorder **Unlabeled uses:** • Schizophrenia	Tabs: 1, 2

Action
- Blocks postsynaptic dopamine receptors in the hypothalamus, limbic system, and reticular formation
- Demonstrates varying affinity for cholinergic, alpha$_1$-adrenergic, and histaminic receptors

Contraindications and Precautions
Contraindicated in: • Hypersensitivity to the drug • Coadministration with other drugs that prolong the QT interval • Coadministration with drugs that inhibit CYP3A enzymes (**pimozide**) • Treatment of tics other than those associated with Tourette's disorder (**pimozide**) • Coadministration with other drugs that may cause tics (e.g., pemoline, methylphenidate, amphetamines) until it has been determined whether the tics are caused by the medications or Tourette's disorder (**pimozide**) • Parkinson disease (**haloperidol**) • In comatose or severely CNS-depressed clients • Clients with blood dyscrasias or bone marrow depression • Narrow-angle glaucoma • Clients with liver, renal, or cardiac insufficiency • Pregnancy and lactation (*safety not established*)

Use Cautiously in: • Elderly and debilitated clients • Diabetic clients • Depressed clients • Clients with history of seizures • Clients with respiratory insufficiency • Prostatic hypertrophy • Children • Elderly patients with dementia-related psychosis (**black box warning**)

Adverse Reactions and Side Effects
- Dry mouth
- Blurred vision
- Constipation
- Urinary retention
- Nausea
- Skin rash
- Sedation
- Orthostatic hypotension
- Photosensitivity
- Decreased libido
- Amenorrhea
- Retrograde ejaculation

Antipsychotic Agents ● **479**

* Gynecomastia
* Weight gain
* Reduction of seizure threshold
* Agranulocytosis
* Extrapyramidal symptoms
* Tardive dyskinesia
* Neuroleptic malignant syndrome
* Prolongation of QT interval

Interactions

* Decreased serum concentrations of haloperidol, worsening schizophrenic symptoms, and tardive dyskinesia with concomitant use of **anticholinergic agents**
* Increased plasma concentrations when administered with drugs that inhibit CYP3A enzymes (**azole antifungal agents; macrolide antibiotics**) and CYP1A2 enzymes (**fluoxetine; fluvoxamine**)
* Decreased therapeutic effects of haloperidol with **carbamazepine**; increased effects of **carbamazepine**
* Additive hypotension with **antihypertensives**
* Additive CNS depression with **alcohol** or other **CNS depressants**
* Coadministration of haloperidol and **lithium** may result in alterations in consciousness, encephalopathy, extrapyramidal effects, fever, leukocytosis, and increased serum enzymes.
* Decreased therapeutic effects of haloperidol with **rifamycins**
* Concurrent use with **epinephrine** or **dopamine** may result in severe hypotension.
* Additive effects with other drugs that prolong QT interval (e.g., **phenothiazines, tricyclic antidepressants, antiarrhythmic agents**)

Route and Dosage

HALOPERIDOL **(Haldol)**

Psychotic Disorders: *Adults:* **PO:** *(Moderate symptoms or geriatric or debilitated patients):* 0.5 to 2 mg 2 or 3 times a day. *(Severe symptoms or chronic or resistant patients):* 3 to 5 mg 2 or 3 times a day. Some patients may require dosages up to 100 mg/day.

Children (3 to 12 years; weight range 15 to 40 kg): Initial dose: 0.5 mg/day (25 to 50 mcg/kg/day). May increase in 0.5 mg increments at 5- to 7-day intervals up to 0.15 mg/kg/day or until therapeutic effect is obtained. Administer in 2 or 3 divided doses.

Control of Acutely Agitated Schizophrenic Patient: *Adults:* **IM (lactate):** 2 to 5 mg. May be repeated every 1 to 8 hours, not to exceed 100 mg/day.

***Chronic Psychosis Requiring Prolonged Antipsychotic
Therapy:*** *Adults:* **IM (decanoate):** 10 to 15 times the
previous daily oral dose, not to exceed 100 mg initially.
Repeat every 4 weeks, or adjust interval to patient response.
For maintenance, titrate dosage upward or downward based
on therapeutic response.

Tourette's Disorder: *Adults:* **PO:** Initial dosage: 0.5 to 1.5 mg
3 times a day. Increase dose gradually as determined by patient
response. Up to 10 mg/day may be required.

Children (3 to 12 years; 15 to 40 kg): **PO:** 0.05 to 0.075 mg/
kg/day.

Behavioral Disorders/Hyperactivity: *Children (3 to 12 years;
15 to 40 kg):* **PO:** 0.05 to 0.075 mg/kg/day.

PIMOZIDE **(Orap)**

Tourette's Disorder: *Adults:* **PO:** Initial dose: 1 to 2 mg/day
in divided doses. Thereafter, increase dose every other day.
Maintenance dose: Less than 0.2 mg/kg/day or 10 mg/day,
whichever is less. Doses greater than 0.2 mg/kg/day or 10 mg/
day are not recommended.

Children (12 years and older): Initial dose: 0.05 mg/kg, preferably
taken once at bedtime. The dose may be increased every third
day to a maximum of 0.2 mg/kg, not to exceed 10 mg/day.

● **CHEMICAL CLASS: DIHYDROINDOLONES**
Examples

Generic (Trade) Name	Pregnancy Categories/ Half-life (hr)	Indications	Available Forms (mg)
Molindone (Moban)	C/12	• Schizophrenia	Caps: 5, 10, 25, 50

Action
- The exact mechanism of action is not fully understood.
- It is thought that molindone exerts its effect on the ascending
  reticular activating system.

Contraindications and Precautions
- **Contraindicated in** hypersensitivity, comatose or severely
  CNS-depressed patients, children under 12 (safety not established), lactation
- **Use cautiously in** patients with history of seizures; respiratory,
  renal, hepatic, thyroid, or cardiovascular disorders; elderly or
  debilitated patients, pregnancy.

Adverse Reactions and Side Effects

- Drowsiness
- Depression
- Hyperactivity/euphoria
- Extrapyramidal symptoms
- Blurred vision
- Tachycardia
- Nausea
- Dry mouth
- Salivation
- Urinary retention
- Constipation

Interactions

- Additive hypotension with **antihypertensive agents**
- Additive CNS effects with **CNS depressants**
- Additive anticholinergic effects with drugs that have anticholinergic properties

Route and Dosage

MOLINDONE **(Moban)**

Schizophremna: Adults: PO: Initial dosage: 50 to 75 mg/day. May increase to 100 mg in 3 or 4 days, up to 225 mg/day if required.

Maintenance Therapy: Adults (mild symptoms): PO: 5 to 15 mg 3 or 4 times a day. *(Moderate symptoms): PO:* 10 to 25 mg 3 or 4 times a day. *(Severe symptoms): PO:* Up to 225 mg/day may be required.

● CHEMICAL CLASS: DIBENZEPINES
Examples

Generic (Trade) Name	Pregnancy Categories/ Half-life (hr)	Indications	Available Forms (mg)
Loxapine (Loxitane)	C/8	• Schizophrenia	Caps: 5, 10, 25, 50
Clozapine (Clozaril)	B/8 (single dose); 12 (at steady state)	• Treatment-resistant schizophrenia • Recurrent suicidal behavior **Unlabeled uses:** • Acute manic episodes associated with bipolar disorder	Tabs: 12.5, 25, 50, 100, 200 Tabs (orally disintegrating): 12.5, 25, 50, 100

Continued

Generic (Trade) Name	Pregnancy Categories/ Half-life (hr)	Indications	Available Forms (mg)
Olanzapine (Zyprexa)	C/21–54	• Schizophrenia • Bipolar mania • Acute agitation in schizophrenia (IM) • Acute agitation associated with bipolar mania (IM) **Unlabeled uses:** • Obsessive-compulsive disorder (refractory to SSRIs)	Tabs: 2.5, 5, 7.5, 10, 15, 20 Tabs (orally disintegrating): 5, 10, 15, 20 Inj: 10/vial
Quetiapine (Seroquel)	C/~6	• Schizophrenia • Bipolar mania	Tabs: 25, 50, 100, 200, 300, 400 Tabs (XR): 200, 300, 400

Action

Loxapine
• Mechanism of action has not been fully established.
• Exerts strong antagonistic effects on dopamine D_2 and D_4 and serotonin $5-HT_2$ receptors

Clozapine
• Exerts an antagonistic effect on dopamine receptors, with a particularly high affinity for the D_4 receptor
• It appears to be more active at limbic than at striatal dopamine receptors.
• Also acts as an antagonist at adrenergic, cholinergic, histaminergic, and serotonergic receptors

Olanzapine
• Efficacy in schizophrenia is mediated through a combination of dopamine and $5-HT_2$ antagonism.
• Also shows antagonism for muscarinic, histaminic, and adrenergic receptors
• The mechanism of action of olanzapine in the treatment of bipolar mania is unknown.

Quetiapine
• Antipsychotic activity is thought to be mediated through a combination of dopamine type 2 (D_2) and serotonin type 2 ($5-HT_2$) antagonism. Other effects may be due to antagonism of histamine H_1 receptors and alpha$_1$-adrenergic receptors.

Contraindications and Precautions:

Loxapine

- **Contraindicated in:** hypersensitivity; comatose or severe drug-induced depressed states; clients with blood dyscrasias; hepatic, renal, or cardiac insufficiency; severe hypotension or hypertension; children, pregnancy, and lactation (*safety not established*)
- **Use cautiously in:** patients with epilepsy or history of seizures; glaucoma; urinary retention; respiratory insufficiency; prostatic hypertrophy; elderly patients with dementia-related psychosis (**black box warning**).

Clozapine

- **Contraindicated in:** hypersensitivity; myeloproliferative disorders; history of clozapine-induced agranulocytosis or severe granulocytopenia; concomitant use with other drugs that have the potential to suppress bone marrow function; severe CNS depression or comatose states; uncontrolled epilepsy; lactation; children (*safety not established*)
- **Use cautiously in:** patients with hepatic, renal, respiratory, or cardiac insufficiency; diabetes mellitus or risk factors for diabetes; prostatic enlargement; narrow-angle glaucoma; pregnancy; elderly patients with dementia-related psychosis (**black box warning**).

Olanzapine

- **Contraindicated in:** hypersensitivity; lactation. *Orally disintegrating tablets only:* Phenylketonuria (orally disintegrating tablets contain aspartame)
- **Use cautiously in:** hepatic insufficiency, elderly clients (reduce dosage), pregnancy and children (*safety not established*), cardiovascular or cerebrovascular disease, history of glaucoma, history of seizures, history of attempted suicide, prostatic hypertrophy, diabetes or risk factors for diabetes, narrow angle glaucoma, history of paralytic ileus; elderly patients with dementia-related psychosis (**black box warning**).

Quetiapine

- **Contraindicated in:** hypersensitivity; lactation
- **Use cautiously in:** cardiovascular or cerebrovascular disease; dehydration or hypovolemia (increased risk of hypotension); hepatic impairment; hypothyroidism; history of suicide attempt; pregnancy or children (*safety not established*); patients with diabetes or risk factors for diabetes; elderly patients with dementia-related psychosis (**black box warning**).

Adverse Reactions and Side Effects

Loxapine
- Drowsiness, dizziness
- Anticholinergic effects (dry mouth, blurred vision, urinary retention, constipation, paralytic ileus)
- Nausea and vomiting
- Extrapyramidal symptoms
- Seizures
- Hypotension; hypertension; tachycardia
- Blood dyscrasias
- Neuroleptic malignant syndrome

Clozapine
- Drowsiness, dizziness, sedation
- Nausea and vomiting
- Dry mouth; blurred vision
- Agranulocytosis
- Seizures (appear to be dose-related)
- Salivation
- Myocarditis; cardiomyopathy
- Tachycardia
- Constipation
- Fever
- Weight gain
- Orthostatic hypotension
- Neuroleptic malignant syndrome
- Hyperglycemia

Olanzapine
- Drowsiness, dizziness, weakness
- Dry mouth, constipation, increased appetite
- Nausea; weight gain
- Orthostatic hypotension, tachycardia
- Restlessness; insomnia
- Rhinitis
- Tremor
- Headache
- Hyperglycemia

Quetiapine
- Drowsiness, dizziness
- Hypotension, tachycardia
- Headache
- Nausea, dry mouth, constipation
- Weight gain
- Hyperglycemia

Interactions

The effects of:	Are increased by:	Are decreased by:	Concurrent use may result in:
Loxapine			Additive CNS depression with alcohol or other CNS depressants. Increased hypotension with antihypertensive agents. Additive anticholinergic effects with anticholinergic agents. Concomitant use with lorazepam (and possibly other benzodiazepines) may result in respiratory depression, stupor, hypotension, and/or respiratory or cardiac arrest.
Clozapine	Caffeine, citalopram, cimetidine, fluoxetine, fluvoxamine, sertraline, CYP3A4-inhibiting drugs (e.g., ketoconazole), risperidone, ritonavir	CYP1A2 inducers (e.g., carbamazepine, omeprazole, rifampin), phenobarbital, phenytoin, nicotine	Additive CNS depression with alcohol or other CNS depressants. Increased hypotension with antihypertensive agents. Additive anticholinergic effects with anticholinergic agents. Concomitant use with benzodiazepines may result in respiratory depression, stupor, hypotension, and/or respiratory or cardiac arrest. Increased effects of risperidone with chronic coadministration.
Olanzapine	Fluvoxamine, fluoxetine	Carbamazepine, omeprazole, rifampin	Decreased effects of levodopa and dopamine agonists. Increased hypotension with antihypertensives. Increased CNS depression with alcohol or other CNS depressants. Increased anticholinergic effects with anticholinergic agents.
Quetiapine	Cimetidine; ketoconazole, itraconazole, fluconazole, erythromycin, or other CYP3A4 inhibitors	Phenytoin, thioridazine	Decreased effects of levodopa and dopamine agonists. Increased CNS depression with alcohol or other CNS depressants. Increased hypotension with antihypertensives. Additive anticholinergic effects with anticholinergic agents.

Route and Dosage

LOXAPINE (Loxitane)

Schizophrenia: *Adults:* **PO:** Initial dosage: 10 mg 2 times a day, although some severely disturbed patients may require up to 50 mg/day. Increase dosage fairly rapidly over the first 7 to 10 days until symptoms are controlled. The usual therapeutic and maintenance dosage range is 60 mg to 100 mg/day. Doses higher than 250 mg/day are not recommended. Dosage should be maintained at the lowest level effective for controlling symptoms.

CLOZAPINE (Clozaril)

Schizophrenia and Recurrent Suicidal Behavior: *Adults:* **PO**: Initial dose: 12.5 mg once or 2 times a day. May increase dosage by 25 to 50 mg/day over a period of 2 weeks to a target dose of 300 to 450 mg/day. If required, make additional increases in increments of 100 mg not more than once or twice weekly to a maximum dosage of 900 mg/day in 3 divided doses. The mean and median doses are approximately 600 mg/day for schizophrenia and 300 mg/day for reducing recurrent suicidal behavior. Titrate dosage slowly to observe for possible seizures and agranulocytosis.

NOTE: A baseline white blood cell (WBC) count and absolute neutrophil count (ANC) must be taken before initiation of treatment with clozapine and weekly for the first 6 months of treatment. Because of the risk of agranulocytosis, clozapine is available only in a 1-week supply through the Clozaril Patient Management System, which combines WBC testing, patient monitoring, and controlled distribution through participating pharmacies. If the counts remain within the acceptable levels (i.e., WBC at least 3,500/mm^3 and the AMC at least 2,000/mm^3) during the 6-month period, blood counts may be monitored biweekly, and a 2-week supply of medication may then be dispensed. If for a 6-month period the counts remain within the acceptable level for the biweekly period, counts may then be monitored every 4 weeks thereafter. When the medication is discontinued, weekly WBC counts are continued for an additional 4 weeks.

OLANZAPINE (Zyprexa)

Schizophrenia: *Adults:* **PO:** 5 to 10 mg/day initially; may increase at weekly intervals by 5 mg/day (not to exceed 20 mg/day).

Bipolar Disorder: *Adults:* **PO:** 10 to 15 mg/day initially; may increase every 24 hours by 5 mg/day (not to exceed 20 mg/day).

Agitation Associated with Schizophrenia or Mania: *Adults:* **IM:** 2.5 to 10 mg, administered slowly, deep into muscle mass. May repeat in 2 hours and again 4 hours later, if needed.

QUETIAPINE (Seroquel)

Schizophrenia: Adults: **PO:** 25 mg 2 times a day initially, increased by 25 to 50 mg 2 to 3 times daily over 3 days, up to 300 to 400 mg/day in 2 to 3 divided doses by the fourth day (not to exceed 800 mg/day).

Bipolar Mania: Adults: **PO:** 100 mg/day in 2 divided doses on day 1; increase dose by 100 mg/day up to 400 mg/day by day 4 given in 2 divided doses. May increase in 200 mg/day increments up to 800 mg/day on day 6 if required.

● CHEMICAL CLASS: BENZISOXAZOLE
Examples

Generic (Trade) Name	Pregnancy Categories/ Half-life (hr)	Indications	Available Forms (mg)
Risperidone (Risperdal)	C/~3–20	• Schizophrenia • Bipolar mania • Irritability associated with autistic disorder in children **Unlabeled uses:** • Obsessive-compulsive disorder (refractory to SSRIs)	Tabs: 0.25, 0.5, 1, 2, 3, 4 Tabs (orally disintegrating): 0.5, 1, 2, 3, 4 Oral Solu: 1/mL Powder for injection: 12.5/vial, 25/vial, 37.5/vial, 50/vial
Paliperidone (Invega)	C/23	• Schizophrenia	Tabs (ER): 3, 6, 9 Inj (ER): 39/0.25 mL, 78/0.5 mL, 117/0.75 mL, 156/mL, 234/1.5 mL
Iloperidone (Fanapt)	C/18–33	• Schizophrenia	Tabs: 1, 2, 4, 6, 8, 10, 12
Ziprasidone (Geodon)	C/~7 (oral) 2–5 (IM)	• Schizophrenia • Bipolar mania • Acute agitation in schizophrenia (IM)	Caps: 20, 40, 60, 80 Powder for injection: 20/vial

Action

• Exerts antagonistic effects on dopamine type 2 (D_2), serotonin type 2 (5-HT_2), alpha$_1$- and alpha$_2$-adrenergic, and H_1 histaminergic receptors

Contraindications and Precautions:

Contraindicated in: • Known hypersensitivity • Comatose or severely depressed patients • Bradycardia, recent myocardial infarction (MI), or uncompensated heart failure • Lactation

• Patients with history of QT prolongation or cardiac arrhythmias
• Concurrent use with drugs known to cause QT prolongation

Use Cautiously in: • Clients with hepatic or renal impairment • Clients with history of seizures • Clients with diabetes or risk factors for diabetes • Clients exposed to temperature extremes • Elderly or debilitated clients • Clients with history of suicide attempt • Pregnancy and children (*safety not established*) • Elderly patients with dementia-related psychosis (**black box warning**) • Conditions that increase risk of hypotension (e.g., dehydration [including from diuretic therapy or diarrhea], hypovolemia, concurrent antihypertensive therapy).

Adverse Reactions and Side Effects

• Anxiety
• Agitation
• Dry mouth
• Weight gain
• Orthostatic hypotension
• Insomnia
• Sedation
• Extrapyramidal symptoms
• Dizziness
• Headache
• Constipation
• Diarrhea
• Nausea
• Rhinitis
• Rash
• Tachycardia
• Hyperglycemia
• Prolonged QT interval

Interactions

• Increased effects of risperidone with **clozapine, fluoxetine, paroxetine,** or **ritonavir**
• Decreased effects of **levodopa** and **other dopamine agonists** with risperidone, paliperidone, and ziprasidone
• Decreased effectiveness of risperidone with **carbamazepine**
• Additive CNS depression with **CNS depressants,** such as **alcohol, antihistamines, sedative/hypnotics,** or **opioid analgesics**
• Increased effects of **clozapine** and **valproate** with risperidone
• Additive hypotension with **antihypertensive agents**
• Additive orthostatic hypotension with coadministration of other drugs that result in this adverse reaction
• Additive anticholinergic effects with **anticholinergic agents**

- Serious life-threatening arrhythmias with drugs known to prolong QT interval (e.g., **antiarrhythmics** [e.g., **quinidine, procainamide, amiodarone, sotalol**], **chlorpromazine, thiroidazine, gatifloxacin, moxifloxacin, pentamidine, levomethadyl**)

Route and Dosage

RISPERIDONE **(Risperdal)**

Bipolar Mania: *Adults:* **PO:** 2 to 3 mg/day as a single daily dose; dose may be increased at 24-hour intervals by 1 mg (range 1 to 6 mg/day).

Children: Initial dose: 0.5 mg once daily as a single daily dose. May increase at 24-hour intervals by 0.5 or 1 mg/day, to a recommended dose of 2.5 mg/day.

Schizophrenia: *Adults:* **PO:** Initial dose: 2 mg/day administered in a single dose or in 2 divided doses. May increase in increments of 1 to 2 mg/day at intervals of 24 hours to a recommended dose of 4 to 8 mg/day.

Adolescents (13 to 17 years): Initial dose: 0.5 mg once daily as a single dose. May increase in increments of 0.5 or 1 mg/day at intervals of 24 hours to a recommended dose of 3 mg/day. **IM:** 25 mg every 2 weeks; some patients may require larger dose of 37.5 or 50 mg every 2 weeks.

Irritability Associated with Autistic Disorder: **PO:** *Children and adolescents (5 to 16 years weighing <20 kg):* 0.25 mg/day initially. After at least 4 days of therapy, may increase to 0.5 mg/day. Dose increases in increments of 0.25 mg/day may be considered at 2 week or longer intervals. May be as a single or divided dose.

Children and adolescents (5 to 16 years weighing >20 kg): 0.5 mg/day initially. After at least 4 days of therapy, may increase to 1.0 mg/day. Dose increases in increments of 0.5 mg/day may be considered at 2-week or longer intervals. May be as a single or divided dose.

PALIPERIDONE **(Invega)**

Schizophrenia: *Adults:* **PO:** 6 mg as a single daily dose. After clinical assessment, dose increases may be made at intervals of more than 5 days. When dose increases are indicated, small increments of 3 mg/day are recommended. Maximum recommended dose: 12 mg/day.

ILOPERIDONE **(Fanapt)**

Schizophrenia: *Adults:* **PO:** Initiate treatment with 1 mg 2 times a day on the first day, then 2 mg 2 times a day the second day, then increase by 2 mg/day every day until a target dose of 12 to 24 mg/day given in two divided doses is reached.

ZIPRASIDONE **(Geodon)**

Schizophrenia: *Adults:* **PO:** Initial dosage: 20 mg 2 times a day with food. May increase dosage by intervals of at least 2 days up to a dosage of 80 mg 2 times a day.

Bipolar Mania: *Adults:* **PO:** Initial dosage: 40 mg 2 times a day with food. On the second day of treatment, increase dose to 60 or 80 mg 2 times a day. Adjust dosage on the basis of toleration and efficacy within the range of 40 to 80 mg 2 times a day.

Acute Agitation in Schizophrenia: *Adults:* **IM:** 10 to 20 mg as needed up to a maximum of 40 mg/day. May be given as 10 mg every 2 hours or 20 mg every 4 hours.

● **CHEMICAL CLASS: QUINOLINONES**
Example

Generic (Trade) Name	Pregnancy Categories/ Half-life (hr)	Indications	Available Forms (mg)
Aripiprazole (Abilify)	C/75 (aripiprazole); 94 (metabolite)	• Schizophrenia • Bipolar mania • Major depression, adjunctive therapy • Agitation associated with schizophrenia or bipolar mania (IM)	Tabs: 2, 5, 10, 15, 20, 30 Tabs (orally disintegrating): 10, 15 Oral solution: 1/mL Inj: 7.5 mL

Action
• The efficacy of aripiprazole is thought to occur through a combination of partial agonist activity at D_2 and $5-HT_{1A}$ receptors and antagonist activity at $5-HT_{2A}$ receptors.
• Also exhibits antagonist activity at adrenergic α_1 receptors.

Contraindications and Precautions
Contraindicated in: • Hypersensitivity • Lactation
Use Cautiously in: • History of seizures • Hepatic or renal impairment • Known cardiovascular or cerebrovascular disease • Conditions that cause hypotension (dehydration, hypovolemia, treatment with antihypertensive medication) • Conditions that increase the core body temperature (excessive exercise, exposure to extreme heat, dehydration) • Patients with diabetes or risk factors for diabetes • Pregnancy (weigh benefits of the drug to potential risk to fetus) • Children and adolescents (*safety and effectiveness not established*) • Elderly patients with dementia-related psychosis (**black box warning**)

Adverse Reactions and Side Effects
- Headache
- Nausea and vomiting
- Constipation
- Anxiety, restlessness
- Insomnia
- Lightheadedness
- Drowsiness, sedation, somnolence
- Weight gain
- Blurred vision
- Increased salivation
- Extrapyramidal symptoms
- Hyperglycemia
- Disruption in the body's ability to reduce core body temperature

Interactions
- Decreased plasma levels of aripiprazole with **carbamazepine** and other **CYP3A4 inducers**
- Increased plasma levels and potential for aripiprazole toxicity with **CYP2D6 inhibitors**, such as **quinidine, fluoxetine,** and **paroxetine**
- Decreased metabolism and increased effects of aripiprazole with **ketoconazole** or **other CYP3A4 inhibitors**
- Additive hypotensive effects with **antihypertensive drugs**
- Additive CNS effects with **alcohol** and other **CNS depressants**

Route and Dosage
Bipolar Mania: *Adults:* **PO:** Initial dose: 15 mg once daily. May increase to 30 mg/day based on clinical response. Maximum dosage: 30 mg/day.
Children (10 to 17 years): **PO:** Initial dose: 2 mg/day. May increase to 5 mg after 2 days and to 10 mg after 2 more days. If required, additional dose increases may be made in 5 mg/day increments. Maintenance dosage: 10 to 30 mg/day (maintain at lowest effective dose for symptom remission).

Schizophrenia: *Adults:* **PO:** Initial dose: 10 or 15 mg/day as a single dose. Doses up to 30 mg have been used. Dosage increases should not be made before 2 weeks, the time required to achieve steady state.
Children (13 to 17 years): **PO:** Initial dose: 2 mg/day. May increase to 5 mg after 2 days and to 10 mg after 2 more days. If required, additional dose increases may be made in 5 mg/day increments. Maintenance dosage: 10 to 30 mg/day (maintain at lowest effective dose for symptom remission).

Major Depression, Adjunctive Therapy: Adults: **PO:** Initial
dose: 2 to 5 mg as adjunctive treatment for patients already
taking an antidepressant. May increase dosage in increments
of 5 mg/day at intervals of at least 1 week. Maintenance dosage:
2 to 15 mg/day.

*Agitation Associated with Schizophrenia or Bipolar
Mania: Adults:* **IM:** Usual dose: 9.75 mg. May use a dose of
5.25 mg, based on clinical situation. May give additional doses
up to a maximum of 30 mg/day if needed for agitation.

● CHEMICAL CLASS: DIBENZO-OXEPINO
 PYRROLE
Example

Generic (Trade) Name	Pregnancy Categories/ Half-life (hr)	Indications	Available Forms (mg)
Asenapine (Saphris)	C/24	● Schizophrenia ● Bipolar mania	Tabs (Sublingual): 5,10

Action
- Efficacy in schizophrenia is achieved through a combination
  of dopamine and serotonin type 2 (5-HT$_2$) antagonism.
- Mechanism of action in the treatment of acute manic episodes
  is unknown.

Contraindications and Precautions:
Contraindicated in: ● Hypersensitivity ● Lactation ● History
of QT prolongation or arrhythmias ● Concurrent use of other
drugs known to prolong QT interval
Use Cautiously in: ● Patients with hepatic, renal, or cardiovascular insufficiency ● Diabetes or risk factors for diabetes ● Patients with preexisting low WBC count and/or history
of drug-induced leukopenia/neutropenia ● History of seizures
● History of suicide attempt ● Patients at risk for aspiration pneumonia ● Pregnancy and children (*safety not established*) ● Elderly
patients with dementia-related psychosis (**black box warning**)

Adverse Reactions and Side Effects
- Constipation
- Dry mouth
- Nausea and vomiting
- Weight gain

- Restlessness
- Extrapyramidal symptoms
- Drowsiness, dizziness
- Insomnia
- Headache

Interactions

- Increased effects of asenapine with **fluvoxamine, imipramine,** or **valproate**
- Decreased effects of asenapine with **carbamazepine, cimetidine,** or **paroxetine**
- Increased effects of **paroxetine** or **dextromethorphan** with asenapine
- Increased CNS depression with **alcohol** or other **CNS depressants**
- Increased hypotension with **antihypertensives**
- Additive effects on QT interval prolongation with **quinidine, dofetilide,** other **Class Ia** and **III antiarrhythmics, pimozide, sotalol, thioridazine, chlorpromazine, floquine, pentamadine, arsenic trioxide, mefloquine, dolasetron, tacrolimus, droperidol, gatifloxacin,** or **moxifloxacin**

Route and Dosage

ASENAPINE **(Saphris)**

Schizophrenia: *Adults:* **PO:** Usual starting and target dose: 5 mg 2 times a day. The safety of doses above 10 mg 2 times a day has not been evaluated in clinical trials.

Bipolar Disorder: *Adults:* **PO:** Recommended initial dose: 10 mg 2 times a day. The dose can be decreased to 5 mg 2 times a day if there are adverse effects. The safety of doses above 10 mg 2 times a day has not been evaluated in clinical trials.

● NURSING DIAGNOSES RELATED TO ALL ANTIPSYCHOTIC AGENTS

1. Risk for other-directed violence related to panic anxiety and mistrust of others.
2. Risk for injury related to medication side effects of sedation, photosensitivity, reduction of seizure threshold, agranulocytosis, extrapyramidal symptoms, tardive dyskinesia, neuroleptic malignant syndrome, and/or QT prolongation.
3. Risk for activity intolerance related to medication side effects of sedation, blurred vision, and/or weakness.
4. Noncompliance with medication regimen related to suspiciousness and mistrust of others.

● NURSING IMPLICATIONS
FOR ANTIPSYCHOTIC AGENTS

The plan of care should include monitoring for the following side effects from antipsychotic medications. Nursing implications related to each side effect are designated by an asterisk (*). A profile of side effects comparing various antipsychotic medications is presented in Table 28-1.

1. **Anticholinergic effects** (see Table 28-1 for differences between typicals and atypicals)
   a. **Dry mouth**
      * Provide the client with sugarless candy or gum, ice, and frequent sips of water.
      * Ensure that client practices strict oral hygiene.
   b. **Blurred vision**
      * Explain that this symptom will most likely subside after a few weeks.
      * Advise client not to drive a car until vision clears.
      * Clear small items from pathway to prevent falls.
   c. **Constipation**
      * Order foods high in fiber; encourage increase in physical activity and fluid intake if not contraindicated.
   d. **Urinary retention**
      * Instruct client to report any difficulty urinating; monitor intake and output.
2. **Nausea; gastrointestinal (GI) upset** (may occur with all classifications)
   * Tablets or capsules may be administered with food to minimize GI upset.
   * Concentrates may be diluted and administered with fruit juice or other liquid; they should be mixed immediately before administration.
3. **Skin rash** (may occur with all classifications)
   * Report appearance of any rash on skin to physician.
   * Avoid spilling any of the liquid concentrate on skin; contact dermatitis can occur.
4. **Sedation** (see Table 28-1 for differences between typicals and atypicals)
   * Discuss with physician possibility of administering drug at bedtime.
   * Discuss with physician possible decrease in dosage or order for less sedating drug.
   * Instruct client not to drive or operate dangerous equipment while experiencing sedation.
5. **Orthostatic hypotension** (see Table 28-1 for differences between typicals and atypicals)
   * Instruct client to rise slowly from a lying or sitting position

TABLE 28–1 Comparison of Side Effects Among Antipsychotic Agents

Class	Generic (Trade) Name	EPS†	Sedation	Anti-cholinergic	Orthostatic Hypotension	Weight Gain
Typicals	Chlorpromazine	3	4	3	4	*
	Fluphenazine	5	2	2	2	
	Haloperidol (Haldol)	5	2	2	2	*
	Loxapine (Loxitane)	3	2	2	2	*
	Molindone (Moban)	3	2	2	2	*
	Perphenazine	4	2	2	2	*
	Pimozide (Orap)	4	2	3	2	*
	Prochlorperazine	3	2	2	2	*
	Thioridazine	2	4	4	4	*
	Thiothixene (Navane)	4	2	2	2	*
	Trifluoperazine	4	2	2	2	*

Continued

TABLE 28–1 Comparison of Side Effects Among Antipsychotic Agents—cont'd

Class	Generic (Trade) Name	EPS†	Sedation	Anti-cholinergic	Orthostatic Hypotension	Weight Gain
Atypicals	Aripiprazole (Abilify)	1	2	1	3	2
	Asenapine (Saphris)	1	3	1	3	4
	Clozapine (Clozaril)	1	5	5	4	5
	Iloperidone (Fanapt)	1	3	2	3	3
	Olanzapine (Zyprexa)	1	3	2	2	5
	Paliperidone (Invega)	1	2	1	3	2
	Quetiapine (Seroquel)	1	3	1	3	4
	Risperidone (Risperdal)	1	2	1	3	4
	Ziprasidone (Geodon)	1	3	1	2	2

Key: 1=Very low; 2=Low; 3=Moderate; 4=High; 5=Very high
† EPS=Extrapyramidal Symptoms
* Weight gain occurs, but incidence is unknown

SOURCE: Adapted from Black & Andreasen (2011); *Drug Facts and Comparisons* (2010); and Schatzberg, Cole, & DeBattista (2010).

        * Monitor blood pressure (lying and standing) each shift; document and report significant changes.

6. **Photosensitivity** (may occur with all classifications)
   * Ensure that client wears protective sunblock lotion, clothing, and sunglasses while spending time outdoors.

7. **Hormonal effects** (may occur with all classifications, but more common with typicals)
   a. **Decreased libido, retrograde ejaculation, gynecomastia** (men)
      * Provide explanation of the effects and reassurance of reversibility. If necessary, discuss with physician possibility of ordering alternate medication.
   b. **Amenorrhea** (women)
      * Offer reassurance of reversibility; instruct client to continue use of contraception, because amenorrhea does not indicate cessation of ovulation.
   c. **Weight gain** (may occur with all classifications; has been problematic with the atypicals)
      * Weigh client every other day; order calorie-controlled diet; provide opportunity for physical exercise; provide diet and exercise instruction.

8. **ECG Changes.** ECG changes, including prolongation of the QT interval, are possible with most of the antipsychotics. This is particularly true with ziprasidone, thioridazine, pimozide, haloperidol, paliperidone, iloperidone, asenapine, and clozapine. Caution is advised in prescribing these medications to individuals with history of arrhythmias. Conditions that produce hypokalemia and/or hypomagnesemia, such as diuretic therapy or diarrhea, should be taken into consideration when prescribing. Routine ECG should be taken before initiation of therapy and periodically during therapy. Clozapine has also been associated with other cardiac events, such as ischemic changes, arrhythmias, congestive heart failure, myocarditis, and cardiomyopathy.
   * Monitor vital signs every shift.
   * Observe for symptoms of dizziness, palpitations, syncope, weakness, dyspnea, and peripheral edema.

9. **Reduction of seizure threshold** (more common with typicals than the atypicals, with the exception of clozapine)
   * Closely observe clients with history of seizures.
   * **NOTE:** This is particularly important with clients taking clozapine (Clozaril), with which seizures have been frequently associated. Dose appears to be an important predictor, with a greater likelihood of seizures occurring at higher doses. Extreme caution is advised in prescribing clozapine for clients with history of seizures.

10. **Agranulocytosis** (more common with typicals than the atypicals, with the exception of clozapine)
    * It usually occurs within the first 3 months of treatment. Observe for symptoms of sore throat, fever, malaise. A complete blood count should be monitored if these symptoms appear.
    * **EXCEPTION:** There is a significant risk of agranulocytosis with clozapine (Clozaril). Agranulocytosis is a potentially fatal blood disorder in which the client's white blood cell (WBC) count can drop to extremely low levels. A baseline WBC count and absolute neutrophil count (ANC) must be taken before initiation of treatment with clozapine and weekly for the first 6 months of treatment. Only a 1-week's supply of medication is dispensed at a time. If the counts remain within the acceptable levels (i.e., WBC at least 3,500/mm^3 and the ANC at least 2,000/mm^3) during the 6-month period, blood counts may be monitored biweekly, and a 2-week supply of medication may then be dispensed. If for a 6-month period the counts remain within the acceptable level for the biweekly period, counts may then be monitored every 4 weeks thereafter. When the medication is discontinued, weekly WBC counts are continued for an additional 4 weeks.
11. **Hypersalivation** (most common with clozapine)
    * A significant number of clients receiving clozapine (Clozaril) therapy experience extreme salivation. Offer support to the client, as this may be an embarrassing situation. It may even be a safety issue (e.g., risk of aspiration), if the problem is very severe. Management has included the use of sugar-free gum to increase the swallowing rate, as well as the prescription of medications such as an anticholinergic (e.g., scopolamine patch) or alpha$_2$-adrenoceptor agonist (e.g., clonidine).
12. **Extrapyramidal symptoms** (EPS) (see Table 28-1 for differences between typicals and atypicals)
    * Observe for symptoms and report; administer antiparkinsonian drugs, as ordered (see Chapter 29)
    a. **Pseudoparkinsonism** (tremor, shuffling gait, drooling, rigidity)
       * Symptoms may appear 1 to 5 days following initiation of antipsychotic medication; occurs most often in women, the elderly, and dehydrated clients.
    b. **Akinesia** (muscular weakness)
       * Same as pseudoparkinsonism.
    c. **Akathisia** (continuous restlessness and fidgeting)
       * This occurs most frequently in women; symptoms may occur 50 to 60 days following initiation of therapy.

d. **Dystonia** (involuntary muscular movements [spasms] of face, arms, legs, and neck)
  * This occurs most often in men and in people younger than 25 years.
e. **Oculogyric crisis** (uncontrolled rolling back of the eyes)
  * This may appear as part of the syndrome described as dystonia. It may be mistaken for seizure activity. Dystonia and oculogyric crisis should be treated as an emergency situation. The physician should be contacted, and intravenous benztropine mesylate (Cogentin) is commonly administered. Stay with the client and offer reassurance and support during this frightening time.

13. **Tardive dyskinesia** (bizarre facial and tongue movements, stiff neck, and difficulty swallowing) (may occur with all classifications, but more common with typical antipsychotics)
  * All clients receiving long-term (months or years) antipsychotic therapy are at risk.
  * Symptoms are potentially irreversible.
  * Drug should be withdrawn at first sign, which is usually vermiform movements of the tongue; prompt action may prevent irreversibility.

14. **Neuroleptic malignant syndrome** (NMS) (more common with the typicals than the atypicals)
  * This is a relatively rare, but potentially fatal, complication of treatment with neuroleptic drugs. Routine assessments should include temperature and observation for parkinsonian symptoms.
  * Onset can occur within hours or even years after drug initiation, and progression is rapid over the following 24 to 72 hours.
  * Symptoms include severe parkinsonian muscle rigidity, very high fever, tachycardia, tachypnea, fluctuations in blood pressure, diaphoresis, and rapid deterioration of mental status to stupor and coma.
  * Discontinue neuroleptic medication immediately.
  * Monitor vital signs, degree of muscle rigidity, intake and output, level of consciousness.
  * The physician may order bromocriptine (Parlodel) or dantrolene (Dantrium) to counteract the effects of NMS.

15. **Hyperglycemia and diabetes** (more common with atypicals)
  * studies have suggested an increased risk of treatment-emergent hyperglycemia-related adverse events in clients using atypical antipsychotics (e.g., risperidone, clozapine, olanzapine, quetiapine, ziprasidone, asenapine, and aripiprazole). The FDA recommends that clients with diabetes starting on atypical antipsychotic drugs be monitored

regularly for worsening of glucose control. Clients with risk factors for diabetes should undergo fasting blood glucose testing at the beginning of treatment and periodically thereafter. All clients taking these medications should be monitored for symptoms of hyperglycemia (polydipsia, polyuria, polyphagia, and weakness). If these symptoms appear during treatment, the client should undergo fasting blood glucose testing.

16. **Increased risk of mortality in elderly patients with dementia-related psychosis.**
   * Recent studies have indicated that elderly patients with dementia-related psychosis who are treated with antipsychotic drugs are at increased risk of death, compared with placebo. Causes of death are most commonly related to infections or cardiovascular problems. All antipsychotic drugs now carry black box warnings to this effect. They are not approved for treatment of elderly patients with dementia-related psychosis.

● **CLIENT/FAMILY EDUCATION RELATED TO ALL ANTIPSYCHOTICS**

- Use caution when driving or operating dangerous machinery. Drowsiness and dizziness can occur.
- Do not stop taking the drug abruptly after long-term use. To do so might produce withdrawal symptoms, such as nausea, vomiting, dizziness, gastritis, headache, tachycardia, insomnia, and tremulousness.
- Use sunblock lotion and wear protective clothing when spending time outdoors. Skin is more susceptible to sunburn, which can occur in as little as 30 minutes.
- Report weekly (if receiving clozapine therapy) to have blood levels drawn and to obtain a weekly supply of the drug.
- Report occurrence of any of the following symptoms to the physician immediately: sore throat, fever, malaise, unusual bleeding, easy bruising, persistent nausea and vomiting, severe headache, rapid heart rate, fainting, difficulty urinating, muscle twitching, tremors, darkly colored urine, excessive urination, excessive thirst, excessive hunger, weakness, pale stools, yellow skin or eyes, muscular incoordination, or skin rash.
- Rise slowly from a sitting or lying position to prevent a sudden drop in blood pressure.
- Take frequent sips of water, chew sugarless gum, or suck on hard candy, if experiencing a problem with dry mouth. Good oral care (frequent brushing, flossing) is very important.

- Consult the physician regarding smoking while taking this medication. Smoking increases the metabolism of some antipsychotics, possibly requiring adjustment in dosage to achieve therapeutic effect.
- Dress warmly in cold weather and avoid extended exposure to very high or low temperatures. Body temperature is harder to maintain with this medication.
- Do not drink alcohol while on antipsychotic therapy. These drugs potentiate each other's effects.
- Do not consume other medications (including over-the-counter products) without physician's approval. Many medications contain substances that interact with antipsychotics in a way that may be harmful.
- Be aware of possible risks of taking antipsychotic medication during pregnancy. Safe use during pregnancy and lactation has not been established. Antipsychotics are thought to readily cross the placental barrier; if so, a fetus could experience adverse effects of the drug. Inform the physician immediately if pregnancy occurs, is suspected, or is planned.
- Be aware of side effects of antipsychotic drugs. Refer to written materials furnished by health care providers for safe self-administration.
- Continue to take medication, even if feeling well and as though it is not needed. Symptoms may return if medication is discontinued.
- Carry card or other identification at all times describing medications being taken.

 INTERNET REFERENCES

a. http://www.rxlist.com
b. http://www.nimh.nih.gov/publicat/medicate.cfm
c. http://www.fadavis.com/townsend
d. http://www.mentalhealth.com/
e. http://www.nlm.nih.gov/medlineplus/druginformation.html

C H A P T E R 29

Antiparkinsonian Agents*

● CHEMICAL CLASS: ANTICHOLINERGICS
Examples

Generic (Trade) Name	Pregnancy Categories/ Half-life (hours)	Indications	Available Forms (mg)
Benztropine (Cogentin)	C/Unknown	• Parkinsonism • Drug-induced extrapyramidal symptoms	Tabs: 0.5, 1, 2 Inj: 1/mL
Biperiden (Akineton)	C/18.4–24.3	• Parkinsonism • Drug-induced extrapyramidal symptoms	Tabs: 2
Trihexyphenidyl	C/5.6–10.2	• Parkinsonism • Drug-induced extrapyramidal symptoms	Tabs: 2, 5 Elixir: 2/5 mL
Diphenhydramine (Benadryl)	B/4–15	• Parkinsonism • Drug-induced extrapyramidal symptoms • Motion sickness • Allergy reactions • Nighttime sleep aid • Cough suppressant	Tabs and Caps: 25, 50 Tabs (orally disintegrating): 12.5 Tabs, chewable: 12.5, 25 Strips (orally disintegrating): 12.5, 25 Elixir/syrup/oral solu: 12.5/5 mL Inj: 50/mL

---

* This chapter includes only those antiparkinsonian agents indicated for the treatment of antipsychotic-induced extrapyramidal symptoms or neuroleptic malignant syndrome (bromocriptine).

Action

- Blocks acetylcholine receptors to diminish excess cholinergic effects. May also inhibit the reuptake and storage of dopamine at central dopamine receptors, thereby prolonging the action of dopamine.
- Diphenhydramine also blocks histamine release by competing with histamine for H_1-receptor sites. Decreased allergic response and somnolence are effected by diminished histamine activity.

Contraindications and Precautions

Contraindicated in: ● Hypersensitivity ● Angle-closure glaucoma ● Pyloric or duodenal obstruction ● Peptic ulcers ● Prostatic hypertrophy ● Bladder neck obstructions ● Megaesophagus ● Megacolon ● Myasthenia gravis ● Lactation ● Children (*except* diphenhydramine)

Use Cautiously in: ● Tachycardia ● Cardiac arrhythmias ● Hypertension ● Hypotension ● Tendency toward urinary retention ● Clients exposed to high environmental temperatures ● Pregnancy

Adverse Reactions and Side Effects

- Dry mouth
- Blurred vision
- Constipation
- Paralytic ileus
- Urinary retention
- Tachycardia
- Agitation, nervousness
- Decreased sweating
- Elevated temperature
- Nausea/vomiting
- Sedation
- Dizziness
- Exacerbation of psychoses
- Orthostatic hypotension

Interactions

- *(Diphenhydramine):* Additive sedative effects with **central nervous system (CNS) depressants**
- Increased effects of **beta-blockers** with diphenhydramine
- Additive anticholinergic effects with other drugs that have anticholinergic properties
- Anticholinergic drugs counteract the cholinergic effects of **bethanechol.**
- Possible increased **digoxin** levels with anticholinergics

- Concomitant use of anticholinergics with **haloperidol** may result in worsening of psychotic symptoms, decreased haloperidol serum levels, and development of tardive dyskinesia.
- Possible decreased efficacy of **phenothiazines** and increased incidence of anticholinergic side effects with concomitant use
- Decreased effects of **levodopa** with concomitant use

Route and Dosage

BENZTROPINE **(Cogentin)**

Parkinsonism: *Adults:* **PO**: 1 to 2 mg/day in 1 to 2 divided doses (range 0.5 to 6 mg/day).

Drug-induced Extrapyramidal Symptoms: *Adults*: **PO**: 1 to 4 mg given 1 or 2 times a day.

Acute Dystonic Reactions: *Adults*: **IM, IV**: 1 to 2 mg, then 1 to 2 mg PO 2 times a day.

BIPERIDEN **(Akineton)**

Parkinsonism: *Adults*: **PO**: 2 mg 3 or 4 times a day, not to exceed 16 mg/24 hours.

Drug-induced Extrapyramidal Symptoms: *Adults*: **PO**: 2 mg 1 to 3 times a day.

TRIHEXYPHENIDYL

Parkinsonism: *Adults:* **PO**: Initial dose: 1 mg on day 1; increase by 2 mg increments at 3- to 5-day intervals, up to a daily dose of 6 to 10 mg in 3 divided doses taken at mealtimes.

Drug-induced Extrapyramidal Symptoms: *Adults*: **PO**: Initial dosage: 1 mg. Repeat dosage every few hours until symptoms are controlled. Maintenance or prophylactic use: 5 to 15 mg/day.

DIPHENHYDRAMINE **(Benadryl)**

Parkinsonism and Drug-induced Extrapyramidal Symptoms/Motion Sickness/Allergy Reactions: *Adults and children ≥12 years*: **PO:** 25 to 50 mg every 4 to 6 hours. Maximum dosage: 300 mg/day. **IM/IV:** *Adults:* 10 to 50 mg IV or 100 mg IM. Maximum daily dose: 400 mg.

Children 6 to 12 years: **PO:** 12.5 to 25 mg every 4 to 6 hours, not to exceed 150 mg/day.

Nighttime Sleep Aid: *Adults and children ≥12 years:* 50 mg at bedtime.

Cough Suppressant: *Adults and children ≥12 years:* **PO Liquid**: 25 to 50 mg every 4 hours, not to exceed 300 mg/day. **PO Syrup:** 25 mg every 4 hours, not to exceed 150 mg/day.

Children 6 to 12 years: **PO Liquid:** 12.5 to 25 mg every 4 hours, not to exceed 150 mg/day.

PO Syrup: 12.5 mg every 4 hours, not to exceed 75 mg/day.
Children 2 to 6 years: **PO Syrup**: 6.25 mg every 4 hours, not to exceed 25 mg/day.

● CHEMICAL CLASS: DOPAMINERGIC
   AGONISTS
Examples

Generic (Trade) Name	Pregnancy Categories/ Half-life (hr)	Indications	Available Forms (mg)
Amantadine (Symmetrel)	C/10–25	• Parkinsonism • Drug-induced extrapyramidal symptoms • Prophylaxis and treatment of Influenza A viral infection	Tabs, Caps: 100 Syrup: 50/5 mL
Bromocriptine (Parlodel)	B/8–20	• Parkinsonism • Hyperprolactinemia-associated dysfunctions • Acromegaly • Neuroleptic malignant syndrome	Tabs: 2.5 Caps: 5

Action
• Amantadine increases dopamine at the receptor either by releasing intact striatal dopamine stores or by blocking neuronal dopamine reuptake. It also inhibits the replication of influenza A virus isolates from each of the subtypes.
• Bromocriptine increases dopamine by direct stimulation of dopamine receptors.

Contraindications and Precautions
Contraindicated in:
Amantadine
• Hypersensitivity to the drug
• Pregnancy, lactation, and in children under 1 year (*safety not established*)
• Angle closure glaucoma

Bromocriptine
• Hypersensitivity to this drug, other ergot alkaloids, or sulfites (contained in some preparations)
• Uncontrolled hypertension
• Pregnancy and lactation; children younger than 15 years (*safety not established*)

Use Cautiously in: • Hepatic or renal impairment • Uncontrolled psychiatric disturbances • History of congestive heart failure, myocardial infarction, or ventricular arrhythmia • Elderly or debilitated clients • Orthostatic hypotension

Amantadine

- Clients with a history of seizures
- Concurrent use of CNS stimulants

Bromocriptine

- Clients with history of peptic ulcer or gastrointestinal bleeding

Adverse Reactions and Side Effects

Amantadine

- Nausea
- Dizziness
- Insomnia; somnolence
- Depression; anxiety
- Hallucinations
- Arrhythmia; tachycardia
- Dry mouth
- Blurred vision

Bromocriptine

- Nausea and vomiting
- Headache; dizziness; drowsiness
- Orthostatic hypotension
- Confusion
- Constipation; diarrhea
- Skin mottling
- Exacerbation of Raynaud syndrome
- Ataxia

Interactions

The effects of:	Are increased by:	Are decreased by:	Concurrent use may result in:
Amantadine	Quinidine, quinine, triamterene, thiazine diuretics, trimethoprim/ sulfamethoxazole, thioridazine		Potentiation of anticholinergic side effects with anticholinergic agents; increased effects of CNS stimulants with concurrent use.
Bromocriptine	Erythromycin, sympathomimetics, isometheptene, phenylpropanolamine	Phenothiazines (and other antipsychotics), metoclopramide	

Route and Dosage
AMANTADINE **(Symmetrel)**

Parkinsonism: *Adults:* **PO**: 100 mg 1 to 2 times/day (up to 400 mg/day).

Drug-induced Extrapyramidal Symptoms: *Adults*: **PO**: 100 mg 2 times a day (up to 300 mg/day in divided doses).

Influenza A Viral Infection: *Adults and children >12 years:* **PO**: 200 mg/day as a single dose or 100 mg 2 times a day.

Children 9 to 12 years: **PO**: 200 mg as a single dose or 100 mg 2 times a day.

Children 1 to 9 years: **PO**: 4.4 to 8.8 mg/kg/day given once daily or divided 2 times a day, not to exceed 150 mg/day.

BROMOCRIPTINE **(Parlodel)**

Parkinsonism: *Adults*: **PO**: Initial dose: 1.25 mg 2 times a day with meals. May increase dosage every 2 to 4 weeks by 2.5 mg/day with meals. Usual range is 10 to 40 mg/day. If adverse reactions necessitate reduction in dosage, reduce dose gradually in 2.5 mg increments.

Hyperprolactinemia-associated Dysfunctions: *Adults*: **PO**: Initial dose: 1.25 to 2.5 mg/day with meals. May increase by 2.5 mg every 2 to 7 days. Usual therapeutic dosage range: 2.5 to 15 mg/day.

Acromegaly: *Adults*: **PO**: Initial dose: 1.25 to 2.5 mg for 3 days (with food) at bedtime. May increase by 1.25 to 2.5 mg/day every 3 to 7 days. Usual therapeutic dosage range: 20 to 30 mg/day. Maximum dosage: 100 mg/day.

Neuroleptic Malignant Syndrome: *Adult*: **PO**: 5 mg every 4 hours.

● **NURSING DIAGNOSES RELATED TO ANTIPARKINSONIAN AGENTS**

1. Risk for injury related to symptoms of Parkinson's disease or drug-induced EPS.
2. Hyperthermia related to anticholinergic effect of decreased sweating.
3. Activity intolerance related to side effects of drowsiness, dizziness, ataxia, weakness, confusion.
4. Deficient knowledge related to medication regimen.

● **NURSING IMPLICATIONS FOR ANTIPARKINSONIAN AGENTS**

The plan of care should include monitoring for the following side effects from antiparkinsonian medications. Nursing implications related to each side effect are designated by an asterisk (*).

1. **Anticholinergic Effects**. These side effects are identical to those produced by antipsychotic drugs. Taking both medications compounds these effects. For this reason, the physician may elect to prescribe an antiparkinsonian agent only at the onset of EPS, rather than as routine adjunctive therapy.
    a. **Dry Mouth**
        * Offer sugarless candy or gum, ice, frequent sips of water.
        * Ensure that client practices strict oral hygiene.
    b. **Blurred Vision**
        * Explain that symptom will most likely subside after a few weeks.
        * Offer to assist with tasks requiring visual acuity.
    c. **Constipation**
        * Order foods high in fiber; encourage increase in physical activity and fluid intake, if not contraindicated.
    d. **Paralytic Ileus**
        * A rare, but potentially very serious side effect of anticholinergic drugs. Monitor for abdominal distension, absent bowel sounds, nausea, vomiting, epigastric pain.
        * Report any of these symptoms to physician immediately.
    e. **Urinary Retention**
        * Instruct client to report any difficulty urinating; monitor intake and output.
    f. **Tachycardia, Decreased Sweating, Elevated Temperature**
        * Assess vital signs each shift; document and report significant changes to physician.
        * Ensure that client remains in cool environment, because the body is unable to cool itself naturally with this medication.
2. **Nausea, Gastrointestinal (GI) Upset**
    * May administer tablets or capsules with food to minimize GI upset.
3. **Sedation, Drowsiness, Dizziness**
    * Discuss with physician possibility of administering drug at bedtime.
    * Discuss with physician possible decrease in dosage or order for less sedating drug.
    * Instruct client not to drive or use dangerous equipment while experiencing sedation or dizziness.
4. **Exacerbation of Psychoses**
    * Assess for signs of loss of contact with reality.
    * Intervene during a hallucination; talk about real people and real events; reorient client to reality.
    * Stay with client during period of agitation and delirium; remain calm and reassure client of his or her safety.

* Discuss with physician possible decrease in dosage or change in medication.
5. **Orthostatic Hypotension**
    * Instruct client to rise slowly from a lying or sitting position; monitor blood pressure (lying and standing) each shift; document and report significant changes.

● CLIENT/FAMILY EDUCATION RELATED TO ALL ANTIPARKINSONIAN AGENTS

* Take the medication with food if GI upset occurs.
* Use caution when driving or operating dangerous machinery. Drowsiness and dizziness can occur.
* Do not stop taking the drug abruptly. To do so might produce unpleasant withdrawal symptoms.
* Report occurrence of any of the following symptoms to the physician immediately: pain or tenderness in area in front of ear; extreme dryness of mouth; difficulty urinating; abdominal pain; constipation; fast, pounding heart beat; rash; visual disturbances; mental changes.
* Rise slowly from a sitting or lying position to prevent a sudden drop in blood pressure.
* Stay inside in air-conditioned room when weather is very hot. Perspiration is decreased with antiparkinsonian agents, and the body cannot cool itself as well. There is greater susceptibility to heat stroke. Inform physician if air-conditioned housing is not available.
* Take frequent sips of water, chew sugarless gum, or suck on hard candy if dry mouth is a problem. Good oral care (frequent brushing, flossing) is very important.
* Do not drink alcohol while on antiparkinsonian therapy.
* Do not consume other medications (including over-the-counter products) without physician's approval. Many medications contain substances that interact with antiparkinsonian agents in a way that may be harmful.
* Be aware of possible risks of taking antiparkinsonian agents during pregnancy. Safe use during pregnancy and lactation has not been fully established. It is thought that antiparkinsonian agents readily cross the placental barrier; if so, fetus could experience adverse effects of the drug. Inform physician immediately if pregnancy occurs, is suspected, or is planned.
* Be aware of side effects of antiparkinsonian agents. Refer to written materials furnished by health-care providers for safe self-administration.
* Continue to take medication, even if feeling well and as though it is not needed. Symptoms may return if medication is discontinued.

● Carry card or other identification at all times describing medications being taken.

 INTERNET REFERENCES

a. http://www.rxlist.com
b. http://www.nimh.nih.gov/publicat/medicate.cfm
c. http://www.fadavis.com/townsend
d. http://www.mentalhealth.com
e. http://www.nlm.nih.gov/medlineplus/druginformation
.html

CHAPTER 30

Sedative-Hypnotics

● **CHEMICAL CLASS: BENZODIAZEPINES**
Examples

Generic (Trade) Name	Controlled/ Pregnancy Categories	Half-life (hr)	Indications	Available Forms (mg)
Estazolam	CIV/X	8–28	• Insomnia	Tabs: 1, 2
Flurazepam (Dalmane)	CIV/(Contraindicated in pregnancy)	2–3 (active metabolite, 47–100)	• Insomnia	Caps: 15, 30
Quazepam (Doral)	CIV/X	41 (active metabolite, 47–100)	• Insomnia	Tabs: 7.5, 15
Temazepam (Restoril)	CIV/X	9–15	• Insomnia	Caps: 7.5, 15, 22.5, 30
Triazolam (Halcion)	CIV/X	1.5–5.5	• Insomnia	Tabs: 0.125, 0.25

Action
- Potentiate gamma-aminobutyric acid (GABA) neuronal inhibition
- The sedative effects involve GABA receptors in the limbic, neocortical, and mesencephalic reticular systems.

Contraindications and Precautions:

Contraindicated in: • Hypersensitivity to these or other benzodiazepines • Pregnancy and lactation • Respiratory depression and sleep apnea • *(Triazolam):* concurrent use with ketoconazole, itraconazole, or nefazodone, medications that impair the metabolism of triazolam by cytochrome P450 3A (CYP3A) • *(Flurazepam):* Children younger than age 15 • *(Estazolam, quazepam, temazepam, triazolam):* Children younger than age 18

Use Cautiously in: • Elderly and debilitated patients • Hepatic or renal dysfunction • Patients with history of drug abuse and dependence • Depressed or suicidal patients

Adverse Reactions and Side Effects

- Drowsiness
- Headache
- Confusion
- Lethargy
- Tolerance
- Physical and psychological dependence
- Potentiates the effects of other central nervous system (CNS) depressants
- May aggravate symptoms in depressed persons
- Palpitations; tachycardia; hypotension
- Paradoxical excitement
- Dry mouth
- Nausea and vomiting
- Blood dyscrasias

Interactions

- Additive CNS depression with **alcohol** and **other CNS depressants**
- Decreased clearance and increased effects of benzodiazepines with **cimetidine, oral contraceptives, disulfiram,** and **isoniazid**
- More rapid onset or more prolonged benzodiazepine effect with **probenecid**
- Increased clearance and decreased half-life of benzodiazepines with **rifampin**
- Increased benzodiazepine clearance with **cigarette smoking**
- Decreased pharmacological effects of benzodiazepines with **theophylline**
- Increased bioavailability of triazolam with **macrolides**
- Benzodiazepines may increase serum levels of **digoxin** and **phenytoin** and increase risk of toxicity

Route and Dosage

ESTAZOLAM

Insomnia: *Adults*: **PO:** 1 to 2 mg at bedtime.
Healthy elderly: **PO:** 1 mg at bedtime. Increase with caution.
Debilitated or small elderly patients: **PO:** 0.5 mg at bedtime.

FLURAZEPAM **(Dalmane)**

Insomnia: *Adults*: **PO:** 15 to 30 mg at bedtime.
Elderly or debilitated: **PO:** 15 mg at bedtime.

QUAZEPAM **(Doral)**

Insomnia: *Adults*: **PO:** 7.5 to 15 mg at bedtime.
Elderly or debilitated: **PO:** Initial dose: 7.5 mg at bedtime. If not effective after 1 or 2 nights, may increase to 15 mg.

TEMAZEPAM **(Restoril)**
Insomnia: *Adults*: **PO**: 15 to 30 mg at bedtime. 7.5 mg may be
  sufficient for some patients.
Elderly or debilitated: **PO:** 7.5 mg at bedtime.

TRIAZOLAM **(Halcion)**
Insomnia: *Adults*: **PO**: 0.125 to 0.5 mg at bedtime.
Elderly or debilitated: **PO**: 0.125 to 0.25 mg at bedtime.

● **CHEMICAL CLASS: BARBITURATES**
Examples

Generic (Trade) Name	Controlled/ Pregnancy Categories	Half-life (hr)	Indications	Available Forms (mg)
Amobarbital	CII/D	16–40	• Sedation • Insomnia	Injection: powder, 500/vial
Butabarbital (Butisol)	CIII/D	66–140	• Sedation • Insomnia	Tabs: 15, 30, 50 Elixir: 30/5 mL
Mephobarbital (Mebaral)	CIV/D	11–67	• Sedation • Epilepsy	Tabs: 32, 50, 100
Pentobarbital (Nembutal)	CII/D	15–50	• Sedation • Insomnia • Preanesthetic • Acute convulsive episodes	Inj: 50/mL
Phenobarbital (Solfoton; Luminal)	CIV/D	53–118	• Sedation • Epilepsy	Tabs: 15, 16, 30, 60, 90, 100 Caps: 16 Elixir: 15/5 mL; 20/5 mL Inj (mg/mL): 30, 60, 65, 130
Secobarbital (Seconal)	CII/D	15–40	• Preoperative sedation • Insomnia	Caps: 100

Action
- Depress the sensory cortex, decrease motor activity, and alter cerebellar function
- All levels of CNS depression can occur, from mild sedation to hypnosis to coma to death
- Can induce anesthesia in sufficiently high therapeutic doses

Contraindications and Precautions
Contraindicated in: • Hypersensitivity to barbiturates • Severe
hepatic, renal, cardiac, or respiratory disease • Individuals with

history of drug abuse or dependence • Porphyria • Uncontrolled severe pain • Intra-arterial or subcutaneous administration • Lactation

Use Cautiously in: • Elderly and debilitated patients • Patients with hepatic, renal, cardiac, or respiratory impairment • Depressed or suicidal patients • Pregnancy • Children

Adverse Reactions and Side Effects

- Bradycardia
- Hypotension
- Somnolence
- Agitation
- Confusion
- Nausea, vomiting
- Constipation
- Skin rashes
- Respiratory depression
- Physical and psychological dependence

Interactions

- Additive CNS depression with **alcohol** and **other CNS depressants**
- Decreased effects of barbiturates with **rifampin**
- Increased effects of barbiturates with monoamine oxidase (**MAO) inhibitors** or **valproic acid**
- Decreased effects of the following drugs with concurrent use of barbiturates: **anticoagulants, beta-blockers, carbamazepine, clonazepam, oral contraceptives, corticosteroids, digitoxin, doxorubicin, doxycycline, felodipine, fenoprofen, griseofulvin, metronidazole, phenylbutazone, quinidine, theophylline, chloramphenicol,** and **verapamil**
- Concomitant use with **methoxyflurane** may enhance renal toxicity.

Route and Dosage

AMOBARBITAL

Sedation: *Adults:* **IM:** 30 to 50 mg, 2 or 3 times a day.

Insomnia: *Adults:* **IM:** 65 to 200 mg at bedtime.

NOTE: Do not inject a volume >5 mL **IM** at any one site regardless of drug concentration. Tissue irritation can occur.

BUTABARBITAL **(Butisol)**

Daytime Sedation: Adults: **PO**: 15 to 30 mg, 3 or 4 times a day.

Insomnia: Adults: **PO**: 50 to 100 mg at bedtime.

Preoperative Sedation: Adults: **PO**: 50 to 100 mg, 60 to 90 minutes before surgery.

Children: **PO**: 2 to 6 mg/kg; maximum 100 mg.

MEPHOBARBITAL **(Mebaral)**

Sedation: Adults: **PO**: 32 to 100 mg 3 or 4 times a day. Optimum dose: 50 mg 3 or 4 times a day.

Children: **PO**: 16 to 32 mg 3 or 4 times a day.

Epilepsy: Adults: **PO**: 400 to 600 mg daily.

Children <5 yr: **PO**: 16 to 32 mg 3 or 4 times a day.

Children >5 yr: **PO**: 32 to 64 mg 3 or 4 times a day.

PENTOBARBITAL **(Nembutal)**

Sedation, Insomnia, Preanesthetic: **IM:** *Adults*: Usual dosage: 150 to 200 mg.

Children: 2 to 6 mg/kg as a single IM injection, not to exceed 100 mg.

NOTE: Inject deeply into large muscle mass. Do not exceed a volume of 5 mL at any one site because of possible tissue irritation.

PHENOBARBITAL **(Luminal)**

Sedation: Adults: **PO or IM**: 30 to 120 mg/day in 2 to 3 divided doses not to exceed 400 mg/day

Children: **PO**: 2 mg/kg 3 times daily.

Preoperative Sedation: Adults: **IM only**: 100 to 200 mg, 60 to 90 minutes before the procedure

Children: **PO, IM or IV:** 1 to 3 mg/kg 60 to 90 minutes before the procedure.

Insomnia: Adults: **PO**: 100 to 200 mg at bedtime.

IM or IV: 100 to 320 mg.

Children: Route and dosage determined by age and weight.

Epilepsy: Adults: **PO**: 60 to 200 mg/day.

Children: **PO**: 3 to 6 mg/kg/day.

SECOBARBITAL **(Seconal)**

Preoperative Sedation: Adults: **PO**: 200 to 300 mg 1 to 2 hours before surgery.

Children: **PO**: 2 to 6 mg/kg, not to exceed 100 mg.

Insomnia: Adults: **PO**: 100 mg at bedtime.

● CHEMICAL CLASS: MISCELLANEOUS
Examples

Generic (Trade) Name	Controlled/ Pregnancy Categories	Half-life (hr)	Indications	Available Forms (mg)
Chloral hydrate	CIV/C	7–10	• Sedation • Insomnia	Caps: 500 Syrup: 250/5 mL; 500/5 mL
Eszopiclone (Lunesta)	CIV/C	6	• Insomnia	Tabs: 1, 2, 3
Ramelteon (Rozerem)	Not controlled/ C	1–2.6	• Insomnia	Tabs: 8
Zaleplon (Sonata)	CIV/C	1	• Insomnia	Caps: 5, 10
Zolpidem (Ambien)	CIV/B	2–3	• Insomnia	Tabs: 5, 10 Tabs CR: 6.25, 12.5 Tabs sublingual: 5, 10 Spray solution, lingual: 5 per actuation

Action

Zolpidem and Zaleplon
• Bind to GABA receptors in the CNS. Appear to be selective for the omega$_1$-receptor subtype.

Eszopiclone
• Action as a hypnotic is unclear but thought to interact with GABA-receptor complexes near benzodiazepine receptors

Chloral Hydrate
• Action unknown. Produces a calming effect through depression of the CNS.
• Has generally been replaced by safer and more effective agents.

Ramelteon
• Ramelteon is a melatonin receptor agonist with high affinity for melatonin MT$_1$ and MT$_2$ receptors.

Contraindications and Precautions

Contraindicated in: • Hypersensitivity • In combination with other CNS depressants • Pregnancy and lactation

Zolpidem, Zaleplon, Eszopiclone, Ramelteon
• Children (*safety not established*)

Chloral Hydrate
• Severe hepatic, renal, or cardiac impairment
• Esophagitis, gastritis, or peptic ulcer disease

Ramelteon
- Severe hepatic function impairment
- Concomitantly with fluvoxamine

Use Cautiously in: • Elderly or debilitated patients • Depressed or suicidal patients • Patients with history of drug abuse or dependence • Patients with hepatic, renal, or respiratory dysfunction • Patients susceptible to acute intermittent porphyria (**chloral hydrate**)

Adverse Reactions and Side Effects
- Headache
- Drowsiness
- Dizziness
- Lethargy
- Amnesia
- Nausea
- Dry mouth
- Rash
- Paradoxical excitement
- Physical and/or psychological dependence

Chloral hydrate, eszopiclone
- Unpleasant taste

Interactions

The effects of:	Are increased by:	Are decreased by:	Concurrent use may result in:
Chloral hydrate	**Alcohol** and other **CNS depressants** including **antihistamines, antidepressants, opioids, sedative/ hypnotics, antipsychotics**		Increased effects of **oral anticoagulants;** symptoms of sweating, hot flashes, tachycardia, hypertension, weakness, and nausea with **IV furosemide;** decreased effects of **phenytoin**
Eszopiclone	Drugs that inhibit the CYP3A4 enzyme system, including **ketoconazole, itraconazole, clarithromycin, nefazodone, ritonavir, nelfinavir**	**Lorazepam;** drugs that induce the CYP3A4 enzyme system, such as **rifampin;** taking eszopiclone with or immediately after **a high-fat or heavy meal**	Additive CNS depression with **alcohol** and other **CNS depressants,** including **antihistamines, antidepressants, opioids, sedative/ hypnotics, antipsychotics;** decreased effects of **lorazepam**
Ramelteon	**Alcohol, azole antifungals, fluoxetine**	**Rifampin;** taking ramelteon with or immediately after a **high-fat or heavy meal**	

Continued

The effects of:	Are increased by:	Are decreased by:	Concurrent use may result in:
Zaleplon	Cimetidine	Drugs that induce the CYP3A4, enzyme system, including **rifampin, phenytoin, carbamazepine,** and **phenobarbital;** taking zaleplon with or immediately after a **high-fat or heavy meal**	Additive CNS depression with **alcohol** and other **CNS depressants,** including **antihistamines, antidepressants, opioids, sedative/ hypnotics, antipsychotics**
Zolpidem	**Azole antifungals, ritonavir, SSRIs**	**Flumazenil; rifampin;** administration with **food**	Risk of life-threatening cardiac arrhythmias with **amiodarone; additive** CNS depression with **alcohol** and other **CNS depressants,** including antihistamines, antidepressants, opioids, sedative/hypnotics, antipsychotics

Route and Dosage

CHLORAL HYDRATE

Sedation: Adults: **PO**: 250 mg 3 times a day after meals. Maximum daily dose: 2 g.

Children: **PO**: 25 mg/kg/day, not to exceed 500 mg per single dose. May be given in divided doses.

Insomnia: Adults: **PO**: 500 mg to 1 g 15 to 30 minutes before bedtime.

Children: **PO**: 50 mg/kg/day, up to 1 g per single dose. May give in divided doses.

ESZOPICLONE **(Lunesta)**

Insomnia: Adults: **PO**: 2 mg immediately before bedtime; may be increased to 3 mg if needed (3 mg dose is more effective for sleep maintenance).

Elderly patients: **PO**: 1 mg immediately before bedtime for patients who have difficulty falling asleep; 2 mg immediately before bedtime for patients who have difficulty staying asleep.

RAMELTEON **(Rozerem)**

Insomnia: Adults: **PO**: 8 mg within 30 minutes of bedtime. It is recommended that ramelteon not be taken with or immediately after a high-fat meal.

ZALEPLON **(Sonata)**

Insomnia: Adults: **PO**: 10 mg (range 5 to 20 mg) at bedtime.
   Elderly and debilitated patients: **PO**: 5 mg at bedtime, not to exceed 10 mg.

ZOLPIDEM **(Ambien)**

Insomnia: Adults: **PO**: 10 mg at bedtime. *Extended-release tablets:* 12.5 mg at bedtime.

Elderly or debilitated patients and patients with hepatic impairment: **PO**: 5 mg at bedtime. *Extended-release tablets:* 6.25 mg at bedtime.

● NURSING DIAGNOSES RELATED TO ALL SEDATIVE-HYPNOTICS

1. Risk for injury related to abrupt withdrawal from long-term use or decreased mental alertness caused by residual sedation.
2. Disturbed sleep pattern related to situational crises, physical condition, or severe level of anxiety.
3. Risk for activity intolerance related to side effects of lethargy, drowsiness, and dizziness.
4. Risk for acute confusion related to action of the medication on the central nervous system.

● NURSING IMPLICATIONS FOR SEDATIVE-HYPNOTICS

The nursing care plan should include monitoring for the following side effects from sedative-hypnotics. Nursing implications related to each side effect are designated by an asterisk (*):

1. **Drowsiness, dizziness, lethargy (most common side effects)**
   * Instruct client not to drive or operate dangerous machinery while taking the medication.
2. **Tolerance, physical and psychological dependence**
   * Instruct client to take the medication exactly as directed. Do not take more than the amount prescribed because of the habit-forming potential. Recommended for short-term use only. Abrupt withdrawal after long-term use may result in serious, even life-threatening, symptoms. *Exception:* **Ramelteon** is not considered to be a drug of abuse or dependence. It is not classified as a controlled substance. It has, however, been associated with cases of rebound insomnia after abrupt discontinuation following long-term use.
3. **Potentiates the effects of other CNS depressants**
   * Instruct client not to drink alcohol or take other medications that depress the CNS while taking this medication.
4. **May aggravate symptoms in depressed persons**
   * Assess mood daily.
   * Take necessary precautions for potential suicide.
5. **Orthostatic hypotension, palpitations, tachycardia**
   * Monitor lying and standing blood pressure and pulse every shift.

* Instruct client to arise slowly from a lying or sitting position.
* Monitor pulse rate and rhythm and report any significant change to the physician.

6. **Paradoxical excitement**
   * Withhold drug and notify the physician.

7. **Dry mouth**
   * Have client take frequent sips of water or ice chips, suck on hard candy, or chew sugarless gum.

8. **Nausea and vomiting**
   * Have client take drug with food or milk (unless it is a drug in which taking with food is not recommended).

9. **Blood dyscrasias**
   * Symptoms of sore throat, fever, malaise, easy bruising, or unusual bleeding should be reported to the physician immediately.

● CLIENT/FAMILY EDUCATION RELATED TO ALL SEDATIVE-HYPNOTICS

* Do not drive or operate dangerous machinery. Drowsiness and dizziness can occur.
* Do not stop taking the drug abruptly after prolonged use. Can produce serious withdrawal symptoms, such as depression, insomnia, anxiety, abdominal and muscle cramps, tremors, vomiting, sweating, convulsions, and delirium.
* Do not consume other CNS depressants (including alcohol).
* Do not take nonprescription medication without approval from physician.
* Rise slowly from the sitting or lying position to prevent a sudden drop in blood pressure.
* Report to physician immediately symptoms of sore throat, fever, malaise, easy bruising, unusual bleeding, or motor restlessness.
* Be aware of risks of taking these drugs during pregnancy. (Congenital malformations have been associated with use during the first trimester.) If pregnancy is suspected or planned, notify the physician of the desirability to discontinue the drug.
* Be aware of possible side effects. Refer to written materials furnished by health-care providers regarding the correct method of self-administration.
* Carry card or piece of paper at all times stating names of medications being taken.

INTERNET REFERENCES

a. http://www.rxlist.com/
b. http://www.drugguide.com/
c. http://www.nimh.nih.gov/publicat/medicate.cfm
d. http://www.fadavis.com/townsend
e. http://www.nlm.nih.gov/medlineplus/druginformation
   .html

Chapter 31

Agents Used to Treat Attention-Deficit/ Hyperactivity Disorder

● **CHEMICAL CLASS: CENTRAL NERVOUS SYSTEM (CNS) STIMULANTS (AMPHETAMINES)**

Examples

Generic (Trade) Name	Controlled/ Pregnancy Categories	Half-life (hr)	Indications	Available Forms (mg)
Amphetamine/ dextroam- phetamine mixtures (Adderall; Adderall XR)	C-II/C	9–13	• ADHD • Narcolepsy	Tabs: 5, 7.5, 10, 12.5, 15, 20, 30 Caps (XR): 5, 10, 15, 20, 25, 30
Dextroamphet- amine sulfate (Dexedrine; Dextrostat)	C-II/C	~12	• ADHD • Narcolepsy	Tabs: 5, 10 Caps (ER): 5, 10, 15 Oral solu: 5 mg/5 mL
Metham- phetamine (Desoxyn)	C-II/C	4–5	• ADHD • Exogenous obesity	Tabs: 5
Lisdexam- fetamine (Vyvanse)	C-II/C	<1	• ADHD	Caps: 20, 30, 40 50, 60, 70

Action
• Central nervous system (CNS) stimulation is mediated by release of norepinephrine from central noradrenergic neurons in cerebral cortex, reticular activating system, and brainstem.

- At higher doses, dopamine may be released in the mesolimbic system.
- Action in the treatment of attention-deficit/hyperactivity disorder (ADHD) is unclear.

Contraindications and Precautions

Contraindicated in: • Advanced arteriosclerosis • Symptomatic cardiovascular disease • Moderate to severe hypertension • Hyperthyroidism • Hypersensitivity or idiosyncrasy to the sympathomimetic amines • Glaucoma • Agitated states • History of drug abuse • During or within 14 days following administration of monoamine oxidase (MAO) inhibitors (*hypertensive crisis may occur*) • Children younger than 3 years (**dextroamphetamine, lisdexamfetamine,** and **mixtures**) • Children younger than 12 years (**methamphetamine**) • Pregnancy and lactation

Use Cautiously in: • Patients with mild hypertension • Children with psychoses (*may exacerbate symptoms*) • Tourette's disorder (may exacerbate tics) • Anorexia • Insomnia • Elderly, debilitated, or asthenic patients • Patients with suicidal or homicidal tendencies

Adverse Reactions and Side Effects

- Overstimulation
- Restlessness
- Dizziness
- Insomnia
- Headache
- Palpitations
- Tachycardia
- Elevation of blood pressure
- Anorexia
- Weight loss
- Dry mouth
- Tolerance
- New or worsened psychiatric symptoms
- Physical and psychological dependence
- Suppression of growth in children (with long-term use)

Interactions

- Increased sensitivity to amphetamines with **furazolidone**
- Use of amphetamines with **MAO inhibitors** can result in hypertensive crisis.
- Increased effects of amphetamines and risk of serotonin syndrome with **selective serotonin reuptake inhibitors (SSRIs)**
- Prolonged effects of amphetamines with **urinary alkalinizers**

- Hastened elimination of amphetamines with **urinary acidifiers**
- Amphetamines may reverse the hypotensive effects of **guanethidine and other antihypertensives.**
- Concomitant use of amphetamines and **tricyclic antidepressants** may increase blood levels of both drugs.
- Patients with diabetes mellitus who take amphetamines may require **insulin** adjustment.

Route and Dosage

AMPHETAMINE/DEXTROAMPHETAMINE MIXTURES **(Adderall; Adderall XR)**

ADHD: Adults and children ≥6 years: **PO:** Initial dose: 5 mg 1 or 2 times a day. May be increased in increments of 5 mg at weekly intervals until optimal response is obtained. Maximum dose: 40 mg/day. *Extended-release caps:* Initial dosage: 10 mg once daily in the morning. May increase in increments of 10 mg at weekly intervals. Maximum dose: 30 mg/day.

Children 3 to 5 years: **PO:** Initial dose: 2.5 mg/day. May increase in increments of 2.5 mg/day at weekly intervals.

Narcolepsy: Adults and children ≥12 years: **PO**: Initial dose: 10 mg/day; may increase in increments of 10 mg/day at weekly intervals up to a maximum of 60 mg/day.

Children 6 to 12 years of age: **PO:** Narcolepsy is rare in children younger than 12 years. When it does occur, initial dose is 5 mg/day. May increase in increments of 5 mg/day at weekly intervals up to a maximum of 60 mg/day.

DEXTROAMPHETAMINE SULFATE **(Dexedrine; Dextrostat)**

ADHD: Adults and children ≥6 years: **PO:** Initial dosage: 5 mg once or 2 times a day. May be increased in increments of 5 mg at weekly intervals. More than 40 mg/day is seldom required. (Sustained-release capsules should not be used as initial therapy.)

Children 3 to 5 years: **PO:** Initial dose: 2.5 mg/day. May increase in increments of 2.5 mg/day at weekly intervals until optimal response is achieved.

Narcolepsy: Adults: **PO:** 5 to 60 mg/day in single or divided doses. Sustained-release capsules should not be used as initial therapy.

Children ≥12 years: **PO:** 10 mg/day. May increase by 10 mg/day at weekly intervals until response is obtained or 60 mg is reached.

Children 6 to 12 years: **PO:** 5 mg/day. May increase by 5 mg/day at weekly intervals until response is obtained or 60 mg is reached.

METHAMPHETAMINE **(Desoxyn)**

ADHD: 5 mg once or 2 times a day. May increase in increments of 5 mg at weekly intervals. Usual effective dose is 20 to 25 mg/day in divided doses.

Exogenous Obesity: 5 mg 1 to 3 times/day 30 minutes before meals.

LISDEXAMFETAMINE **(Vyvanse)**

ADHD: *Children 6 to 12 years of age:* **PO:** 20 or 30 mg once daily in the morning. Dosage may be increased in increments of 10 or 20 mg/day at weekly intervals. Maximum dosage: 70 mg/day.

● CHEMICAL CLASS: CNS STIMULANTS (MISCELLANEOUS AGENTS)

Examples

Generic (Trade) Name	Controlled/ Pregnancy Categories	Half-life (hr)	Indications	Available Forms (mg)
Dexmethylphenidate (Focalin; Focalin XR)	C-II/C	2.2	• ADHD	Tabs: 2.5, 5, 10 Caps (ER): 5, 10, 15, 20
Methylphenidate (Ritalin; Ritalin-SR; Ritalin LA; Methylin; Methylin ER; Metadate ER; Metadate CD; Concerta; Daytrana)	C-II/C	2–4	• ADHD • Narcolepsy (except Concerta, Metadate CD, and Ritalin LA)	Immediate Release Tabs (Methylin, Ritalin): 5, 10, 20 Chewable tabs (Methylin): 2.5, 5, 10 Metadate ER, Methylin ER: Tabs 10, 20 Concerta: Tabs ER: 18, 27, 36, 54 Ritalin-SR: Tabs SR: 20 Metadate CD, Ritalin LA: Caps ER: 10, 20, 30, 40, (50, 60—*Metadate CD only*) Oral Solu (Methylin): 5/5 mL, 10/5 mL Transdermal Patch (Daytrana): 10, 15, 20, 30

ER, CD, LA=extended release forms; SR=sustained release.

Actions

- Dexmethylphenidate blocks the reuptake of norepinephrine and dopamine into the presynaptic neuron and increases the release of these monoamines into the extraneuronal space.
- Methylphenidate activates the brain stem arousal system and cortex to produce its stimulant effect.
- Action in the treatment of ADHD is unknown.

Contraindications and Precautions

Contraindicated in: • Hypersensitivity • Pregnancy, lactation, and children younger than 6 years (*safety has not been established*) • Clients with marked anxiety, tension, or agitation • History of glaucoma • Motor tics or family history or diagnosis of Tourette's disorder • During or within 14 days of treatment with MAO inhibitors (*hypertensive crisis can occur*) • Clients with structural cardiac abnormalities, cardiomyopathy, arrhythmias, recent myocardial infarction (MI), or other serious cardiac problems

Use Cautiously in: • Patients with history of seizure disorder and/or electroencephalographic (EEG) abnormalities • Hypertension • History of drug or alcohol dependence • Emotionally unstable patients • Renal or hepatic insufficiency • Clients with preexisting psychotic disorder

Adverse Reactions and Side Effects

- Headache
- Nausea
- Rhinitis
- Fever
- Anorexia
- Insomnia
- Tachycardia; palpitations; hypertension
- Nervousness
- Abdominal pain
- Growth suppression in children (with long-term use)
- Skin redness or itching at site of transdermal patch (*Daytrana*)

Interactions

- Decreased effectiveness of **antihypertensive agents**
- Increased serum levels of **anticonvulsants** (e.g., **phenobarbital, phenytoin,** and **primidone**), **tricyclic antidepressants, selective serotonin reuptake inhibitors [SSRIs], warfarin**
- Increased effects of **vasopressor agents** with concurrent use
- Hypertensive crisis may occur with concurrent use (or within 2 weeks use) of **MAO inhibitors**

- Concurrent use with **clonidine** may result in serious electro-cardiographic (ECG) abnormalities
- Increased sympathomimetic effects with other **adrenergics**, including **vasoconstrictors** and **decongestants**

Route and Dosage

DEXMETHYLPHENIDATE **(Focalin; Focalin XR)**
ADHD: *(Immediate release tabs):*
Adults and children ≥6 years: Patients not previously taking methylphenidate: **PO:** 2.5 mg 2 times a day. May be increased weekly as needed up to 10 mg 2 times a day. *Patients currently taking methylphenidate:* Starting dose is ½ of the methylphenidate dose, up to 10 mg 2 times a day.
(Extended-release capsules):
Adults: Patients not previously taking methylphenidate: **PO:** 10 mg once daily. May be increased by 10 mg after 1 week to 20 mg/day. *Patients currently taking methylphenidate:* Starting dose is ½ of the methylphenidate dose, up to 20 mg/day given as a single daily dose. *Patients currently taking dexmethylphenidate:* Give same daily dose as a single dose.
Children ≥6 years: PO: *Patients not previously taking methylphenidate:* 5 mg once daily. May be increased by 5 mg weekly up to 20 mg/day. *Patients currently taking methylphenidate:* Starting dose is ½ of the methylphenidate dose, up to 20 mg/day, given as a single daily dose. *Patients currently taking dexmethylphenidate:* Give same daily dose as a single dose.

METHYLPHENIDATE **(Ritalin; Ritalin-SR; Ritalin LA; Methylin; Methylin ER; Metadate ER; Metadate CD; Concerta; Daytrana)**
ADHD: *(Immediate release forms):*
Adults: **PO**: Range 10 to 60 mg/day, in divided doses 2 or 3 times/day, preferably 30 to 45 minutes before meals. Average dose is 20 to 30 mg/day. To prevent interruption of sleep, take last dose of the day before 6 p.m.
Children ≥6 yr: **PO**: Individualize dosage. May start with low dose of 5 mg 2 times a day before breakfast and lunch. May increase dosage in 5 to 10 mg increments at weekly intervals. Maximum daily dosage: 60 mg.
(Extended-release forms):
Ritalin-SR, Methylin ER, and Metadate ER: Adults and children ≥6 years: **PO**: May be used in place of the immediate-release tablets when the 8-hour dosage corresponds to the titrated 8-hour dosage of the immediate-release tablets. Must be swallowed whole.
Ritalin LA and Metadate CD: Adults and children ≥6 years: Initial dosage: 20 mg once daily in the morning. May increase

dosage in 10 to 20 mg increments at weekly intervals to a maximum of 60 mg taken once daily in the morning. Capsules may be swallowed whole with liquid or opened and contents sprinkled on soft food (e.g., applesauce). Ensure that entire contents of capsule are consumed when taken in this manner. **NOTE:** Ritalin LA may be used in place of 2 times a day regimen given once daily at same total dose, or in place of SR product at same dose.

Concerta: Adults and children ≥6 years: **PO**: Should be taken once daily in the morning. Must be swallowed whole and not chewed, divided, or crushed.

Clients new to methylphenidate: 18 mg once daily in the morning. May adjust dosage at weekly intervals to maximum of 54 mg/day for children 6 to 12 years, and to a maximum of 72 mg/day (not to exceed 2 mg/kg/day) for adolescents 13 to 17 years.

Clients currently using methylphenidate: Should use following conversion table:

Previous Methylphenidate Dose	Recommended Concerta Dose
5 mg 2 or 3 times/day or 20 mg (SR)	18 mg every morning
10 mg 2 or 3 times/day or 40 mg (SR)	36 mg every morning
15 mg 2 or 3 times/day or 60 mg (SR)	54 mg every morning

Daytrana (Transdermal Patch): Adults and children ≥6 years: Patch should be applied to hip area 2 hours before an effect is needed and should be removed 9 hours after application. Alternate hips with additional doses. Dosage for patients new to methylphenidate should be titrated to desired effect according to the following recommended schedule:

	Week 1	Week 2	Week 3	Week 4
Nominal delivered dose (mg/9 hr)	10 mg	15 mg	20 mg	30 mg
Delivery rate (based on 9-hr wear period)	1.1 mg/hr	1.6 mg/hr	2.2 mg/hr	3.3 mg/hr

Patients converting from another formulation of methylphenidate should follow the above titration schedule due to differences in bioavailability of Daytrana compared to other products.

Narcolepsy: *Adults*: **PO**: *Ritalin, Methylin, Methylin ER, Ritalin-SR, and Metadate ER* indicated for this use. 10 mg 2 to 3 times/day. Maximum dose 60 mg/day.

● CHEMICAL CLASS: ALPHA-ADRENERGIC AGONISTS

Examples

Generic (Trade) Name	Pregnancy Categories/ Half-life (hr)	Indications	Available Forms (mg)
Clonidine (Catapres)	C/12–16	• Hypertension **Unlabeled use:** • ADHD	Tabs: 0.1, 0.2, 0.3 Transdermal patches: 0.1/24 hr, 0.2/24 hr, 0.3/24 hr
Guanfacine (Tenex; Intuniv)	B/16–18	• Hypertension *(Tenex)* • ADHD *(Intuniv)* **Unlabeled use:** • ADHD *(Tenex)*	Tabs *(Tenex)*: 1, 2 Tabs (ER) *(Intuniv)*: 1, 2, 3, 4

Action

- Stimulates alpha-adrenergic receptors in the brain, thereby reducing sympathetic outflow from the CNS resulting in decreases in peripheral vascular resistance, heart rate, and blood pressure.
- Mechanism of action in the treatment of ADHD is unknown.

Contraindications and Precautions

Contraindicated in: • Hypersensitivity to the drug or any of its inactive ingredients

Use Cautiously in: • Coronary insufficiency • Recent myocardial infarction • Cerebrovascular disease • History of hypotension, bradycardia, or syncope • Chronic renal or hepatic failure • Elderly • Pregnancy and lactation

Adverse Reactions and Side Effects

- Orthostatic hypotension
- Bradycardia
- Palpitations
- Syncope
- Dry mouth
- Constipation
- Nausea
- Fatigue
- Sedation
- Rebound syndrome with abrupt withdrawal

Interactions

- Increased effects of clonidine with **verapamil** and **beta-blockers**
- Decreased effects of clonidine with **prazosin** and **tricyclic antidepressants**
- Decreased effects of **levodopa** with clonidine
- Additive CNS effects with **CNS depressants**, including alcohol**, antihistamines, opioid analgesics,** and **sedative/ hypnotics**
- Decreased effects of guanfacine with **barbiturates, rifampin,** or **phenytoin**
- Increased effects of guanfacine with **ketoconazole**
- Increased effects of **valproic acid** with guanfacine

Route and Dosage

CLONIDINE **(Catapres)**

Hypertension: *Adults:* **PO:** Initial dosage: 0.1 mg 2 times a day. May increase dosage in increments of 0.1 mg/day at weekly intervals until desired response is achieved. Maximum dose: 2.4 mg/day. *Transdermal system:* Transdermal system delivering 0.1 mg to 0.3 mg/24 hr applied every 7 days. Initiate with 0.1 mg/24 hr system. Dosage increments may be made every 1 to 2 weeks when system is changed.

ADHD: *Adults and children ≥12 years:* **PO:** Initial dosage: 0.05 mg/day. May increase in increments of 0.05 mg at intervals of 3 to 7 days to a maximum dose of 0.3 mg/day in divided doses.

GUANFACINE **(Tenex; Intuniv)**

Hypertension (Tenex): *Adults:* **PO:** 1 mg daily at bedtime. If satisfactory results are not achieved after 3 to 4 weeks, may increase to 2 mg.

ADHD (Intuniv): *Adults and children ≥6 years:* **PO:** Initial dosage: 1 mg once daily. May increase dose in increments of 1 mg/day at weekly intervals until desired response is achieved. Maximum dose: 4 mg/day. Tablets should not be chewed, crushed, or broken before swallowing, and should not be administered with high-fat meals.

● CHEMICAL CLASS: MISCELLANEOUS AGENTS FOR ADHD

Examples

Generic (Trade) Name	Pregnancy Categories/ Half-life (hr)	Indications	Available Forms (mg)
Atomoxatine (Strattera)	C/5.2 hr (metabolites 6–8 hr)	● ADHD	Caps: 10, 18, 25, 40, 60, 80, 100

Generic (Trade) Name	Pregnancy Categories/ Half-life (hr)	Indications	Available Forms (mg)
Bupropion (Wellbutrin; Wellbutrin SR; Wellbutrin XL)	B/8–24 hr	• Depression **Unlabeled use :** • ADHD	Tabs: 75, 100 Tabs SR: 100, 150, 200 Tabs XL: 150, 300

SR = 12-hour tablets; XL = 24-hour tablets.

Action

- Atomoxetine selectively inhibits the reuptake of the neurotransmitter norepinephrine.
- Bupropion is a weak inhibitor of the neuronal uptake of norepinephrine, serotonin, and dopamine.
- Action in the treatment of ADHD is unclear.

Contraindications and Precautions

Contraindicated in: • Hypersensitivity • Coadministration with or within 2 weeks after discontinuing an MAO inhibitor • Lactation

Atomoxetine
- Narrow-angle glaucoma

Bupropion
- Known or suspected seizure disorder
- Acute phase of myocardial infarction
- Clients with bulimia or anorexia nervosa
- Clients undergoing abrupt discontinuation of alcohol or sedatives (increased risk of seizures)

Use Cautiously in: • Clients with suicidal ideation • Clients with urinary retention • Hypertension • Hepatic, renal, or cardiovascular insufficiency • Pregnancy (*use only if benefits outweigh possible risks to fetus*) • Children and adolescents (*may increase suicidal risk*) • Elderly and debilitated patients

Atomoxetine
- Children younger than 6 years (*safety not established*)

Adverse Reactions and Side Effects

- Dry mouth
- Anorexia
- Nausea and vomiting
- Constipation
- Urinary retention
- Sexual dysfunction
- Headache
- Dizziness
- Insomnia or sedation

- Palpitations; tachycardia
- Weight loss
- Abdominal pain
- Increased sweating

Atomoxetine
- Fatigue
- Cough
- New or worsened psychiatric symptoms
- Severe liver damage

Bupropion
- Weight gain
- Tremor
- Seizures
- Blurred vision

Interactions

The effects of:	Are increased by:	Are decreased by:	Concurrent use may result in:
Atomoxetine	Concomitant use of **CYP2D6 inhibitors (paroxetine, fluoxetine, quinidine)**		Increased risk of cardiovascular effects with **albuterol** or **vasopressors;** potentially fatal reactions with concurrent use (or use within 2 weeks of discontinuation) of **MAO inhibitors;** increased cardiovascular effects of **albuterol** with concurrent use
Bupropion	**Amantadine, levodopa, cimetidine, triclopidine, guanfacine, ritonavir**	**Carbamazepine**	Increased risk of acute toxicity with **MAO inhibitors;** increased risk of hypertension with **nicotine replacement agent;** adverse neuropsychiatric events with **alcohol** (alcohol tolerance is reduced); increased anticoagulant effect of **warfarin;** increased effects of drugs metabolized by CYP2D6 (e.g., **nortriptyline, imipramine, desipramine, paroxetine, fluoxetine, sertraline, haloperidol, risperidone, thioridazine, metoprolol, propafenone,** and **flecainide**); increased risk of seizures with drugs that lower the seizure threshold (antidepressants, antipsychotics, theophylline, corticosteroids, stimulants/anorectics)

Route and Dosage

ATOMOXETINE **(Strattera)**

ADHD: *Adults, adolescents, and children weighing more than 70 kg (154 lb):* **PO**: Initial dose: 40 mg/day. Increase after a minimum of 3 days to a target total daily dose of 80 mg, as a single dose in the morning or 2 evenly divided doses in the morning and late afternoon or early evening. After 2 to 4 weeks, total dosage may be increased to a maximum of 100 mg, if needed.

Children weighing 70 kg (154 lb) or less: **PO**: Initial dose: 0.5 mg/kg/day. Increase after a minimum of 3 days to a target total daily dose of about 1.2 mg/kg taken either as a single dose in the morning or 2 evenly divided doses in the morning and late afternoon or early evening. Maximum daily dose: 1.4 mg/kg or 100 mg daily, whichever is less.

Adjusted Dosing: Hepatic impairment: In clients with moderate hepatic impairment, reduce to 50% of usual dose. In clients with severe hepatic impairment, reduce to 25% of usual dose.

Adjusted dosing: Coadministration with strong CYP2D6 inhibitors: Adults, adolescents, and children weighing more than 70 kg: Initiate dosage at 40 mg/day and only increase to the usual target dose of 80 mg/day if symptoms fail to improve after 4 weeks and the initial dose is well tolerated.

Children and adolescents up to 70 kg: Initiate dosage at 0.5 mg/kg/day and only increase to the usual target dose of 1.2 mg/kg/day if symptoms fail to improve after 4 weeks and the initial dose is well tolerated.

BUPROPION **(Wellbutrin; Wellbutrin SR; Wellbutrin XL)**

ADHD: *Children and adolescents:* **PO:** Initial dose: 3 mg/kg/day. May titrate to a maximum dose of 6 mg/kg/day. Single dose should not exceed 150 mg. Usually given daily in 2 or 3 divided doses.

Adults: 150 to 450 mg/day. No single dose of bupropion should exceed 150 mg. To prevent the risk of seizures, administer with 4 to 6 hours between doses.

Depression (Wellbutrin): **PO**: *Adults (immediate release tabs):* 100 mg 2 times/day. May increase after 3 days to 100 mg given 3 times/day. For patients who do not show improvement after several weeks of dosing at 300 mg/day, an increase in dosage up to 450 mg/day may be considered. No single dose of bupropion should exceed 150 mg. To prevent the risk of seizures, administer with 4 to 6 hours between doses.

Sustained release tabs: Give as a single 150 mg dose in the morning. May increase to twice a day (total 300 mg), with 8 hours between doses.

Extended release tabs: Begin dosing at 150 mg/day, given as a single daily dose in the morning. May increase after 3 days to 300 mg/day, given as a single daily dose in the morning.

Seasonal Affective Disorder (Wellbutrin XL): PO: 150 mg administered each morning beginning in the autumn prior to the onset of depressive symptoms. Dose may be uptitrated to the target dose of 300 mg/day after 1 week. Therapy should continue through the winter season before being tapered to 150 mg/day for 2 weeks prior to discontinuation in early spring.

● NURSING DIAGNOSES RELATED TO AGENTS FOR ADHD

1. Risk for injury related to overstimulation and hyperactivity (CNS stimulants) or seizures (possible side effect of bupropion).
2. Risk for suicide secondary to major depression related to abrupt withdrawal after extended use (CNS stimulants).
3. Imbalanced nutrition, less than body requirements, related to side effects of anorexia and weight loss (CNS stimulants).
4. Disturbed sleep pattern related to side effects of overstimulation or insomnia.
5. Nausea related to side effects of atomoxetine or bupropion.
6. Pain related to side effect of abdominal pain (atomoxetine, bupropion) or headache (all agents).
7. Risk for activity intolerance related to side effects of sedation or dizziness (atomoxetine or bupropion)

● NURSING IMPLICATIONS FOR ADHD AGENTS

The plan of care should include monitoring for the following side effects from agents for ADHD. Nursing implications related to each side effect are designated by an asterisk (*).

1. **Overstimulation, restlessness, insomnia** (CNS stimulants)
   * Assess mental status for changes in mood, level of activity, degree of stimulation, and aggressiveness.
   * Ensure that the client is protected from injury.
   * Keep stimuli low and environment as quiet as possible to discourage overstimulation.
   * To prevent insomnia, administer the last dose at least 6 hours before bedtime. Administer sustained-release forms in the morning.
2. **Palpitations, tachycardia** (CNS stimulants; atomoxetine; bupropion; clonidine) or **bradycardia** (clonidine, guanfacine)
   * Monitor and record vital signs at regular intervals (two or three times a day) throughout therapy. Report significant changes to the physician immediately.

NOTE: The U.S. Food and Drug Administration recently issued warnings associated with CNS stimulants and atomoxetine of the risk for sudden death in patients who have cardiovascular disease. A careful personal and family history of heart disease, heart defects, or hypertension should be obtained before these medications are prescribed. Careful monitoring of cardiovascular function during administration must be ongoing.

3. **Anorexia, weight loss** (CNS stimulants; atomoxetine; bupropion)
   * To reduce anorexia, the medication may be administered immediately after meals. The client should be weighed regularly (at least weekly) when receiving therapy with CNS stimulants, atomoxetine, or bupropion because of the potential for anorexia and weight loss, and temporary interruption of growth and development.

4. **Tolerance, physical and psychological dependence** (CNS stimulants)
   * Tolerance develops rapidly.
   * In children with ADHD, a drug "holiday" should be attempted periodically under direction of the physician to determine the effectiveness of the medication and the need for continuation.
   * The drug should not be withdrawn abruptly. To do so could initiate the following syndrome of symptoms: nausea, vomiting, abdominal cramping, headache, fatigue, weakness, mental depression, suicidal ideation, increased dreaming, and psychotic behavior.

5. **Nausea and vomiting** (atomoxetine and bupropion)
   * May be taken with food to minimize GI upset.

6. **Constipation** (atomoxetine, bupropion, clonidine, guanfacine)
   * Increase fiber and fluid in diet, if not contraindicated.

7. **Dry mouth** (clonidine and guanfacine)
   * Offer the client sugarless candy, ice, frequent sips of water
   * Strict oral hygiene is very important.

8. **Sedation** (clonidine and guanfacine)
   * Warn client that this effect is increased by concomitant use of alcohol and other CNS drugs.
   * Warn clients to refrain from driving or performing hazardous tasks until response has been established.

9. **Potential for seizures** (bupropion)
   * Protect client from injury if seizure should occur. Instruct family and significant others of clients on bupropion therapy how to protect client during a seizure if one should occur. Ensure that doses of the immediate release medication are administered 4 to 6 hours apart, and doses of the sustained release medication at least 8 hours apart.

10. **Severe liver damage** (with atomoxetine)
    * Monitor for the following side effects and report to physician immediately: itching, dark urine, right upper quadrant pain, yellow skin or eyes, sore throat, fever, malaise.

11. **New or worsened psychiatric symptoms** (with CNS stimulants and atomoxetine)
    * Monitor for psychotic symptoms (e.g., hearing voices, paranoid behaviors, delusions).
    * Monitor for manic symptoms, including aggressive and hostile behaviors.

12. **Rebound syndrome** (with clonidine and guanfacine)
    * Client should be instructed not to discontinue therapy abruptly. To do so may result in symptoms of nervousness, agitation, headache, and tremor, and a rapid rise in blood pressure. Dosage should be tapered gradually under the supervision of the physician.

● CLIENT/FAMILY EDUCATION RELATED TO AGENTS FOR ADHD

* Use caution in driving or operating dangerous machinery. Drowsiness, dizziness, and blurred vision can occur.
* Do not stop taking CNS stimulants abruptly. To do so could produce serious withdrawal symptoms.
* Avoid taking CNS stimulants late in the day to prevent insomnia. Take no later than 6 hours before bedtime.
* Do not take other medications (including over-the-counter drugs) without physician's approval. Many medications contain substances that, in combination with agents for ADHD, can be harmful.
* Diabetic clients should monitor blood sugar 2 or 3 times a day or as instructed by the physician. Be aware of the need for possible alteration in insulin requirements because of changes in food intake, weight, and activity.
* Avoid consumption of large amounts of caffeinated products (coffee, tea, colas, chocolate), as they may enhance the CNS stimulant effect.
* Notify physician if symptoms of restlessness, insomnia, anorexia, or dry mouth become severe or if rapid, pounding heartbeat becomes evident. Report any of the following side effects to the physician immediately: shortness of breath, chest pain, jaw/left arm pain, fainting, seizures, sudden vision changes, weakness on one side of the body, slurred speech, confusion, itching, dark urine, right upper quadrant pain, yellow skin or eyes, sore throat, fever, malaise, increased hyperactivity, believing things that are not true, or hearing voices.

- Be aware of possible risks of taking agents for ADHD during pregnancy. Safe use during pregnancy and lactation has not been established. Inform the physician immediately if pregnancy is suspected or planned.
- Be aware of potential side effects of agents for ADHD. Refer to written materials furnished by health-care providers for safe self-administration.
- Carry a card or other identification at all times describing medications being taken.

 INTERNET REFERENCES
   a. http://www.rxlist.com
   b. http://www.drugguide.com
   c. http://www.nimh.nih.gov/publicat/medicate.cfm
   d. http://www.fadavis.com/townsend
   e. http://www.nlm.nih.gov/medlineplus/druginformation
      .html

A PPENDIX **A**

Comparison of Development Theories

Age	Stage	Major Developmental Tasks
FREUD'S STAGES OF PSYCHOSEXUAL DEVELOPMENT		
Birth–18 months	Oral	Relief from anxiety through oral gratification of needs
18 months–3 years	Anal	Learning independence and control, with focus on the excretory function
3–6 years	Phallic	Identification with parent of same gender; development of sexual identity; focus is on genital organs
6–12 years	Latency	Sexuality is repressed; focus is on relationships with same-gender peers
13–20 years	Genital	Libido is reawakened as genital organs mature; focus is on relationships with members of the opposite gender

STAGES OF DEVELOPMENT IN H.S. SULLIVAN'S INTERPERSONAL THEORY

Birth–18 months	Infancy	Relief from anxiety through oral gratification of needs
18 months–6 years	Childhood	Learning to experience a delay in personal gratification without undue anxiety
6–9 years	Juvenile	Learning to form satisfactory peer relationships
9–12 years	Preadolescence	Learning to form satisfactory relationships with persons of the same gender; the initiation of feelings of affection for another person
12–14 years	Early adolescence	Learning to form satisfactory relationships with persons of the opposite gender; developing a sense of identity
14–21 years	Late adolescence	Establishing self-identity; experiencing satisfying relationships; working to develop a lasting, intimate opposite-gender relationship

STAGES OF DEVELOPMENT IN ERIC ERIKSON'S PSYCHOSOCIAL THEORY

Infancy (Birth–18 months)	Trust vs. mistrust	To develop a basic trust in the mothering figure and be able to generalize it to others
Early childhood (18 months–3 years)	Autonomy vs. shame and doubt	To gain some self-control and independence within the environment
Late childhood. (3–6 years)	Initiative vs. guilt	To develop a sense of purpose and the ability to initiate and direct own activities
School age (6–12 years)	Industry vs. inferiority	To achieve a sense of self-confidence by learning, competing, performing successfully, and receiving recognition from significant others, peers, and acquaintances
Adolescence (12–20 years)	Identity vs. role confusion	To integrate the tasks mastered in the previous stages into a secure sense of self
Young adulthood (20–30 years)	Intimacy vs. isolation	To form an intense, lasting relationship or a commitment to another person, a cause, an institution, or a creative effort
Adulthood while (30–65 years)	Generativity vs. stagnation	To achieve the life goals established for oneself, also considering the welfare of future generations
Old age (65 years–death)	Ego integrity vs. despair	To review one's life and derive meaning from both positive and negative events, while achieving a positive sense of self-worth

STAGES OF DEVELOPMENT IN M. MAHLER'S THEORY
OF OBJECT RELATIONS

Birth–1 month	I. Normal autism	Fulfillment of basic needs for survival and comfort
1–5 months	II. Symbiosis	Developing awareness of external source of need fulfillment
	III. Separation-Individuation	
5–10 months	a. Differentiation	Commencement of a primary recognition of separateness from the mothering figure
10–16 months	b. Practicing	Increased independence through locomotor functioning; increased sense of separateness of self
16–24 months	c. Rapprochement	Acute awareness of separateness of self; learning to seek "emotional refueling" from mothering figure to maintain feeling of security
24–36 months	d. Consolidation	Sense of separateness established; on the way to object constancy (i.e., able to internalize a sustained image of loved object/person when it is out of sight); resolution of separation anxiety

PIAGET'S STAGES OF COGNITIVE DEVELOPMENT

Birth–2 years	Sensorimotor	With increased mobility and awareness, develops a sense of self as separate from the external environment; the concept of object permanence emerges as the ability to form mental images evolves
2–6 years	Preoperational	Learning to express self with language; develops understanding of symbolic gestures; achievement of object permanence
6–12 years	Concrete operations	Learning to apply logic to thinking; development of understanding of reversibility and spatiality; learning to differentiate and classify; increased socialization and application of rules
12–15+ years	Formal operations	Learning to think and reason in abstract terms; making and testing hypotheses; capability of logical thinking and reasoning expand and are refined; cognitive maturity achieved

KOHLBERG'S STAGES OF MORAL DEVELOPMENT

I. Preconventional (common from ages 4 to 10 years)	1. Punishment and obedience orientation	Behavior is motivated by fear of punishment
	2. Instrumental relativist orientation	Behavior is motivated by egocentrism and concern for self

KOHLBERG'S STAGES OF MORAL DEVELOPMENT

II. Conventional (common from ages 10 to 13 years and into adulthood)	3. Interpersonal concordance orientation	Behavior is motivated by the expectations of others; strong desire for approval and acceptance
	4. Law and order orientation	Behavior is motivated by respect for authority
III. Postconventional (can occur from adolescence on)	5. Social contract legalistic orientation	Behavior is motivated by respect for universal laws and moral principles and guided by an internal set of values
	6. Universal ethical principle orientation	Behavior is motivated by internalized principles of honor, justice, and respect for human dignity and guided by the conscience

STAGES OF DEVELOPMENT IN H. PEPLAU'S INTERPERSONAL THEORY

Infancy	Learning to count on others	Learning to communicate in various ways to the primary caregiver in order to have comfort needs fulfilled

Continued

STAGES OF DEVELOPMENT IN H. PEPLAU'S INTERPERSONAL THEORY

Toddlerhood	Learning to delay gratification	Learning the satisfaction of pleasing others by delaying self-gratification in small ways
Early childhood	Identifying oneself	Learning appropriate roles and behaviors by acquiring the ability to perceive the expectations of others
Late childhood	Developing skills in participation	Learning the skills of compromise, competition, and cooperation with others; establishment of a more realistic view of the world and a feeling of one's place in it.

Source: Adapted from Townsend, M.C. (2009). *Psychiatric/mental health nursing: Concepts of care in evidence-based practice* (6th ed.). Philadelphia: FA Davis, pp. 33, 35, 36, 38, 40, 41, 43.

Ego Defense Mechanisms

Defense Mechanisms	Example	Defense Mechanisms	Example
Compensation: Covering up a real or perceived weakness by emphasizing a trait one considers more desirable.	A physically handicapped boy is unable to participate in football, so he compensates by becoming a great scholar.	**Rationalization:** Attempting to make excuses or formulate logical reasons to justify unacceptable feelings or behaviors.	John tells the rehab nurse, "I drink because it's the only way I can deal with my bad marriage and my worse job."
Denial: Refusing to acknowledge the existence of a real situation or the feelings associated with it.	A woman who drinks alcohol every day and cannot stop fails to acknowledge that she has a problem.	**Reaction Formation:** Preventing unacceptable or undesirable thoughts or behaviors from being expressed by exaggerating opposite thoughts or types of behaviors	Jane hates nursing. She attended nursing school to please her parents. During career day, she speaks to prospective students about the excellence of nursing as a career.

Continued

Defense Mechanisms	*Example*	*Defense Mechanisms*	*Example*
Displacement: The transfer of feelings from one target to another that is considered less threatening or that is neutral.	A client is angry at his physician, does not express it, but becomes verbally abusive with the nurse.	**Regression:** Retreating in response to stress to an earlier level of development and the comfort measures associated with that level of functioning.	When 2-year-old Jay is hospitalized for tonsillitis he will drink only from a bottle, even though his mom states he has been drinking from a cup for 6 months.
Identification: An attempt to increase self-worth by acquiring certain attributes and characteristics of an individual one admires.	A teenager who required lengthy rehabilitation after an accident decides to become a physical therapist as a result of his experiences.	**Repression:** Involuntarily blocking unpleasant feelings and experiences from one's awareness.	An accident victim can remember nothing about his accident.
Intellectualization: An attempt to avoid expressing actual emotions associated with a stressful situation by using	S's husband is being transferred with his job to a city far away from her parents. She hides anxiety by explaining to her parents the advantages	**Sublimation:** Rechanneling of drives or impulses that are personally or socially unacceptable into activities that are constructive.	A mother whose son was killed by a drunk driver channels her anger and energy into being the president of the local chapter of

Defense Mechanisms	*Example*	*Defense Mechanisms*	*Example*
the intellectual processes of logic, reasoning, and analysis.	associated with the move.		Mothers Against Drunk Drivers.
Introjection: Integrating the beliefs and values of another individual into one's own ego structure.	Children integrate their parents' value system into the process of conscience formation. A child says to friend, "Don't cheat. It's wrong."	**Suppression:** The voluntary blocking of unpleasant feelings and experiences from one's awareness.	Scarlett O'Hara says, "I don't want to think about that now. I'll think about that tomorrow."
Isolation: Separating a thought or memory from the feeling tone or emotion associated with it.	A young woman describes being attacked and raped, without showing any emotion.	**Undoing:** Symbolically negating or canceling out an experience that one finds intolerable.	Joe is nervous about his new job and yells at his wife. On his way home he stops and buys her some flowers.
Projection Attributing feelings or impulses unacceptable to one's self to another person.	Sue feels a strong sexual attraction to her track coach and tells her friend, "He's coming on to me!"		

Source: Townsend, M.C. (2009). *Psychiatric/mental health nursing: Concepts of care in evidence-based practice* (6th ed.). Philadelphia: FA Davis, p. 18.

Appendix C

Levels of Anxiety

Level	Perceptual Field	Ability to Learn	Physical Characteristics	Emotional/Behavioral Characteristics
Mild	Heightened perception (e.g., noises may seem louder; details within the environment are clearer) Increased awareness Increased alertness	Learning is enhanced.	Restlessness Irritability	May remain superficial with others Rarely experienced as distressful Motivation is increased.
Moderate	Reduction in perceptual field Reduced alertness to environmental events (e.g., someone talking may not be heard; part of the room may not be noticed)	Learning still occurs, but not at optimal ability. Decreased attention span Decreased ability to concentrate	Increased restlessness Increased heart and respiration rate Increased perspiration Gastric discomfort Increased muscular tension Increase in speech rate, volume, and pitch	A feeling of discontent May lead to a degree of impairment in interpersonal relationships as individual begins to focus on self and the need to relieve personal discomfort *Continued*

Level	Perceptual Field	Ability to Learn	Physical Characteristics	Emotional/Behavioral Characteristics
Severe	Greatly diminished. Only extraneous details are perceived, or fixation on a single detail may occur. May not take notice of an event even when attention is directed by another	Extremely limited attention span Unable to concentrate or problem-solve Effective learning cannot occur.	Headaches Dizziness Nausea Trembling Insomnia Palpitations Tachycardia Hyperventilation Urinary frequency Diarrhea	Feelings of dread, loathing, horror Total focus on self and intense desire to relieve the anxiety

Level	Perceptual Field	Ability to Learn	Physical Characteristics	Emotional/Behavioral Characteristics
Panic	Unable to focus on even one detail within the environment Misperceptions of the environment are common (e.g., a perceived detail may be elaborated and out of proportion).	Learning cannot occur. Unable to concentrate Unable to comprehend even simple directions	Dilated pupils Labored breathing Severe trembling Sleeplessness Palpitations Diaphoresis and pallor Muscular incoordination Immobility or purposeless hyperactivity Incoherence or inability to verbalize	Sense of impending doom Terror Bizarre behavior, including shouting, screaming, running about wildly, clinging to anyone or anything from which a sense of safety and security is derived Hallucinations; delusions Extreme withdrawal into self

Source: From Townsend, M.C. (2009). *Psychiatric/mental health nursing: Concepts of care in evidence-based practice* (6th ed.). Philadelphia: FA Davis, p. 16.

Stages of Grief

APPENDIX D ● 553

A Comparison of Models by Elisabeth Kübler-Ross, John Bowlby, George Engel, and William Worden

	Stages/Tasks			Possible Time Dimension	Behaviors
Kübler-Ross	*Bowlby*	*Engel*	*Worden*		
I. Denial	I. Numbness/ protest	I. Shock/disbelief	I. Accepting the reality of the loss	Occurs immediately on experiencing the loss. Usually lasts no more than a few weeks.	Individual refuses to acknowledge that the loss has occurred.
II. Anger	II. Disequilibrium	II. Developing awareness		In most cases begins within hours of the loss; peaks within a few weeks.	Anger is directed toward self or others. Ambivalence and guilt may be felt toward the lost object.
III. Bargaining					The individual fervently seeks alternatives to improve current situation. *Continued*

A Comparison of Models by Elisabeth Kübler-Ross, John Bowlby, George Engel, and William Worden

	Stages/Tasks				
Kübler-Ross	Bowlby	Engel	Worden	Possible Time Dimension	Behaviors
		III. Restitution			Attends to various rituals associated with the culture in which the loss has occurred.
IV. Depression	III. Disorganization and despair	IV. Resolution of the loss	II. Processing the pain of grief	Very individual. Commonly 6 to 12 months. Longer for some.	The actual work of grieving. Preoccupation with the lost entity. Feelings of helplessness and loneliness occur in response to realization of the loss. Feelings associated with the loss are confronted.

A Comparison of Models by Elisabeth Kübler-Ross, John Bowlby, George Engel, and William Worden

	Stages/Tasks				Possible Time Dimension	Behaviors
Kübler-Ross	Bowlby	Engel	Worden			
			III. Adjusting to a world without the lost entity.		Ongoing	How the environment changes depends on the roles the lost entity played in the life of the bereaved person. Adaptations will have to be made as the changes are presented in daily life. New coping skills will have to be developed. *Continued*

A Comparison of Models by Elisabeth Kübler-Ross, John Bowlby, George Engel, and William Worden

Stages/Tasks					
Kübler-Ross	Bowlby	Engel	Worden	Possible Time Dimension	Behaviors
V. Acceptance	IV. Reorganization	V. Recovery	IV. Finding an enduring connection with the lost entity in the midst of embarking on a new life.		Resolution is complete. The bereaved person experiences a reinvestment in new relationships and new goals. The lost entity is not purged or replaced, but relocated in the life of the bereaved. At this stage, terminally ill persons express a readiness to die.

Source: Adapted from Townsend, M.C. (2009). *Psychiatric/mental health nursing: Concept of care in evidence-based practice* (6rh ed.). Philadelphia: FA Davis.

Relationship Development and Therapeutic Communication

● PHASES OF A THERAPEUTIC NURSE-CLIENT RELATIONSHIP

Psychiatric nurses use interpersonal relationship development as the primary intervention with clients in various psychiatric and mental health settings. This is congruent with Peplau's (1962) identification of counseling as the major subrole of nursing in psychiatry. If Sullivan's (1953) belief is true, that is, that all emotional problems stem from difficulties with interpersonal relationships, then this role of the nurse in psychiatry becomes especially meaningful and purposeful. It becomes an integral part of the total therapeutic regimen.

The therapeutic interpersonal relationship is the means by which the nursing process is implemented. Through the relationship, problems are identified and resolution is sought. Tasks of the relationship have been categorized into four phases: the preinteraction phase, the orientation (introductory) phase, the working phase, and the termination phase. Although each phase is presented as specific and distinct from the others, there may be some overlapping of tasks, particularly when the interaction is limited.

The Preinteraction Phase

The preinteraction phase involves preparation for the first encounter with the client. Tasks include the following:

1. Obtaining available information about the client from the chart, significant others, or other health-team members. From this information, the initial assessment is begun. From

this initial information, the nurse may also become aware of personal responses to knowledge about the client.

2. Examining one's feelings, fears, and anxieties about working with a particular client. For example, the nurse may have been reared in an alcoholic family and have ambivalent feelings about caring for a client who is alcohol dependent. All individuals bring attitudes and feelings from prior experiences to the clinical setting. The nurse needs to be aware of how these preconceptions may affect his or her ability to care for individual clients.

The Orientation (Introductory) Phase

During the orientation phase, the nurse and client become acquainted. Tasks include the following:

1. Creating an environment for the establishment of trust and rapport
2. Establishing a contract for intervention that details the expectations and responsibilities of both the nurse and client
3. Gathering assessment information to build a strong client database
4. Identifying the client's strengths and limitations
5. Formulating nursing diagnoses
6. Setting goals that are mutually agreeable to the nurse and client
7. Developing a plan of action that is realistic for meeting the established goals
8. Exploring feelings of both the client and the nurse in terms of the introductory phase. Introductions are often uncomfortable, and the participants may experience some anxiety until a degree of rapport has been established. Interactions may remain on a superficial level until the anxiety subsides. Several interactions may be required to fulfill the tasks associated with this phase.

The Working Phase

The therapeutic work of the relationship is accomplished during this phase. Tasks include the following:

1. Maintaining the trust and rapport that was established during the orientation phase
2. Promoting the client's insight and perception of reality
3. Problem-solving in an effort to bring about change in the client's life
4. Overcoming resistance behaviors on the part of the client as the level of anxiety rises in response to discussion of painful issues
5. Continuously evaluating progress toward goal attainment

The Termination Phase

Termination of the relationship may occur for a variety of reasons: the mutually agreed-upon goals may have been reached, the client may be discharged from the hospital, or in the case of a student nurse, the clinical rotation may come to an end. Termination can be a difficult phase for both the client and nurse. Tasks include the following:

1. Bringing a therapeutic conclusion to the relationship. This occurs when:
   a. Progress has been made toward attainment of mutually set goals.
   b. A plan for continuing care or for assistance during stressful life experiences is mutually established by the nurse and client.
   c. Feelings about termination of the relationship are recognized and explored. Both the nurse and client may experience feelings of sadness and loss. The nurse should share his or her feelings with the client. Through these interactions, the client learns that it is acceptable to undergo these feelings at a time of separation. Through this knowledge, the client experiences growth during the process of termination.

   Note: When the client feels sadness and loss, behaviors to delay termination may become evident. If the nurse experiences the same feelings, he or she may allow the client's behaviors to delay termination. For therapeutic closure, the nurse must establish the reality of the separation and resist being manipulated into repeated delays by the client.

● THERAPEUTIC COMMUNICATION TECHNIQUES

Technique	Explanation/ Rationale	Examples
Using silence	Gives the client the opportunity to collect and organize thoughts, to think through a point, or to consider introducing a topic of greater concern than the one being discussed.	

Continued

Technique	Explanation/ Rationale	Examples
Accepting	Conveys an attitude of reception and regard.	"Yes, I understand what you said." Eye contact; nodding.
Giving recognition	Acknowledging; indicating awareness; better than complimenting, which reflects the nurse's judgment.	"Hello, Mr. J. I notice that you made a ceramic ash tray in OT." "I see you made your bed."
Offering self	Making oneself available on an unconditional basis, increasing the client's feelings of self-worth.	"I'll stay with you a while." "We can eat our lunch together." "I'm interested in you."
Giving broad openings	Allows the client to take the initiative in introducing the topic; emphasizes the importance of the client's role in the interaction.	"What would you like to talk about today?" "Tell me what you are thinking."
Offering general leads	Offers the client encouragement to continue.	"Yes, I see." "Go on." "And after that?"
Placing the event in time or sequence	Clarifies the relationship of events in time so that the nurse and client can view them in perspective.	"What seemed to lead up to...?" "Was this before or after...?" "When did this happen?"
Making observations	Verbalizing what is observed or perceived. This encourages the client to recognize specific behaviors and compare perceptions with the nurse.	"You seem tense." "I notice you are pacing a lot." "You seem uncomfortable when you..."

Technique	Explanation/ Rationale	Examples
Encouraging description of perceptions	Asking the client to verbalize what is being perceived; often used with clients experiencing hallucinations.	"Tell me what is happening now." "Are you hearing the voices again?" "What do the voices seem to be saying?"
Encouraging comparison	Asking the client to compare similarities and differences in ideas, experiences, or interpersonal relationships. Helps the client recognize life experiences that tend to recur as well as those aspects of life that are changeable.	"Was this something like...?" "How does this compare with the time when...?" "What was your response the last time this situation occurred?"
Restating	The main idea of what the client has said is repeated; lets the client know whether an expressed statement has been understood and gives him or her the chance to continue, or to clarify if necessary.	Cl: "I can't study. My mind keeps wandering." Ns: "You have difficulty concentrating." Cl: "I can't take that new job. What if I can't do it?" Ns: "You're afraid you will fail in this new position."
Reflecting	Questions and feelings are referred back to the client so that they may be recognized and accepted and so that the client may recognize that his or her point of view has value. A good technique to use when the client asks the nurse for advice.	Cl: "What do you think I should do about my wife's drinking problem?" Ns: "What do *you* think you should do?" Cl: "My sister won't help a bit toward my mother's care. I have to do it all!" Ns: "You feel angry when she doesn't help."

Continued

Technique	Explanation/ Rationale	Examples
Focusing	Taking notice of a single idea or even a single word. Works especially well with a client who is moving rapidly from one thought to another. This technique is *not* therapeutic, however, with the client who is very anxious. Focusing should not be pursued until the anxiety level has subsided.	"This point seems worth looking at more closely. Perhaps you and I can discuss it together."
Exploring	Delving further into a subject, idea, experience, or relationship. Especially helpful with clients who tend to remain on a superficial level of communication. However, if the client chooses not to disclose further information, the nurse should refrain from pushing or probing in an area that obviously creates discomfort.	"Please explain that situation in more detail." "Tell me more about that particular situation."
Seeking clarification and validation	Striving to explain that which is vague or incomprehensible and searching for mutual understanding; clarifying the meaning of what has been said facilitates and increases understanding for both client and nurse.	"I'm not sure that I understand. Would you please explain?" "Tell me if my understanding agrees with yours." "Do I understand correctly that you said...?"

Technique	Explanation/ Rationale	Examples
Presenting reality	When the client has a misperception of the environment, the nurse defines reality or indicates his or her perception of the situation for the client.	"I understand that the voices seem real to you, but I do not hear any voices." "There is no one else in the room but you and me."
Voicing doubt	Expressing uncertainty as to the reality of the client's perceptions. Often used with clients experiencing delusional thinking.	"I find that hard to believe (or accept)." "That seems rather doubtful to me."
Verbalizing the implied	Putting into words what the client has only implied or said indirectly; can also be used with the client who is mute or is otherwise experiencing impaired verbal communication. This clarifies that which is *implicit* rather than *explicit*.	Cl: "It's a waste of time to be here. I can't talk to you or anyone." Ns: "Are you feeling that no one understands?" Cl: (Mute) Ns: "It must have been very difficult for you when your husband died in the fire."
Attempting to translate words into feelings	When feelings are expressed indirectly, the nurse tries to "desymbolize" what has been said and to find clues to the underlying true feelings.	Cl: "I'm way out in the ocean." Ns: "You must be feeling very lonely now."

Continued

Technique	Explanation/ Rationale	Examples
Formulating a plan of action	When a client has a plan in mind for dealing with what is considered to be a stressful situation, it may serve to prevent anger or anxiety from escalating to an unmanageable level.	"What could you do to let your anger out harmlessly?" "Next time this comes up, what might you do to handle it more appropriately?"

Source: Adapted from Hays, J.S., and Larson, K.H. (1963). *Interacting with patients.* New York: Holt, Rinehart, and Winston.

● NONTHERAPEUTIC COMMUNICATION TECHNIQUES

Technique	Explanation/ Rationale	Examples
Giving reassurance	Indicates to the client that there is no cause for anxiety, thereby devaluing the client's feelings. May discourage the client from further expression of feelings if he or she believes they will only be downplayed or ridiculed.	"I wouldn't worry about that if I were you." "Everything will be all right." **Better to say:** "We will work on that together."
Rejecting	Refusing to consider or showing contempt for the client's ideas or behavior. This may cause the client to discontinue interaction with the nurse for fear of further rejection.	"Let's not discuss..." "I don't want to hear about..." **Better to say:** "Let's look at that a little closer."

Technique	Explanation/ Rationale	Examples
Giving approval or disapproval	Sanctioning or denouncing the client's ideas or behavior. Implies that the nurse has the right to pass judgment on whether the client's ideas or behaviors are "good" or "bad," and that the client is expected to please the nurse. The nurse's acceptance of the client is then seen as conditional depending on the client's behavior.	"That's good. I'm glad that you..." "That's bad. I'd rather you wouldn't..." **Better to say:** "Let's talk about how your behavior invoked anger in the other clients at dinner."
Agreeing/ disagreeing	Indicating accord with or opposition to the client's ideas or opinions. Implies that the nurse has the right to pass judgment on whether the client's ideas or opinions are "right" or "wrong." Agreement prevents the client from later modifying his or her point of view without admitting error. Disagreement implies inaccuracy, provoking the need for defensiveness on the part of the client.	"That's right. I agree." "That's wrong. I disagree." "I don't believe that." **Better to say:** "Let's discuss what you feel is unfair about the new community rules."
Giving advice	Telling the client what to do or how to behave implies that the nurse knows what is best and that the client is incapable of any self-direction. It nurtures the client in the dependent role by discouraging independent thinking.	"I think you should..." "Why don't you..." **Better to say:** "What do you think you should do?" or "What do you think would be best for you?"

Continued

Technique	Explanation/ Rationale	Examples
Probing	Persistent questioning of the client. Pushing for answers to issues the client does not wish to discuss. This causes the client to feel used and valued only for what is shared with the nurse, and places the client on the defensive.	"Tell me how your mother abused you when you were a child." "Tell me how you feel toward your mother now that she is dead." "Now tell me about..." **Better technique:** The nurse should be aware of the client's response and discontinue the interaction at the first sign of discomfort.
Defending	Attempting to protect someone or something from verbal attack. To defend what the client has criticized is to imply that he or she has no right to express ideas, opinions, or feelings. Defending does not change the client's feelings and may cause the client to think the nurse is taking sides with those being criticized and against the client.	"No one here would lie to you." "You have a very capable physician. I'm sure he only has your best interests in mind." **Better to say:** "I will try to answer your questions and clarify some issues regarding your treatment."

Technique	Explanation/ Rationale	Examples
Requesting an explanation	Asking the client to provide the reasons for thoughts, feelings, behavior, and events. Asking "why" a client did something or feels a certain way can be very intimidating, and implies that the client must defend his or her behavior or feelings.	"Why do you think that?" "Why do you feel this way?" "Why did you do that?" **Better to say:** "Describe what you were feeling just before that happened."
Indicating the existence of an external source of power	Attributing the source of thoughts, feelings, and behavior to others or to outside influences. This encourages the client to project blame for his or her thoughts or behaviors on others rather than accepting the responsibility personally.	"What makes you say that?" "What made you do that?" "What made you so angry last night?" **Better to say:** "You became angry when your brother insulted your wife."
Belittling feelings expressed	When the nurse misjudges the degree of the client's discomfort, a lack of empathy and understanding may be conveyed. The nurse may tell the client to "perk up" or "snap out of it." This causes the client to feel insignificant or unimportant. When one is experiencing discomfort, it is no relief to hear that others are or have been in similar situations.	Cl: "I have nothing to live for. I wish I were dead." Ns: "Everybody gets down in the dumps at times. I feel that way myself sometimes." **Better to say:** "You must be very upset. Tell me what you are feeling right now."

Continued

Technique	Explanation/ Rationale	Examples
Making stereo-typed comments	Cliches and trite expressions are meaningless in a nurse-client relationship. For the nurse to make empty conversation is to encourage a like response from the client.	"I'm fine, and how are you?" "Hang in there. It's for your own good." "Keep your chin up." **Better to say:** "The therapy must be difficult for you at times. How do you feel about your progress at this point?"
Using denial	When the nurse denies that a problem exists, he or she blocks discussion with the client and avoids helping the client identify and explore areas of difficulty.	Cl: "I'm nothing." Ns: "Of course you're something. Everybody is somebody." **Better to say:** "You're feeling like no one cares about you right now."
Interpreting	With this technique the therapist seeks to make conscious that which is unconscious, to tell the client the meaning of his or her experience.	"What you really mean is..." "Unconsciously you're saying..." **Better to say:** The nurse must leave interpretation of the client's behavior to the psychiatrist. The nurse has not been prepared to perform this technique and, in attempting to do so, may endanger other nursing roles with the client.

Technique	Explanation/ Rationale	Examples
Introducing an unrelated topic	Changing the subject causes the nurse to take over the direction of the discussion. This may occur in order to get to something that the nurse wants to discuss with the client or to get away from a topic that he or she would prefer not to discuss.	Cl: "I don't have anything to live for." Ns: "Did you have visitors this weekend?" **Better technique:** The nurse must remain open and free to hear the client, to take in all that is being conveyed, both verbally and nonverbally.

Source: Adapted from Hays, J.S., and Larson, K.H. (1963). *Interacting with patients.* New York: Holt, Rinehart, and Winston.

Psychosocial Therapies

● GROUP THERAPY

Group therapy is a type of psychosocial therapy with a number of clients at one time. The group is founded in a specific theoretical framework, with the goal being to encourage improvement in interpersonal functioning.

Nurses often lead "therapeutic groups," which are based to a lesser degree in theory. The focus of therapeutic groups is more on group relations, interactions among group members, and the consideration of a selected issue.

Types of groups include *task groups*, in which the function is to accomplish a specific outcome or task; *teaching groups*, in which knowledge or information is conveyed to a number of individuals; *supportive-therapeutic groups*, which help prevent future upsets by teaching participants effective ways of dealing with emotional stress arising from situational or developmental crises; and *self-help groups* of individuals with similar problems who meet to help each other with emotional distress associated with those problems.

Yalom (2005) identified 11 curative factors that individuals can achieve through interpersonal interactions within the group. They include the following:

1. The instillation of hope
2. Universality (individuals come to understand that they are not alone in the problems they experience)
3. The imparting of information
4. Altruism (mutual sharing and concern for each other)
5. The corrective recapitulation of the primary family group
6. The development of socializing techniques
7. Imitative behavior
8. Interpersonal learning
9. Group cohesiveness
10. Catharsis (open expression of feelings)

11. Existential factors (the group is able to help individual members take direction of their own lives and to accept responsibility for the quality of their existence)

● PSYCHODRAMA

Psychodrama is a specialized type of therapeutic group that employs a dramatic approach in which clients become "actors" in life-situation scenarios.

The group leader is called the *director*, group members are the *audience*, and the *set*, or *stage*, may be specially designed or may just be any room or part of a room selected for this purpose. Actors are members from the audience who agree to take part in the "drama" by role-playing a situation about which they have been informed by the director. Usually the situation is an issue with which one individual client has been struggling. The client plays the role of himself or herself and is called the *protagonist*. In this role, the client is able to express true feelings toward individuals (represented by group members) with whom he or she has unresolved conflicts.

In some instances, the group leader may ask for a client to volunteer to be the protagonist for that session. The client may choose a situation he or she wishes to enact and select the audience members to portray the roles of others in the life situation. The psychodrama setting provides the client with a safer and less threatening atmosphere than the real situation in which to express true feelings. Resolution of interpersonal conflicts is facilitated.

When the drama has been completed, group members from the audience discuss the situation they have observed, offer feedback, express their feelings, and relate their own similar experiences. In this way, all group members benefit from the session, either directly or indirectly.

Nurses often serve as actors, or role players, in psychodrama sessions. Leaders of psychodrama have graduate degrees in psychology, social work, nursing, or medicine with additional training in group therapy and specialty preparation to become a psychodramatist.

● FAMILY THERAPY

In family therapy, the nurse-therapist works with the family as a group to improve communication and interaction patterns. Areas of assessment include communication, manner of self-concept reinforcement, family members' expectations, handling differences, family interaction patterns, and the "climate" of the family (a blend of feelings and experiences that are the result of sharing and interacting).

The Family as a System

General systems theory is a way of organizing thought according to the holistic perspective. A system is considered greater than the sum of its parts. A family can be viewed as a system composed of various subsystems. The systems approach to family therapy is composed of eight major concepts: (1) differentiation of self, (2) triangles, (3) nuclear family emotional process, (4) family projection process, (5) multigenerational transmission process, (6) sibling position profiles, (7) emotional cutoff, and (8) societal regression. The goal is to increase the level of differentiation of self, while remaining in touch with the family system.

The Structural Model

In this model, the family is viewed as a social system within which the individual lives and to which the individual must adapt. The individual both contributes to and responds to stresses within the family. Major concepts include systems, subsystems, transactional patterns, and boundaries. The goal of therapy is to facilitate change in the family structure. The therapist does this by joining the family, evaluating the family system, and restructuring the family.

The Strategic Model

This model uses the interactional or communications approach. Functional families are open systems where clear and precise messages, congruent with the situation, are sent and received. Healthy communication patterns promote nurturance and individual self-worth. In dysfunctional families, viewed as partially closed systems, communication is vague, and messages are often inconsistent and incongruent with the situation. Destructive patterns of communication tend to inhibit healthful nurturing and decrease individual feelings of self-worth. Concepts of this model include double-bind communication, pseudomutuality and pseudohostility, marital schism, and marital skew. The goal of therapy is to create change in destructive behavior and communication patterns among family members. This is accomplished by using paradoxical intervention (prescribing the symptom) and reframing (changing the setting or viewpoint in relation to which a situation is experienced and placing it in another more positive frame of reference).

● MILIEU THERAPY

In psychiatry, milieu therapy, or a therapeutic community, constitutes a manipulation of the environment in an effort to create behavioral changes and to improve the psychological health and functioning of the individual. The goal of therapeutic community is for the client to learn adaptive coping, interaction, and relationship skills that can be generalized to other aspects of his or her life. The community environment itself serves as the primary tool of therapy.

According to Skinner (1979), a therapeutic community is based on seven basic assumptions:

1. The health in each individual is to be realized and encouraged to grow.
2. Every interaction is an opportunity for therapeutic intervention.
3. The client owns his or her own environment.
4. Each client owns his or her behavior.
5. Peer pressure is a useful and a powerful tool.
6. Inappropriate behaviors are dealt with as they occur.
7. Restrictions and punishment are to be avoided.

Since the goals of milieu therapy relate to helping the client learn to generalize that which is learned to other aspects of his or her life, the conditions that promote a therapeutic community in the hospital setting are similar to the types of conditions that exist in real-life situations. They include the following:

1. The fulfillment of basic physiological needs.
2. Physical facilities that are conducive to the achievement of the goals of therapy.
3. The existence of a democratic form of self-government.
4. The assignment of unit responsibilities according to client capabilities.
5. A structured program of social and work-related activities.
6. The inclusion of community and family in the program of therapy in an effort to facilitate discharge from the hospital.

The program of therapy on the milieu unit is conducted by the interdisciplinary treatment (IDT) team. The team includes some, or all, of the following disciplines and may include others that are not specified here: psychiatrist, clinical psychologist, psychiatric clinical nurse specialist, psychiatric nurse, mental health technician, psychiatric social worker, occupational therapist, recreational therapist, art therapist, music therapist, psychodramatist, dietitian, and chaplain.

Nurses play a crucial role in the management of a therapeutic milieu. They are involved in the assessment, diagnosis, outcome identification, planning, implementation, and evaluation of all treatment programs. They have significant input into the IDT plans that are developed for all clients. They are responsible for ensuring that clients' basic needs are fulfilled, for continual assessment of physical and psychosocial status, for medication administration, for the development of trusting relationships,

for setting limits on unacceptable behaviors, for client education, and ultimately, for helping clients, within the limits of
their capability, become productive members of society.

Milieu therapy came into its own during the 1960s through
the early 1980s. During this period, psychiatric inpatient treatment provided sufficient time to implement programs of therapy that were aimed at social rehabilitation. Currently, care in
inpatient psychiatric facilities is shorter and more biologically
based, limiting clients' benefit from the socialization that occurs
in a milieu as treatment program. Although strategies for milieu therapy are still used, they have been modified to conform
to the short-term approach to care or to outpatient treatment
programs.

● CRISIS INTERVENTION

A *crisis* is "a sudden event in one's life that disturbs homeo-
stasis, during which usual coping mechanisms cannot resolve
the problem" (Lagerquist, 2006). All individuals experience
crises at one time or another. This does not necessarily indicate psychopathology.

Crises are precipitated by specific, identifiable events and are
determined by an individual's personal perception of the situation. They are acute, not chronic, and generally last no longer
than 4 to 6 weeks.

Crises occur when an individual is exposed to a stressor
and previous problem-solving techniques are ineffective. This
causes the level of anxiety to rise. Panic may ensue when new
techniques are employed and resolution fails to occur.

Six types of crises have been identified. They include disposi-
tional crises, crises of anticipated life transitions, crises resulting
from traumatic stress, maturational or developmental crises, crises reflecting psychopathology, and psychiatric emergencies. The
type of crisis determines the method of intervention selected.

Crisis intervention is designed to provide rapid assistance for
individuals who have an urgent need. Aguilera (1998) suggests
that the "focus is on the supportive, with the restoration of the
individual to his precrisis level of functioning or possibly to a
higher level of functioning."

Nurses regularly respond to individuals in crisis in all types
of settings. Nursing process is the vehicle by which nurses assist
individuals in crisis with a short-term problem-solving approach
to change. A four-phase technique is used: assessment/analysis,
planning of therapeutic intervention, intervention, and evaluation of crisis resolution and anticipatory planning. Through this
structured method of assistance, nurses assist individuals in crisis to develop more adaptive coping strategies for dealing with
stressful situations in the future.

● RELAXATION THERAPY

Stress is a part of our everyday lives. It can be positive or negative, but it cannot be eliminated. Keeping stress at a manageable level is a lifelong process.

Individuals under stress respond with a physiological arousal that can be dangerous over long periods. Indeed, the stress response has been shown to be a major contributor, either directly or indirectly, to coronary heart disease, cancer, lung ailments, accidental injuries, cirrhosis of the liver, and suicide—six of the leading causes of death in the United States.

Relaxation therapy is an effective means of reducing the stress response in some individuals. The degree of anxiety that an individual experiences in response to stress is related to certain predisposing factors, such as characteristics of temperament with which he or she was born, past experiences resulting in learned patterns of responding, and existing conditions, such as health status, coping strategies, and adequate support systems.

Deep relaxation can counteract the physiological and behavioral manifestations of stress. Various methods of relaxation include the following:

Deep-Breathing Exercises: Tension is released when the lungs are allowed to breathe in as much oxygen as possible. Deep-breathing exercises involve inhaling slowly and deeply through the nose, holding the breath for a few seconds, then exhaling slowly through the mouth, pursing the lips as if trying to whistle.

Progressive Relaxation: This method of deep-muscle relaxation is based on the premise that the body responds to anxiety-provoking thoughts and events with muscle tension. Each muscle group is tensed for 5 to 7 seconds and then relaxed for 20 to 30 seconds, during which time the individual concentrates on the difference in sensations between the two conditions. Soft, slow background music may facilitate relaxation. A modified version of this technique (called *passive progressive relaxation*) involves relaxation of the muscles by concentrating on the feeling of relaxation within the muscle, rather than the actual tensing and relaxing of the muscle.

Meditation: The goal of meditation is to gain mastery over attention. It brings on a special state of consciousness as attention is concentrated solely on one thought or object. During meditation, as the individual becomes totally preoccupied with the selected focus, the respiration rate, heart rate, and blood pressure decrease. The overall metabolism declines, and the need for oxygen consumption is reduced.

Mental Imagery: Mental imagery uses the imagination in an effort to reduce the body's response to stress. The frame of reference is very personal, based on what each individual considers to be a relaxing environment. The relaxing scenario is most useful when taped and played back at a time when the individual wishes to achieve relaxation.

Biofeedback: Biofeedback is the use of instrumentation to become aware of processes in the body that usually go unnoticed and to help bring them under voluntary control. Biological conditions, such as muscle tension, skin surface temperature, blood pressure, and heart rate, are monitored by the biofeedback equipment. With special training, the individual learns to use relaxation and voluntary control to modify the biological condition, in turn indicating a modification of the autonomic function it represents. Biofeedback is often used together with other relaxation techniques such as deep breathing, progressive relaxation, and mental imagery.

● ASSERTIVENESS TRAINING

Assertive behavior helps individuals feel better about themselves by encouraging them to stand up for their own basic human rights. These rights have equal representation for all individuals. But along with rights comes an equal number of responsibilities. Part of being assertive includes living up to these responsibilities.

Assertive behavior increases self-esteem and the ability to develop satisfying interpersonal relationships. This is accomplished through honesty, directness, appropriateness, and respecting one's own rights, as well as the rights of others.

Individuals develop patterns of responding in various ways, such as role modeling, by receiving positive or negative reinforcement, or by conscious choice. These patterns can take the form of nonassertiveness, assertiveness, aggressiveness, or passive-aggressiveness.

Nonassertive individuals seek to please others at the expense of denying their own basic human rights. *Assertive* individuals stand up for their own rights while protecting the rights of others. Those who respond *aggressively* defend their own rights by violating the basic rights of others. Individuals who respond in a *passive-aggressive* manner defend their own rights by expressing resistance to social and occupational demands.

Some important behavioral considerations of assertive behavior include eye contact, body posture, personal distance, physical contact, gestures, facial expression, voice, fluency, timing, listening, thoughts, and content. Various techniques have been developed to assist individuals in the process of becoming more assertive. Some of these include the following:

1. **Standing up for one's basic human rights.**
   Example: "I have the right to express my opinion."
2. **Assuming responsibility for one's own statements.**
   Example: "I *don't want* to go out with you tonight," instead of "I *can't* go out with you tonight." The latter implies a lack of power or ability.
3. **Responding as a "broken record."** Persistently repeating in a calm voice what is wanted.
   Example: Telephone salesperson: "I want to help you save money by changing long-distance services."

   Assertive response: "I don't want to change my long-distance service."

   Telephone salesperson: "I can't believe you don't want to save money!"

   Assertive response: "I don't want to change my long-distance service."
4. **Agreeing assertively.** Assertively accepting negative aspects about oneself. Admitting when an error has been made.
   Example:
   Ms. Jones: "You sure let that meeting get out of hand. What a waste of time."
   Ms. Smith: "Yes, I didn't do a very good job of conducting the meeting today."
5. **Inquiring assertively.** Seeking additional information about critical statements.
   Example:
   Male board member: "You made a real fool of yourself at the board meeting last night."
   Female board member: "Oh, really? Just what about my behavior offended you?"
   Male board member: "You were so damned pushy!"
   Female board member: "Were you offended that I spoke up for my beliefs, or was it because my beliefs are in direct opposition to yours?"
6. **Shifting from content to process.** Changing the focus of the communication from discussing the topic at hand to analyzing what is actually going on in the interaction.
   Example:
   Wife: "Would you please call me if you will be late for dinner?"
   Husband: "Why don't you just get off my back! I always have to account for every minute of my time with you!"

Wife: "Sounds to me like we need to discuss some other things here. What are you *really* angry about?"

7. **Clouding/fogging.** Concurring with the critic's argument without becoming defensive and without agreeing to change.
Example:
Nurse No. 1: "You make so many mistakes. I don't know how you ever got this job!"
Nurse No. 2: "You're right. I have made some mistakes since I started this job."

8. **Defusing**. Putting off further discussion with an angry individual until he or she is calmer.
Example:
"You are very angry right now. I don't want to discuss this matter with you while you are so upset. I will discuss it with you in my office at 3 o'clock this afternoon."

9. **Delaying assertively.** Putting off further discussion with another individual until one is calmer.
Example:
"That's a very challenging position you have taken, Mr. Brown. I'll need time to give it some thought. I'll call you later this afternoon."

10. **Responding assertively with irony.**
Example:
Man: "I bet you're one of them so-called 'women's libbers,' aren't you?"
Woman: "Yes, thank you for noticing."

● COGNITIVE THERAPY

Cognitive therapy, developed by Aaron Beck, is commonly used in the treatment of mood disorders. In cognitive therapy, the individual is taught to control thought distortions that are considered to be a factor in the development and maintenance of mood disorders. In the cognitive model, depression is characterized by a triad of negative distortions related to expectations of the environment, self, and future. The environment and activities within it are viewed as unsatisfying, the self is unrealistically devalued, and the future is perceived as hopeless. In the same model, mania is characterized by a positive cognitive triad—the self is seen as highly valued and powerful, experiences within the environment are viewed as overly positive, and the future is seen as one of unlimited opportunity.

The general goals in cognitive therapy are to obtain symptom relief as quickly as possible, to assist the client in identifying dysfunctional patterns of thinking and behaving, and to guide the client to evidence and logic that effectively test the validity of the dysfunctional thinking. Therapy focuses on changing "automatic thoughts" that occur spontaneously and contribute to the distorted affect. Examples of "automatic thoughts" in depression include the following:

1. **Personalizing**: "I'm the only one who failed."
2. **All or nothing:** "I'm a complete failure."
3. **Mind reading:** "He thinks I'm foolish."
4. **Discounting positives:** "The other questions were so easy. Any dummy could have gotten them right."

Examples of "automatic thoughts" in mania include the following:

1. **Personalizing:** "She's this happy only when she's with me."
2. **All or nothing:** "Everything I do is great."
3. **Mind reading:** "She thinks I'm wonderful."
4. **Discounting negatives:** "None of those mistakes are really important."

The client is asked to describe evidence that both supports and disputes the automatic thought. The logic underlying the inferences is then reviewed with the client. Another technique involves evaluating what would most likely happen if the client's automatic thoughts were true. Implications of the consequences are then discussed.

Clients should not become discouraged if one technique seems not to be working. There is no single technique that works with all clients. He or she should be reassured that there are a number of techniques that may be used, and both therapist and client may explore these possibilities. Cognitive therapy has been shown to be an effective treatment for mood disorders, particularly in conjunction with psychopharmacological intervention.

Electroconvulsive Therapy

● DEFINED

Electroconvulsive therapy (ECT) is a type of somatic treatment in which electric current is applied to the brain through electrodes placed on the temples. The current is sufficient to induce a grand mal seizure, from which the desired therapeutic effect is achieved.

● INDICATIONS

ECT is primarily used in the treatment of severe depression. It is sometimes administered in conjunction with antidepressant medication, but most physicians prefer to perform this treatment only after an unsuccessful trial of drug therapy.

ECT may also be used as a fast-acting treatment for very hyperactive manic clients in danger of physical exhaustion, and with individuals who are extremely suicidal.

ECT was originally attempted in the treatment of schizophrenia, but with little success in most instances. There has been evidence, however, of its effectiveness in the treatment of acute schizophrenia, particularly if it is accompanied by catatonic or affective (depression or mania) symptomatology (Black & Andreasen, 2011).

● CONTRAINDICATIONS

ECT should not be used if there is increased intracranial pressure (resulting from a brain tumor, recent cardiovascular accident, or other cerebrovascular lesion). Other conditions, although not considered absolute contraindications, may render clients at high risk for the treatment. They are largely cardiovascular in nature and include myocardial infarction or cerebrovascular accident within the preceding 3 months, aortic or cerebral aneurysm, severe underlying hypertension, and congestive heart failure.

● MECHANISM OF ACTION

The exact mechanism of action is unknown. However, it is thought that ECT produces biochemical changes in the brain—an increase in the levels of norepinephrine, serotonin, and dopamine—similar to the effects of antidepressant medications.

● SIDE EFFECTS AND NURSING IMPLICATIONS

Temporary Memory Loss and Confusion

- These are the most common side effects of ECT. It is important for the nurse to be present when the client awakens, to alleviate the fears that accompany this loss of memory.
- Provide reassurance that memory loss is only temporary.
- Describe to client what has occurred.
- Reorient client to time and place.
- Allow client to verbalize fears and anxieties related to receiving ECT.
- To minimize confusion, provide a good deal of structure for client's routine activities.

● RISKS ASSOCIATED WITH ECT

1. **Death**. The mortality rate from ECT is about 2 per 100,000 treatments (Marangell et al., 2003; Sadock & Sadock, 2007). The major cause is cardiovascular complications, such as acute myocardial infarction or cardiac arrest.
2. **Brain Damage.** Brain damage is considered to be a risk, but evidence is largely unsubstantiated.
3. **Permanent Memory Loss.** Most individuals report no problems with their memory, aside from the time immediately surrounding the ECT treatments. However, some clients have reported retrograde amnesia extending back to months before treatment. In rare instances, more extensive amnesia has occurred, resulting in memory gaps dating back years (Joska & Stein, 2008), Black and Andreasen (2011) suggest that all clients receiving ECT should be informed of the possibility of permanent memory loss.

   Although the potential for these effects appears to be minimal, the client must be made aware of the risks involved before consenting to treatment.

● POTENTIAL NURSING DIAGNOSES ASSOCIATED WITH ECT

1. Risk for injury related to certain risks associated with ECT.
2. Risk for aspiration related to altered level of consciousness immediately following treatment.

3. Decreased cardiac output related to vagal stimulation occurring during the ECT.
4. Disturbed thought processes related to side effects of temporary memory loss and confusion.
5. Deficient knowledge related to necessity for, and side effects and risks of, ECT.
6. Anxiety (moderate to severe) related to impending therapy.
7. Self-care deficit related to incapacitation during postictal stage.
8. Risk for activity intolerance related to post-ECT confusion and memory loss.

● **NURSING INTERVENTIONS FOR CLIENT RECEIVING ECT**

1. Ensure that physician has obtained informed consent and that a signed permission form is on the chart.
2. Ensure that most recent laboratory reports (complete blood count [CBC], urinalysis) and results of ECG and x-ray examination are available.
3. Client should receive nothing by mouth (NPO) on the morning of the treatment.
4. Prior to the treatment, client should void, dress in night clothes (or other loose clothing), and remove dentures and eyeglasses or contact lenses. Bedrails should be raised.
5. Take baseline vital signs and blood pressure.
6. Administer cholinergic blocking agent (e.g., atropine sulfate, glycopyrrolate) approximately 30 minutes before treatment, as ordered by the physician, to decrease secretions and increase heart rate (which is suppressed in response to vagal stimulation caused by the ECT).
7. Assist physician and/or anesthesiologist as necessary in the administration of intravenous medications. A short-acting anesthetic, such as methohexital sodium (Brevital sodium), is given along with the muscle relaxant succinylcholine chloride (Anectine).
8. Administer oxygen and provide suctioning as required.
9. After the procedure, take vital signs and blood pressure every 15 minutes for the first hour. Position client on side to prevent aspiration.
10. Stay with client until he or she is fully awake.
11. Allow client to verbalize fears and anxieties associated with the treatment.
12. Reassure client that memory loss and confusion are only temporary.

Medication Assessment
Tool

Date _____ Client's Name _____ Age _____

Marital Status _____ Children _____

Occupation _____

Presenting Symptoms (subjective & objective) _____

_____

Diagnosis (DSM-IV-TR) _____

Current Vital Signs: Blood Pressure: Sitting _____ / _____ ; Standing _____ / _____ ; Pulse _____ ; Respirations _____

CURRENT/PAST USE OF PRESCRIPTION DRUGS (Indicate with "c" or "p" beside name of drug whether current or past use):

Name	Dosage	How Long Used	Why Prescribed	By Whom	Side Effects/Results
____	____	____	____	____	____
____	____	____	____	____	____
____	____	____	____	____	____

CURRENT/PAST USE OF OVER-THE-COUNTER DRUGS (Indicate with "c" or "p" beside name of drug whether current or past use):

Name	Dosage	How Long Used	Why Prescribed	By Whom	Side Effects/Results

CURRENT/PAST USE OF STREET DRUGS, ALCOHOL, NICOTINE, AND/OR CAFFEINE (Indicate with "c" or "p" beside name of drug whether current or past use):

Name	Amount Used	How Often Used	When Last Used	Effects/Produced

Any allergies to food or drugs? _____

Any special diet considerations? _____

Do you have (or have you ever had) any of the following? If yes, provide explanation on the back of this sheet.

	Yes	No
1. Difficulty swallowing		
2. Delayed wound healing		
3. Constipation problems		
4. Urination problems		
5. Recent change in elimination patterns		
6. Weakness or tremors		
7. Seizures		
8. Headaches		
9. Dizziness		
10. High blood pressure		
11. Palpitations		
12. Chest pain		

	Yes	No
13. Blood clots/pain in legs		
14. Fainting spells		
15. Swollen ankles/legs/hands		
16. Asthma		
17. Varicose veins		
18. Numbness/tingling (location?)		
19. Ulcers		
20. Nausea/vomiting		
21. Problems with diarrhea		
22. Shortness of breath		
23. Sexual dysfunction		

	Yes	No
24. Lumps in your breasts		
25. Blurred or double vision		
26. Ringing in the ears		
27. Insomnia		
28. Skin rashes		
29. Diabetes		
30. Hepatitis (or other liver disease)		
31. Kidney disease		
32. Glaucoma		

Are you pregnant or breast feeding? _____ Date of last menses _____ Type of contraception used _____

Describe any restrictions/limitations that might interfere with your use of medication for your current problem. _____

Patient teaching related to medications prescribed:

Prescription orders:

Lab work ordered:

Nurse's Signature

Client's Signature

Cultural Assessment Tool

Client's Name _____ Ethnic Origin _____

Address _____ Birth Date _____

Name of Significant Other _____ Relationship _____

Primary Language Spoken _____

Second Language Spoken _____

How does client usually communicate with people who speak a different language? _____

Is an interpreter required? _____

Available? _____

Highest level of education achieved _____

Occupation _____

Presenting Problem _____

Has this problem ever occurred before? _____

If so, in what manner was it handled previously? _____

What is client's usual manner of coping with stress? _____

Who is(are) the client's main support system(s)? _____

Describe the family living arrangements _____

Who is the major decision maker in the family? _____

Describe client's/family members' roles within the family _____

Describe religious beliefs and practices _____

Are there any religious requirements or restrictions that place limitations on the client's care? _____

If so, describe _____

Who in the family takes responsibility for health concerns?

_____

Describe any special health beliefs and practices that may vary from the conventional _____

From whom does family usually seek medical assistance in time of need? _____

Describe client's usual emotional/behavioral response to: _____
_____

Anxiety _____

Anger _____

Loss/change/failure _____

Pain _____

Fear _____

Describe any topics that are particularly sensitive or that the client is unwilling to discuss (because of cultural taboos)
_____

Describe any activities in which the client is unwilling to participate (because of cultural customs or taboos) _____

What are the client's personal feelings regarding touch? _____
_____

What are the client's personal feelings regarding eye contact?
_____

What is the client's personal orientation to time? (past, present, future) _____

Describe any particular illnesses to which the client may be bioculturally susceptible (e.g., hypertension and sickle cell anemia in African Americans) _____

Describe any nutritional deficiencies to which the client may be bioculturally susceptible (e.g., lactose intolerance in Native and Asian Americans) _____

Describe client's favorite foods _____

Are there any foods the client requests or refuses because of cultural beliefs related to this illness? (e.g., "hot" and "cold" foods for Hispanic and Asian Americans). If so, please describe
_____

Describe client's perception of the problem and expectations of health care _____
_____

The DSM-IV-TR Multiaxial Evaluation System

The American Psychiatric Association (APA, 2000) endorses case evaluation on a multiaxial system, "to facilitate comprehensive and systematic evaluation with attention to the various mental disorders and general medical conditions, psychosocial and environmental problems, and level of functioning that might be overlooked if the focus were on assessing a single presenting problem." Each individual is evaluated on five axes. They are defined by the *Diagnostic and Statistical Manual of Mental Disorders, Fourth Edition, Text Revision (DSM-IV-TR)* in the following manner:

Axis I—Clinical Disorders and Other Conditions That May Be a Focus of Clinical Attention
> These include all mental disorders (except personality disorders and mental retardation).

Axis II—Personality Disorders and Mental Retardation
> These disorders usually begin in childhood or adolescence and persist in a stable form into adult life.

Axis III—General Medical Conditions
> These include any current general medical condition that is potentially relevant to the understanding or management of the individual's mental disorder.

Axis IV—Psychosocial and Environmental Problems
> These are problems that may affect the diagnosis, treatment, and prognosis of mental disorders named on axes I and II. Examples include: problems related to primary support group, social environment, education, occupation, housing, economics, access to health care services, interaction with the legal system or crime, and other types of psychosocial and environmental problems.

Axis V—Global Assessment of Functioning

This allows the clinician to rate the individual's overall functioning on the Global Assessment of Functioning (GAF) Scale. This scale represents in global terms a single measure of the individual's psychological, social, and occupational functioning. A copy of the GAF Scale appears in Appendix K.

Source: From the *Diagnostic and Statistical Manual of Mental Disorders, 4th Edition, Text Revision, 2000.* Used with permission from the American Psychiatric Association.

Example of a psychiatric diagnosis using the Multiaxial Evaluation System:

Axis I	300.4	Dysthymic Disorder
Axis II	301.6	Dependent Personality Disorder
Axis III	244.9	Hypothyroidism
Axis IV		Unemployed
Axis V	GAF = 65 (current)	

Global Assessment of Functioning (GAF) Scale

Consider psychological, social, and occupational functioning on a hypothetical continuum of mental health-illness. Do not include impairment in functioning due to physical (or environmental) limitations.

Code	(Note: Use intermediate codes when appropriate, e.g., 45, 68, 72)
100–91	Superior functioning in a wide range of activities, life's problems never seem to get out of hand, is sought out by others because of his or her many positive qualities. No symptoms.
90–81	Absent or minimal symptoms (e.g., mild anxiety before an exam), good functioning in all areas, interested and involved in a wide range of activities, socially effective, generally satisfied with life, no more than everyday problems or concerns (e.g., an occasional argument with family members).
80–71	If symptoms are present, they are transient and expectable reactions to psychosocial stressors (e.g., difficulty concentrating after family argument); no more than slight impairment in social, occupational, or school functioning (e.g., temporarily falling behind in schoolwork).

70–61   Some mild symptoms (e.g., depressed mood and mild insomnia) OR some difficulty in social, occupational, or school functioning (e.g., occasional truancy, or theft within the household), but generally functioning pretty well, has some meaningful interpersonal relationships.

60–51   Moderate symptoms (e.g., flat affect and circumstantial speech, occasional panic attacks) OR moderate difficulty in social, occupational, or school functioning (e.g., few friends, conflicts with peers or co-workers).

50–41   Serious symptoms (e.g., suicidal ideation, severe obsessional rituals, frequent shoplifting) OR any serious impairment in social, occupational, or school functioning (e.g., no friends, unable to keep a job).

40–31   Some impairment in reality testing or communication (e.g., speech is at times illogical, obscure, or irrelevant) OR major impairment in several areas, such as work or school, family relations, judgment, thinking, or mood (e.g., depressed man avoids friends, neglects family, and is unable to work; child frequently beats up younger children, is defiant at home, and is failing at school).

30–31   Behavior is considerably influenced by delusions or hallucinations OR serious impairment in communication or judgment (e.g., sometimes incoherent, acts grossly inappropriately, suicidal preoccupation) OR inability to function in almost all areas (e.g., stays in bed all day; no job, home, or friends).

20–11   Some degree of hurting self or others (e.g., suicide attempts without clear expectation of death; frequently violent; manic excitement) OR occasionally fails to maintain minimal personal hygiene (e.g., smears feces) OR gross impairment in communication (e.g., largely incoherent or mute).

Continued

10–1   Persistent danger of severely hurting self or others
         (e.g., recurrent violence) OR persistent inability
         to maintain minimal personal hygiene OR seri-
         ous suicidal act with clear expectation of death.

0   Inadequate information.

Source: *Diagnostic and Statistical Manual of Mental Disorders* (4th ed.). *Text Revision.* Washington, DC: American Psychiatric Publishing (2000). With permission.

DSM-IV-TR Classification: Axes I and II Categories and Codes

● **DISORDERS USUALLY FIRST DIAGNOSED IN INFANCY, CHILDHOOD, OR ADOLESCENCE**

Mental Retardation

Note: These are coded on Axis II.

317	Mild Mental Retardation
318.0	Moderate Retardation
318.1	Severe Retardation
318.2	Profound Mental Retardation
319	Mental Retardation, Severity Unspecified

Learning Disorders

315.00	Reading Disorder
315.1	Mathematics Disorder
315.2	Disorder of Written Expression
315.9	Learning Disorder Not Otherwise Specified (NOS)

Motor Skills Disorder

315.4	Developmental Coordination Disorder

Communication Disorders

315.31	Expressive Language Disorder
315.32	Mixed Receptive-Expressive Language Disorder
315.39	Phonological Disorder
307.0	Stuttering
307.9	Communication Disorder NOS

Pervasive Developmental Disorders

299.00	Autistic Disorder
299.80	Rett's Disorder
299.10	Childhood Disintegrative Disorder
299.80	Asperger's Disorder
299.80	Pervasive Developmental Disorder NOS

Attention-Deficit and Disruptive Behavior Disorders

314.xx	Attention-Deficit/Hyperactivity Disorder
314.01	Combined Type
314.00	Predominantly Inattentive Type
314.01	Predominantly Hyperactive-Impulsive Type
314.9	Attention-Deficit/Hyperactivity Disorder NOS
312.xx	Conduct Disorder
.81	Childhood-Onset Type
.82	Adolescent-Onset Type
.89	Unspecified Onset
313.81	Oppositional Defiant Disorder
312.9	Disruptive Behavior Disorder NOS

Feeding and Eating Disorders of Infancy or Early Childhood

307.52	Pica
307.53	Rumination Disorder
307.59	Feeding Disorder of Infancy or Early Childhood

Tic Disorders

307.23	Tourette's Disorder
307.22	Chronic Motor or Vocal Tic Disorder
307.21	Transient Tic Disorder
307.20	Tic Disorder NOS

Elimination Disorders

—	Encopresis
787.6	With Constipation and Overflow Incontinence
307.7	Without Constipation and Overflow Incontinence
307.6	Enuresis (Not Due to a General Medical Condition)

Other Disorders of Infancy, Childhood, or Adolescence

309.21   Separation Anxiety Disorder
313.23   Selective Mutism
313.89   Reactive Attachment Disorder of Infancy or Early
         Childhood
307.3   Stereotypic Movement Disorder
313.9   Disorder of Infancy, Childhood, or Adolescence NOS

● DELIRIUM, DEMENTIA, AND AMNESTIC AND OTHER COGNITIVE DISORDERS

Delirium

293.0   Delirium Due to... *(Indicate the General Medical Condition)*
—   Substance Intoxication Delirium *(refer to Substance-Related Disorders for substance-specific codes)*
—   Substance Withdrawal Delirium *(refer to Substance-Related Disorders for substance-specific codes)*
—   Delirium Due to Multiple Etiologies *(code each of the specific etiologies)*
780.09   Delirium NOS

Dementia

294.xx   Dementia of the Alzheimer's Type, With Early Onset
.10   Without Behavioral Disturbance
.11   With Behavioral Disturbance
294.xx   Dementia of the Alzheimer's Type, With Late Onset
.10   Without Behavioral Disturbance
.11   With Behavioral Disturbance
290.xx   Vascular Dementia
.40   Uncomplicated
.41   With Delirium
.42   With Delusions
.43   With Depressed Mood
294.1x   Dementia Due to HIV Disease
294.1x   Dementia Due to Head Trauma
294.1x   Dementia Due to Parkinson's Disease
294.1x   Dementia Due to Huntington's Disease
294.1x   Dementia Due to Pick's Disease
294.1x   Dementia Due to Creutzfeldt-Jakob Disease
294.1x   Dementia Due to *(Indicate the General Medical Condition not listed above)*
—   Substance-Induced Persisting Dementia *(refer to Substance-Related Disorders for substance-specific codes)*
—   Dementia Due to Multiple Etiologies *(code each of the specific etiologies)*
294.8   Dementia NOS

Amnestic Disorders

294.0   Amnestic Disorder Due to *(Indicate the General Medical Condition)*

—   Substance-Induced Persisting Amnestic Disorder *(refer to Substance-Related Disorders for substance-specific codes)*

294.8   Amnestic Disorder NOS

Other Cognitive Disorders

294.9   Cognitive Disorder NOS

● MENTAL DISORDERS DUE TO A GENERAL MEDICAL CONDITION NOT ELSEWHERE CLASSIFIED

293.89   Catatonic Disorder Due to *(Indicate the General Medical Condition)*

310.1   Personality Change Due to *(Indicate the General Medical Condition)*

293.9   Mental Disorder NOS Due to *(Indicate the General Medical Condition)*

● SUBSTANCE-RELATED DISORDERS

Alcohol-Related Disorders

Alcohol Use Disorders

303.90   Alcohol Dependence
305.00   Alcohol Abuse

Alcohol-Induced Disorders

303.00   Alcohol Intoxication
291.81   Alcohol Withdrawal
291.0   Alcohol Intoxication Delirium
291.0   Alcohol Withdrawal Delirium
291.2   Alcohol-Induced Persisting Dementia
291.1   Alcohol-Induced Persisting Amnestic Disorder
291.x   Alcohol-Induced Psychotic Disorder
  .5   With Delusions
  .3   With Hallucinations
291.89   Alcohol-Induced Mood Disorder
291.89   Alcohol-Induced Anxiety Disorder
291.89   Alcohol-Induced Sexual Dysfunction
291.89   Alcohol-Induced Sleep Disorder
291.9   Alcohol Related Disorder NOS

Amphetamine (or Amphetamine-Like)-Related Disorders

Amphetamine Use Disorders

304.40   Amphetamine Dependence
305.70   Amphetamine Abuse

Amphetamine-Induced Disorders

292.89	Amphetamine Intoxication
292.0	Amphetamine Withdrawal
292.81	Amphetamine Intoxication Delirium
292.xx	Amphetamine-Induced Psychotic Disorder
.11	With Delusions
.12	With Hallucinations
292.84	Amphetamine-Induced Mood Disorder
292.89	Amphetamine-Induced Anxiety Disorder
292.89	Amphetamine-Induced Sexual Dysfunction
292.89	Amphetamine-Induced Sleep Disorder
292.9	Amphetamine-Related Disorder NOS

Caffeine-Related Disorders
Caffeine-Induced Disorders

305.90	Caffeine Intoxication
292.89	Caffeine-Induced Anxiety Disorder
292.89	Caffeine-Induced Sleep Disorder
292.9	Caffeine-Related Disorder NOS

Cannabis-Related Disorders
Cannabis Use Disorders

304.30	Cannabis Dependence
305.20	Cannabis Abuse

Cannabis-Induced Disorders

292.89	Cannabis Intoxication
292.81	Cannabis Intoxication Delirium
292.xx	Cannabis-Induced Psychotic Disorder
.11	With Delusions
.12	With Hallucinations
292.89	Cannabis-Induced Anxiety Disorder
292.9	Cannabis-Related Disorder NOS

Cocaine-Related Disorders
Cocaine Use Disorders

304.20	Cocaine Dependence
305.60	Cocaine Abuse

Cocaine-Induced Disorders

292.89	Cocaine Intoxication
292.0	Cocaine Withdrawal
292.81	Cocaine Intoxication Delirium
292.xx	Cocaine-Induced Psychotic Disorder
.11	With Delusions
.12	With Hallucinations
292.84	Cocaine-Induced Mood Disorder

292.89   Cocaine-Induced Anxiety Disorder
292.89   Cocaine-Induced Sexual Dysfunction
292.89   Cocaine-Induced Sleep Disorder
292.9   Cocaine-Related Disorder NOS

Hallucinogen-Related Disorders
Hallucinogen Use Disorders

304.50   Hallucinogen Dependence
305.30   Hallucinogen Abuse

Hallucinogen-Induced Disorders

292.89   Hallucinogen Intoxication
292.89   Hallucinogen Persisting Perception Disorder
         (Flashbacks)
292.81   Hallucinogen Intoxication Delirium
292.xx   Hallucinogen-Induced Psychotic Disorder
   .11   With Delusions
   .12   With Hallucinations
292.84   Hallucinogen-Induced Mood Disorder
292.89   Hallucinogen-Induced Anxiety Disorder
292.9   Hallucinogen-Related Disorder NOS

Inhalant-Related Disorders
Inhalant Use Disorders

304.60   Inhalant Dependence
305.90   Inhalant Abuse

Inhalant-Induced Disorders

292.89   Inhalant Intoxication
292.81   Inhalant Intoxication Delirium
292.82   Inhalant-Induced Persisting Dementia
292.xx   Inhalant-Induced Psychotic Disorder
   .11   With Delusions
   .12   With Hallucinations
292.84   Inhalant-Induced Mood Disorder
292.89   Inhalant-Induced Anxiety Disorder
292.9   Inhalant-Related Disorder NOS

Nicotine-Related Disorders
Nicotine Use Disorders

305.1   Nicotine Dependence

Nicotine-Induced Disorders

292.0   Nicotine Withdrawal
292.9   Nicotine-Related Disorder NOS

Opioid-Related Disorders

Opioid Use Disorders

304.00   Opioid Dependence
305.50   Opioid Abuse

Opioid-Induced Disorders

292.89   Opioid Intoxication
292.0   Opioid Withdrawal
292.81   Opioid Intoxication Delirium
292.xx   Opioid-Induced Psychotic Disorder
  .11   With Delusions
  .12   With Hallucinations
292.84   Opioid-Induced Mood Disorder
292.89   Opioid-Induced Sexual Dysfunction
292.89   Opioid-Induced Sleep Disorder
292.9   Opioid-Related Disorder NOS

Phencyclidine (or Phencyclidine-Like)-Related Disorders

Phencyclidine Use Disorders

304.60   Phencyclidine Dependence
305.90   Phencyclidine Abuse

Phencyclidine-Induced Disorders

292.89   Phencyclidine Intoxication
292.81   Phencyclidine Intoxication Delirium
292.xx   Phencyclidine-Induced Psychotic Disorder
  .11   With Delusions
  .12   With Hallucinations
292.84   Phencyclidine-Induced Mood Disorder
292.89   Phencyclidine-Induced Anxiety Disorder
292.9   Phencyclidine-Related Disorder NOS

Sedative-, Hypnotic-, or Anxiolytic-Related Disorders

Sedative, Hypnotic, or Anxiolytic Use Disorders

304.10   Sedative, Hypnotic, or Anxiolytic Dependence
305.40   Sedative, Hypnotic, or Anxiolytic Abuse

Sedative-, Hypnotic-, or Anxiolytic-Induced Disorders

292.89   Sedative, Hypnotic, or Anxiolytic Intoxication
292.0   Sedative, Hypnotic, or Anxiolytic Withdrawal
292.81   Sedative, Hypnotic, or Anxiolytic Intoxication Delirium

292.81	Sedative, Hypnotic, or Anxiolytic Withdrawal Delirium
292.82	Sedative-, Hypnotic-, or Anxiolytic-Induced Persisting Dementia
292.83	Sedative-, Hypnotic-, or Anxiolytic-Induced Persisting Amnestic Disorder
292.xx	Sedative-, Hypnotic-, or Anxiolytic-Induced Psychotic Disorder
.11	With Delusions
.12	With Hallucinations
292.84	Sedative-, Hypnotic-, or Anxiolytic-Induced Mood Disorder
292.89	Sedative-, Hypnotic-, or Anxiolytic-Induced Anxiety Disorder
292.89	Sedative-, Hypnotic-, or Anxiolytic-Induced Sexual Dysfunction
292.89	Sedative-, Hypnotic-, or Anxiolytic-Induced Sleep Disorder
292.9	Sedative-, Hypnotic-, or Anxiolytic-Related Disorder NOS

Polysubstance-Related Disorder
304.80	Polysubstance Dependence

Other (or Unknown) Substance-Related Disorders

Other (or Unknown) Substance Use Disorders
304.90	Other (or Unknown) Substance Dependence
305.90	Other (or Unknown) Substance Abuse

Other (or Unknown) Substance-Induced Disorders
292.89	Other (or Unknown) Substance Intoxication
292.0	Other (or Unknown) Substance Withdrawal
292.81	Other (or Unknown) Substance-Induced Delirium
292.82	Other (or Unknown) Substance-Induced Persisting Dementia
292.83	Other (or Unknown) Substance-Induced Persisting Amnestic Disorder
292.xx	Other (or Unknown) Substance-Induced Psychotic Disorder
.11	With Delusions
.12	With Hallucinations
292.84	Other (or Unknown) Substance-Induced Mood Disorder
292.89	Other (or Unknown) Substance-Induced Anxiety Disorder

292.89   Other (or Unknown) Substance-Induced Sexual Dysfunction
292.89   Other (or Unknown) Substance-Induced Sleep Disorder
292.9   Other (or Unknown) Substance-Related Disorder NOS

● SCHIZOPHRENIA AND OTHER PSYCHOTIC DISORDERS

295.xx   Schizophrenia
   .30   Paranoid type
   .10   Disorganized type
   .20   Catatonic type
   .90   Undifferentiated type
   .60   Residual type
295.40   Schizophreniform Disorder
295.70   Schizoaffective Disorder
297.1   Delusional Disorder
298.8   Brief Psychotic Disorder
297.3   Shared Psychotic Disorder
293.xx   Psychotic Disorder Due to *(Indicate the General Medical Condition)*
   .81   With Delusions
   .82   With Hallucinations
   —   Substance-Induced Psychotic Disorder *(refer to Substance-Related Disorders for substance-specific codes)*
298.9   Psychotic Disorder NOS

● MOOD DISORDERS

(Code current state of Major Depressive Disorder or Bipolar I Disorder in fifth digit: 0 = unspecified; 1 = mild; 2 = moderate; 3 = severe, without psychotic features; 4 = severe, with psychotic features; 5 = in partial remission; 6 = in full remission.)

Depressive Disorders

296.xx   Major Depressive Disorder
   .2x   Single episode
   .3x   Recurrent
300.4   Dysthymic Disorder
311   Depressive Disorder NOS

Bipolar Disorders

296.xx   Bipolar I Disorder
   .0x   Single Manic Episode
   .40   Most Recent Episode Hypomanic
   .4x   Most Recent Episode Manic
   .6x   Most Recent Episode Mixed
   .5x   Most Recent Episode Depressed

.7   Most Recent Episode Unspecified
296.89 Bipolar II Disorder *(Specify current or most recent episode: Hypomanic or Depressed)*
301.13 Cyclothymic Disorder
296.80 Bipolar Disorder NOS
293.83 Mood Disorder Due to *(Indicate the General Medical Condition)*
—   Substance-Induced Mood Disorder *(refer to Substance-Related Disorders for substance-specific codes)*
296.90 Mood Disorder NOS

● ANXIETY DISORDERS

300.01 Panic Disorder Without Agoraphobia
300.21 Panic Disorder With Agoraphobia
300.22 Agoraphobia Without History of Panic Disorder
300.29 Specific Phobia
300.23 Social Phobia
300.3   Obsessive-Compulsive Disorder
309.81 Posttraumatic Stress Disorder
308.3   Acute Stress Disorder
300.02 Generalized Anxiety Disorder
293.89 Anxiety Disorder Due to *(Indicate the General Medical Condition)*
—   Substance-Induced Anxiety Disorder *(refer to Substance-Related Disorders for substance-specific codes)*
300.00 Anxiety Disorder NOS

● SOMATOFORM DISORDERS

300.81 Somatization Disorder
300.82 Undifferentiated Somatoform Disorder
300.11 Conversion Disorder
307.xx Pain Disorder
  .80   Associated with Psychological Factors
  .89   Associated with Both Psychological Factors and a General Medical Condition
300.7   Hypochondriasis
300.7   Body Dysmorphic Disorder
300.82 Somatoform Disorder NOS

● FACTITIOUS DISORDERS

300.xx Factitious Disorder
  .16   With Predominantly Psychological Signs and Symptoms
  .19   With Predominantly Physical Signs and Symptoms
  .19   With Combined Psychological and Physical Signs and Symptoms
300.19 Factitious Disorder NOS

● DISSOCIATIVE DISORDERS

300.12   Dissociative Amnesia
300.13   Dissociative Fugue
300.14   Dissociative Identity Disorder
300.6   Depersonalization Disorder
300.15   Dissociative Disorder NOS

● SEXUAL AND GENDER IDENTITY DISORDERS

Sexual Dysfunctions

Sexual Desire Disorders

302.71   Hypoactive Sexual Desire Disorder
302.79   Sexual Aversion Disorder

Sexual Arousal Disorders

302.72   Female Sexual Arousal Disorder
302.72   Male Erectile Disorder

Orgasmic Disorders

302.73   Female Orgasmic Disorder
302.74   Male Orgasmic Disorder
302.75   Premature Ejaculation

Sexual Pain Disorders

302.76   Dyspareunia (Not Due to a General Medical Condition)
306.51   Vaginismus (Not Due to a General Medical Condition)

Sexual Dysfunction Due to a General Medical Condition

625.8   Female Hypoactive Sexual Desire Disorder Due to *(Indicate the General Medical Condition)*
608.89   Male Hypoactive Sexual Desire Disorder Due to *(Indicate the General Medical Condition)*
607.84   Male Erectile Disorder Due to *(Indicate the General Medical Condition)*
625.0   Female Dyspareunia Due to *(Indicate the General Medical Condition)*
608.89   Male Dyspareunia Due to *(Indicate the General Medical Condition)*
625.8   Other Female Sexual Dysfunction Due to *(Indicate the General Medical Condition)*
608.89   Other Male Sexual Dysfunction Due to *(Indicate the General Medical Condition)*
—   Substance-Induced Sexual Dysfunction *(refer to Substance-Related Disorders for substance-specific codes)*
302.70   Sexual Dysfunction NOS

Paraphilias

302.4   Exhibitionism
302.81   Fetishism
302.89   Frotteurism
302.2   Pedophilia
302.83   Sexual Masochism
302.84   Sexual Sadism
302.3   Transvestic Fetishism
302.82   Voyeurism
302.9   Paraphilia NOS

Gender Identity Disorders

302.xx   Gender Identity Disorder
  .6   In Children
  .85   In Adolescents or Adults
302.6   Gender Identity Disorder NOS
302.9   Sexual Disorder NOS

● EATING DISORDERS

307.1   Anorexia Nervosa
307.51   Bulimia Nervosa
307.50   Eating Disorder NOS

● SLEEP DISORDERS
Primary Sleep Disorders
Dyssomnias

307.42   Primary Insomnia
307.44   Primary Hypersomnia
347   Narcolepsy
780.59   Breathing-Related Sleep Disorder
307.45   Circadian Rhythm Sleep Disorder
307.47   Dyssomnia NOS

Parasomnias

307.47   Nightmare Disorder
307.46   Sleep Terror Disorder
307.46   Sleepwalking Disorder
307.47   Parasomnia NOS

Sleep Disorders Related to Another Mental Disorder

307.42   Insomnia Related to *(Indicate the Axis I or Axis II Disorder)*
307.44   Hypersomnia Related to *(Indicate the Axis I or Axis II Disorder)*

Other Sleep Disorders

780.xx   Sleep Disorder Due to *(Indicate the General Medical Condition)*
  .52   Insomnia type
  .54   Hypersomnia type
  .59   Parasomnia type
  .59   Mixed type
  —   Substance-Induced Sleep Disorder *(refer to Substance-Related Disorders for substance-specific codes)*

● IMPULSE CONTROL DISORDERS NOT ELSEWHERE CLASSIFIED

312.34   Intermittent Explosive Disorder
312.32   Kleptomania
312.33   Pyromania
312.31   Pathological Gambling
312.39   Trichotillomania
312.30   Impulse Control Disorder NOS

● ADJUSTMENT DISORDERS

309.xx   Adjustment Disorder
  .0   With Depressed Mood
  .24   With Anxiety
  .28   With Mixed Anxiety and Depressed Mood
  .3   With Disturbance of Conduct
  .4   With Mixed Disturbance of Emotions and Conduct
  .9   Unspecified

● PERSONALITY DISORDERS

Note: These are coded on Axis II.
301.0   Paranoid Personality Disorder
301.20   Schizoid Personality Disorder
301.22   Schizotypal Personality Disorder
301.7   Antisocial Personality Disorder
301.83   Borderline Personality Disorder
301.50   Histrionic Personality Disorder
301.81   Narcissistic Personality Disorder
301.82   Avoidant Personality Disorder
301.6   Dependent Personality Disorder
301.4   Obsessive-Compulsive Personality Disorder
301.9   Personality Disorder NOS

● OTHER CONDITIONS THAT MAY BE A FOCUS OF CLINICAL ATTENTION

Psychological Factors Affecting Medical Condition

316   *Choose name based on nature of factors:*
         Mental Disorder Affecting Medical Condition
         Psychological Symptoms Affecting Medical Condition
         Personality Traits or Coping Style Affecting Medical Condition
         Maladaptive Health Behaviors Affecting Medical Condition
         Stress-Related Physiological Response Affecting Medical Condition
         Other or Unspecified Psychological Factors Affecting Medical Condition

Medication-Induced Movement Disorders

332.1   Neuroleptic-Induced Parkinsonism
333.92   Neuroleptic Malignant Syndrome
333.7   Neuroleptic-Induced Acute Dystonia
333.99   Neuroleptic-Induced Acute Akathisia
333.82   Neuroleptic-Induced Tardive Dyskinesia
333.1   Medication-Induced Postural Tremor
333.90   Medication-Induced Movement Disorder NOS

Other Medication-Induced Disorder

995.2   Adverse Effects of Medication NOS

Relational Problems

V61.9   Relational Problem Related to a Mental Disorder or General Medical Condition
V61.20   Parent-Child Relational Problem
V61.10   Partner Relational Problem
V61.8   Sibling Relational Problem
V62.81   Relational Problem NOS

Problems Related to Abuse or Neglect

V61.21   Physical Abuse of Child
V61.21   Sexual Abuse of Child
V61.21   Neglect of Child
—   Physical Abuse of Adult
V61.12   (if by partner)
V62.83   (if by person other than partner)
—   Sexual Abuse of Adult

V61.12   (if by partner)
V62.83   (if by person other than partner)

Additional Conditions That May Be a Focus of Clinical Attention

V15.81   Noncompliance with Treatment
V65.2   Malingering
V71.01   Adult Antisocial Behavior
V71.02   Childhood or Adolescent Antisocial Behavior
V62.89   Borderline Intellectual Functioning (coded on Axis II)
780.9   Age-Related Cognitive Decline
V62.82   Bereavement
V62.3   Academic Problem
V62.2   Occupational Problem
313.82   Identity Problem
V62.89   Religious or Spiritual Problem
V62.4   Acculturation Problem
V62.89   Phase of Life Problem

● ADDITIONAL CODES

300.9   Unspecified Mental Disorder (nonpsychotic)
V71.09   No Diagnosis or Condition on Axis I
799.9   Diagnosis or Condition Deferred on Axis I
V71.09   No Diagnosis on Axis II
799.9   Diagnosis Deferred on Axis II

Mental Status Assessment

Gathering the correct information about the client's mental status is essential to the development of an appropriate plan of care. The mental status examination is a description of all the areas of the client's mental functioning. The following are the components that are considered critical in the assessment of a client's mental status. Examples of interview questions and criteria for assessment are included.

● IDENTIFYING DATA

1. Name
2. Gender
3. Age
   a. How old are you?
   b. When were you born?
4. Race/culture
   a. What country did you (your ancestors) come from?
5. Occupational/financial status
   a. How do you make your living?
   b. How do you obtain money for your needs?
6. Educational level
   a. What was the highest grade level you completed in school?
7. Significant other
   a. Are you married?
   b. Do you have a significant relationship with another person?
8. Living arrangements
   a. Do you live alone?
   b. With whom do you share your home?
9. Religious preference
   a. Do you have a religious preference?

10. Allergies
    a. Are you allergic to anything?
    b. Foods? Medications?
11. Special diet considerations
    a. Do you have any special diet requirements?
    b. Diabetic? Low sodium?
12. Chief complaint
    a. For what reason did you come for help today?
    b. What seems to be the problem?
13. Medical diagnosis

● GENERAL DESCRIPTION
Appearance

1. Grooming and dress
    a. Note unusual modes of dress.
    b. Evidence of soiled clothing?
    c. Use of makeup
    d. Neat; unkempt
2. Hygiene
    a. Note evidence of body or breath odor.
    b. Condition of skin, fingernails
3. Posture
    a. Note if standing upright, rigid, slumped over.
4. Height and weight
    a. Perform accurate measurements.
5. Level of eye contact
    a. Intermittent?
    b. Occasional and fleeting?
    c. Sustained and intense?
    d. No eye contact?
6. Hair color and texture
    a. Is hair clean and healthy-looking?
    b. Greasy, matted, tangled?
7. Evidence of scars, tattoos, or other distinguishing skin marks
    a. Note any evidence of swelling or bruises.
    b. Birth marks?
    c. Rashes?
8. Evaluation of client's appearance compared with chronological age.

Motor Activity

1. Tremors
    a. Do hands or legs tremble?
        • Continuously?
        • At specific times?

2. Tics or other stereotypical movements
   a. Any evidence of facial tics?
   b. Jerking or spastic movements?
3. Mannerisms and gestures
   a. Specific facial or body movements during conversation?
   b. Nail biting?
   c. Covering face with hands?
   d. Grimacing?
4. Hyperactivity
   a. Gets up and down out of chair
   b. Paces
   c. Unable to sit still
5. Restlessness or agitation
   a. Lots of fidgeting
   b. Clenching hands
6. Aggressiveness
   a. Overtly angry and hostile
   b. Threatening
   c. Uses sarcasm
7. Rigidity
   a. Sits or stands in a rigid position
   b. Arms and legs appear stiff and unyielding
8. Gait patterns
   a. Any evidence of limping?
   b. Limitation of range of motion?
   c. Ataxia?
   d. Shuffling?
9. Echopraxia
   a. Evidence of mimicking the actions of others?
10. Psychomotor retardation
    a. Movements are very slow.
    b. Thinking and speech are very slow.
    c. Posture is slumped.
11. Freedom of movement (range of motion)
    a. Note any limitation in ability to move.

Speech Patterns

1. Slowness or rapidity of speech
   a. Note whether speech seems very rapid or slower than normal.
2. Pressure of speech
   a. Note whether speech seems frenzied.
   b. Unable to be interrupted?
3. Intonation
   a. Are words spoken with appropriate emphasis?
   b. Are words spoken in monotone, without emphasis?

4. Volume
   a. Is speech very loud? Soft?
   b. Is speech low-pitched? High-pitched?
5. Stuttering or other speech impairments
   a. Hoarseness?
   b. Slurred speech?
6. Aphasia
   a. Difficulty forming words
   b. Use of incorrect words
   c. Difficulty thinking of specific words
   d. Making up words (neologisms)

General Attitude

1. Cooperative/uncooperative
   a. Answers questions willingly
   b. Refuses to answer questions
2. Friendly/hostile/defensive
   a. Is sociable and responsive
   b. Is sarcastic and irritable
3. Uninterested/apathetic
   a. Refuses to participate in interview process
4. Attentive/interested
   a. Actively participates in interview process
5. Guarded/suspicious
   a. Continuously scans the environment
   b. Questions motives of interviewer
   c. Refuses to answer questions

● EMOTIONS
Mood

1. Depressed; despairing
   a. An overwhelming feeling of sadness
   b. Loss of interest in regular activities
2. Irritable
   a. Easily annoyed and provoked to anger
3. Anxious
   a. Demonstrates or verbalizes feeling of apprehension
4. Elated
   a. Expresses feelings of joy and intense pleasure
   b. Is intensely optimistic
5. Euphoric
   a. Demonstrates a heightened sense of elation
   b. Expresses feelings of grandeur ("Everything is wonderful!")
6. Fearful
   a. Demonstrates or verbalizes feeling of apprehension associated with real or perceived danger

7. Guilty
    a. Expresses a feeling of discomfort associated with real or perceived wrongdoing
    b. May be associated with feelings of sadness and despair
8. Labile
    a. Exhibits mood swings that range from euphoria to depression or anxiety

Affect

1. Congruence with mood
    a. Outward emotional expression is consistent with mood (e.g., if depressed, emotional expression is sadness, eyes downcast, may be crying)
2. Constricted or blunted
    a. Minimal outward emotional expression is observed
3. Flat
    a. There is an absence of outward emotional expression
4. Appropriate
    a. The outward emotional expression is what would be expected in a certain situation (e.g., crying upon hearing of a death)
5. Inappropriate
    a. The outward emotional expression is incompatible with the situation (e.g., laughing upon hearing of a death)

● THOUGHT PROCESSES

Form of Thought

1. Flight of ideas
    a. Verbalizations are continuous and rapid, and flow from one to another
2. Associative looseness
    a. Verbalizations shift from one unrelated topic to another
3. Circumstantiality
    a. Verbalizations are lengthy and tedious, and because of numerous details, are delayed reaching the intended point
4. Tangentiality
    a. Verbalizations that are lengthy and tedious, and never reach an intended point
5. Neologisms
    a. The individual is making up nonsensical-sounding words, which only have meaning to him or her
6. Concrete thinking
    a. Thinking is literal; elemental
    b. Absence of ability to think abstractly
    c. Unable to translate simple proverbs

7. Clang associations
   a. Speaking in puns or rhymes; using words that sound alike but have different meanings
8. Word salad
   a. Using a mixture of words that have no meaning together; sounding incoherent
9. Perseveration
   a. Persistently repeating the last word of a sentence spoken to the client. (e.g., Nurse: "George, it's time to go to lunch." George: "lunch, lunch, lunch, lunch")
10. Echolalia
    a. Persistently repeating what another person says
11. Mutism
    a. Does not speak (either cannot or will not)
12. Poverty of speech
    a. Speaks very little; may respond in monosyllables
13. Ability to concentrate and disturbance of attention
    a. Does the person hold attention to the topic at hand?
    b. Is the person easily distractible?
    c. Is there selective attention (e.g., blocks out topics that create anxiety)?

Content of Thought

1. Delusions (Does the person have unrealistic ideas or beliefs?)
   a. Persecutory: A belief that someone is out to get him or her in some way (e.g., "The FBI will be here at any time to take me away.").
   b. Grandiose: An idea that he or she is all-powerful or of great importance (e.g., "I am the king...and this is my kingdom! I can do anything!").
   c. Reference: An idea that whatever is happening in the environment is about him or her (e.g., "Just watch the movie on TV tonight. It is about my life.").
   d. Control or influence: A belief that his or her behavior and thoughts are being controlled by external forces (e.g., "I get my orders from Channel 27. I do only what the forces dictate.").
   e. Somatic: A belief that he or she has a dysfunctional body part (e.g., "My heart is at a standstill. It is no longer beating.").
   f. Nihilistic: A belief that he or she, or a part of the body, or even the world does not exist or has been destroyed (e.g., "I am no longer alive.").
2. Suicidal or homicidal ideas
   a. Is the individual expressing ideas of harming self or others?

3. Obsessions
   a. Is the person verbalizing about a persistent thought or feeling that he or she is unable to eliminate from their consciousness?
4. Paranoia/suspiciousness
   a. Continuously scans the environment
   b. Questions motives of interviewer
   c. Refuses to answer questions
5. Magical thinking
   a. Is the client speaking in a way that indicates his or her words or actions have power? (e.g., "If you step on a crack, you break your mother's back!")
6. Religiosity
   a. Is the individual demonstrating obsession with religious ideas and behavior?
7. Phobias
   a. Is there evidence of irrational fears (of a specific object, or a social situation)?
8. Poverty of content
   a. Is little information conveyed by the client because of vagueness or stereotypical statements or clichés?

● PERCEPTUAL DISTURBANCES

1. Hallucinations (Is the person experiencing unrealistic sensory perceptions?)
   a. Auditory (Is the individual hearing voices or other sounds that do not exist?)
   b. Visual (Is the individual seeing images that do not exist?)
   c. Tactile (Does the individual feel unrealistic sensations on the skin?)
   d. Olfactory (Does the individual smell odors that do not exist?)
   e. Gustatory (Does the individual have a false perception of an unpleasant taste?)
2. Illusions
   a. Does the individual misperceive or misinterpret real stimuli within the environment? (Sees something and thinks it is something else?)
3. Depersonalization (altered perception of the self)
   a. The individual verbalizes feeling "outside the body;" visualizing him- or herself from afar.
4. Derealization (altered perception of the environment)
   a. The individual verbalizes that the environment feels "strange or unreal." A feeling that the surroundings have changed.

APPENDIX M ● **617**

● SENSORIUM AND COGNITIVE ABILITY

1. Level of alertness/consciousness
   a. Is the individual clear-minded and attentive to the environment?
   b. Or is there disturbance in perception and awareness of the surroundings?
2. Orientation. Is the person oriented to the following?
   a. Time
   b. Place
   c. Person
   d. Circumstances
3. Memory
   a. Recent (Is the individual able to remember occurrences of the past few days?)
   b. Remote (Is the individual able to remember occurrences of the distant past?)
   c. Confabulation (Does the individual fill in memory gaps with experiences that have no basis in fact?)
4. Capacity for abstract thought
   a. Can the individual interpret proverbs correctly?
      • "What does 'no use crying over spilled milk' mean?"

● IMPULSE CONTROL

1. Ability to control impulses. (Does psychosocial history reveal problems with any of the following?)
   a. Aggression
   b. Hostility
   c. Fear
   d. Guilt
   e. Affection
   f. Sexual feelings

● JUDGMENT AND INSIGHT

1. Ability to solve problems and make decisions
   a. What are your plans for the future?
   b. What do you plan to do to reach your goals?
2. Knowledge about self
   a. Awareness of limitations
   b. Awareness of consequences of actions
   c. Awareness of illness
      • "Do you think you have a problem?"
      • "Do you think you need treatment?"
3. Adaptive/maladaptive use of coping strategies and ego defense mechanisms (e.g., rationalizing maladaptive behaviors, projection of blame, displacement of anger)

A PPENDIX N

Assigning Nursing Diagnoses to Client Behaviors

Following is a list of client behaviors and the NANDA nursing diagnoses that correspond to the behaviors and that may be used in planning care for the client exhibiting the specific behavioral symptoms.

Behaviors	*NANDA Nursing Diagnoses*
Aggression; hostility	Risk for injury; Risk for other-directed violence
Anorexia or refusal to eat	Imbalanced nutrition: Less than body requirements
Anxious behavior	Anxiety (Specify level)
Confusion; memory loss	Confusion, acute/chronic; Disturbed thought processes; Impaired memory
Delusions	Disturbed thought processes
Denial of problems	Ineffective denial
Depressed mood or anger turned inward	Complicated grieving
Detoxification; withdrawal from substances	Risk for injury

Behaviors	*NANDA Nursing Diagnoses*
Difficulty accepting new diagnosis or recent change in health status	Risk-prone health behavior
Difficulty making important life decision	Decisional conflict (specify)
Difficulty sleeping	Insomnia; Disturbed sleep pattern
Difficulty with interpersonal relationships	Impaired social interaction
Disruption in capability to perform usual responsibilities	Ineffective role performance
Dissociative behaviors (depersonalization; derealization)	Disturbed sensory perception (kinesthetic)
Expresses feelings of disgust about body or body part	Disturbed body image
Expresses anger at God	Spiritual distress
Expresses lack of control over personal situation	Powerlessness
Fails to follow prescribed therapy	Ineffective self-health management; Noncompliance
Flashbacks, nightmares, obsession with traumatic experience	Posttrauma syndrome
Hallucinations	Disturbed sensory perception (auditory; visual)
Highly critical of self or others	Low self-esteem (chronic; situational)
HIV-positive; altered immunity	Ineffective protection

Continued

Behaviors	*NANDA Nursing Diagnoses*
Inability to meet basic needs	Self-care deficit (feeding; bathing; dressing; toileting)
Loose associations or flight of ideas	Impaired verbal communication
Loss of a valued entity, recently experienced	Risk for complicated grieving
Manic hyperactivity	Risk for injury
Manipulative behavior	Ineffective coping
Multiple personalities; gender identity disturbance	Disturbed personal identity
Orgasm, problems with; lack of sexual desire; erectile dysfunction	Sexual dysfunction
Overeating, compulsive	Risk for imbalanced nutrition: More than body requirements
Phobias	Fear
Physical symptoms as coping behavior	Ineffective coping
Potential or anticipated loss of significant entity	Grieving
Projection of blame; rationalization of failures; denial of personal responsibility	Defensive coping
Ritualistic behaviors	Anxiety (severe); Ineffective coping
Seductive remarks; inappropriate sexual behaviors	Impaired social interaction
Self-inflicted injuries (non-life-threatening)	Self-mutilation; Risk for self-mutilation

Behaviors	*NANDA Nursing Diagnoses*
Sexual behaviors (difficulty, limitations, or changes in; reported dissatisfaction)	Ineffective sexuality pattern
Stress from caring for chronically ill person	Caregiver role strain
Stress from locating to new environment	Relocation stress syndrome
Substance use as a coping behavior	Ineffective coping
Substance use (denies use is a problem)	Ineffective denial
Suicidal gestures/threats; suicidal ideation	Risk for suicide; Risk for self-directed violence
Suspiciousness	Disturbed thought processes; Ineffective coping
Vomiting, excessive, self-induced	Risk for deficient fluid volume
Withdrawn behavior	Social isolation

Brief Mental Status Evaluation

Area of Mental Function Evaluated	Evaluation Activity
Orientation to time	"What year is it? What month is it? What day is it? (3 points)
Orientation to place	"Where are you now?" (1 point)
Attention and immediate recall	"Repeat these words now: bell, book, & candle" (3 points) "Remember these words and I will ask you to repeat them in a few minutes."
Abstract thinking	"What does this mean: No use crying over spilled milk." (3 points)
Recent memory	"Say the 3 words I asked you to remember earlier." (3 points)
Naming objects	Point to eyeglasses and ask, "What is this?" Repeat with 1 other item (e.g., calendar, watch, pencil). (2 points possible)
Ability to follow simple verbal command	"Tear this piece of paper in half and put it in the trash container." (2 points)

Ability to follow simple written command	Write a command on a piece of paper (e.g., TOUCH YOUR NOSE), give the paper to the patient and say, "Do what it says on this paper." (1 point for correct action)
Ability to use language correctly	Ask the patient to write a sentence. (3 points if sentence has a subject and a verb, and has valid meaning).
Ability to concentrate	"Say the months of the year in reverse, starting with December." (1 point each for correct answers from November through August. 4 points possible.)
Understanding spatial relationships	Draw a clock; put in all the numbers; and set the hands on 3 o'clock. (clock circle = 1 point; numbers in correct sequence = 1 point; numbers placed on clock correctly = 1 point; two hands on the clock = 1 point; hands set at correct time = 1 point. 5 points possible.)

Scoring: 30 to 21 = normal; 20 to 11 = mild cognitive impairment; 10 to 0 = severe cognitive impairment (scores are not absolute and must be considered within the comprehensive diagnostic assessment).

Sources: *The Merck manual of health and aging* (2005); Folstein, Folstein, and McHugh (1975); Kaufman and Zun (1995); Kokman et al. (1991); and Pfeiffer (1975).

APPENDIX P

U.S. Food and Drug Administration (FDA) Pregnancy Categories

Category A   Adequate, well-controlled studies in pregnant women have not shown an increased risk of fetal abnormalities.

Category B   Animal studies have revealed no evidence of harm to the fetus; however, there are no adequate and well-controlled studies in pregnant women.
OR Animal studies have shown an adverse effect, but adequate and well-controlled studies in pregnant women have failed to demonstrate a risk to the fetus.

Category C   Animal studies have shown an adverse effect and there are no adequate and well-controlled studies in pregnant women.
OR No animal studies have been conducted and there are no adequate and well-controlled studies in pregnant women.

Category D   Studies, adequate well-controlled or observational, in pregnant women have demonstrated a risk to the fetus. However, the benefits of therapy may outweigh the potential risk.

Category X Studies, adequate well-controlled or observational, in animals or pregnant women have demonstrated positive evidence of fetal abnormalities. The use of the product is contraindicated in women who are or may become pregnant.

Source: From Deglin, J.H., & Vallerand, A.H. (2009). *Davis's drug guide for nurses* (11th ed.). Philadelphia: F.D. Davis. With permission.

U.S. Drug Enforcement Agency (DEA) Controlled Substances Schedules

Classes or schedules are determined by the DEA, an arm of the U.S. Justice Department, and are based on the potential for abuse and dependence liability (physical and psychological) of the medication. Some states may have stricter prescription regulations. Physicians, dentists, podiatrists, and veterinarians may prescribe controlled substances. Nurse practitioners and physician's assistants may prescribe controlled substances with certain limitations.

Schedule I (C-I)
Potential for abuse is so high as to be unacceptable. May be used for research with appropriate limitations. Examples are LSD and heroin.

Schedule II (C-II)
High potential for abuse and extreme liability for physical and psychological dependence (amphetamines, opioid analgesics, dronabinol, certain barbiturates). Outpatient prescriptions must be in writing. In emergencies, telephone orders may be acceptable if a written prescription is provided within 72 hours. No refills are allowed.

Schedule III (C-III)
Intermediate potential for abuse (less than C-II) and intermediate liability for physical and psychological dependence (certain non-barbiturate sedatives, certain nonamphetamine CNS stimulants, and limited dosages of certain opioid analgesics). Outpatient

prescriptions can be refilled 5 times within 6 months from date of issue if authorized by prescriber. Telephone orders are acceptable.

Schedule IV (C-IV)

Less abuse potential than Schedule III with minimal liability for physical or psychological dependence (certain sedative/hypnotics, certain antianxiety agents, some barbiturates, benzodiazepines, chloral hydrate, pentazocine, and propoxyphene). Outpatient prescriptions can be refilled 6 times within 6 months from date of issue if authorized by prescriber. Telephone orders are acceptable.

Schedule V (C-V)

Minimal abuse potential. Number of outpatient refills determined by prescriber. Some products (cough suppressants with small amounts of codeine, antidiarrheals containing paregoric) may be available without prescription to patients at least 18 years of age.

Source: From Deglin, J.H., & Vallerand, A.H. (2009). *Davis's drug guide for nurses* (11th ed.). Philadelphia: F.D. Davis. With permission.

Abnormal Involuntary Movement Scale (AIMS)

The AIMS rating scale is a 5- to 10-minute rating scale to assess for tardive dyskinesia (TD). A baseline exam should be administered before instituting pharmacotherapy with antipsychotics, and then every 3 to 6 months thereafter.

There are two parallel procedures, the *Examination Procedure*, which tells the client what to do, and the *Scoring Procedure*, which tells the clinician how to rate what he or she observes.

Examination Procedure

Either before or after completing the Examination Procedure, observe the client unobtrusively, at rest (e.g., in waiting room). The chair to be used in this examination should be a hard, firm one without arms.

1. Ask client to remove shoes and socks.
2. Ask client whether there is anything in his/her mouth (i.e., gum, candy, etc.), and if there is, to remove it.
3. Ask client about the current condition of his/her teeth. Ask client if he/she wears dentures. Do teeth or dentures bother client now?
4. Ask client whether he/she notices any movements in mouth, face, hands, or feet. If yes, ask him/her to describe and to what extent they currently bother client or interfere with his/her activities.
5. Have client sit in chair with both hands on knees, legs slightly apart, and feet flat on floor. (Look at entire body for movements while in this position.)
6. Ask client to sit with hands hanging unsupported. If male, between legs, if female and wearing a dress, hanging over knees. (Observe hands and other body areas.)
7. Ask client to open mouth. (Observe tongue at rest within mouth.) Do this twice.

8. Ask client to protrude tongue. (Observe abnormalities of tongue movement.) Do this twice.
9. Ask client to tap thumb with each finger as rapidly as possible for 10 to 15 seconds; separately with right hand, then with left hand. (Observe facial and leg movements.)
10. Flex and extend client's left and right arms (one at a time). (Note any rigidity.)
11. Ask client to stand up. (Observe in profile. Observe all body areas again, hips included.)
12. Ask client to extend both arms outstretched in front with palms down. (Observe trunk, legs, and mouth.)
13. Have client walk a few paces, turn, and walk back to chair. (Observe hands and gait.) Do this twice.

Scoring Procedure

Instructions: Complete examination procedure before making ratings.
Rate highest severity observed.

Code: 0 None
       1 Minimal, may be extreme normal
       2 Mild
       3 Moderate
       4 Severe

Facial and Oral Movements

1. Muscles of Facial Expression (e.g., movement of forehead, eyebrows, periorbital area, cheeks; include frowning, blinking, smiling, grimacing)

    0 1 2 3 4

2. Lips and Perioral Area (e.g., puckering, pouting, smacking)

    0 1 2 3 4

3. Jaws (e.g., biting, clenching, chewing, mouth opening, lateral movement)

    0 1 2 3 4

4. Tongue (Rate only increase in movement both in and out of mouth, NOT inability to sustain movement.)

    0 1 2 3 4

Extremity Movements

5. Upper (arms, wrists, hands, fingers). Include choreic movements (i.e., rapid, objectively purposeless, irregular, spontaneous), athetoid movements (i.e., slow, irregular, complex, serpentine). Do NOT include tremor (i.e., repetitive, regular, rhythmic).

    0 1 2 3 4

6. Lower (legs, knees, ankles, toes) (e.g., lateral knee movement, foot taping, heel dropping, foot squirming, inversion and eversion of foot)

0 1 2 3 4

Trunk Movements

7. Neck, shoulders, hips (e.g., rocking, twisting, squirming, pelvic gyrations)

0 1 2 3 4

Global Judgments

8. Severity of abnormal movements:
   0 1 2 3 4 (Based on the highest single score on the above items.)
9. Incapacitation due to abnormal movements:
   0 None, normal
   1 Minimal
   2 Mild
   3 Moderate
   4 Severe
10. Client's awareness of abnormal movements (Rate only client's report)
    0 No awareness
    1 Aware, no distress
    2 Aware, mild distress
    3 Aware, moderate distress
    4 Aware, severe distress

Dental Status

11. Current problems with teeth and/or dentures
    0 No
    1 Yes
12. Does client usually wear dentures?
    0 No
    1 Yes

Interpretation of AIMS Score

Add client scores and note areas of difficulty.
Score of:
- 0 to 1 = low risk
- 2 in only ONE of the areas assessed = borderline/observe closely
- 2 in TWO or more of the areas assessed **or** 3 to 4 in ONLY ONE area = indicative of TD

Source: U.S. Department of Health and Human Services. Available for use in the public domain.

Bibliography

Aguilera, D.C. (1998). *Crisis intervention: Theory and methodology* (8th ed.) St. Louis: C.V. Mosby.

American Academy of Child and Adolescent Psychiatry. (2002). *Children of alcoholics.* Retrieved January 13, 2010, from http://www.aacap.org/galleries/FactsForFamilies/17_children_of_alchoholics.pdf

American Nurses' Association (ANA). (2008). *Home health nursing: Scope and standards of practice.* Silver Spring, MD: ANA.

American Nurses' Association (ANA). (2010). *Nursing's social policy statement*: The essence of the profession. Silver Spring, MD: ANA.

American Nurses' Association (ANA). (2010). *Scope and standards of practice.* (2nd ed.). Silver Spring, MD: ANA.

American Psychiatric Association. (2000). *Diagnostic and statistical manual of mental disorders, fourth edition, text revision.* Washington, DC: American Psychiatric Publishing.

Avants, S.K., Margolin, A., Holford, T.R., & Kosten, T.R. (2000). A randomized controlled trial of auricular acupuncture for cocaine dependence. *Archives of Internal Medicine, 160*(15), 2305-2312.

Bagley, C., & Mallick, K. (2000). Spiralling up and spiralling down: Implications of a long-term study of temperament and conduct disorder for social work with children. *Child & Family Social Work 5*(4), 291-301.

Banks, M.R., & Banks, W.A. (2002). The effects of animal-assisted therapy on loneliness in an elderly population in long-term care facilities. *The Journals of Gerontology Series A: Biological Sciences and Medical Sciences, 57*(7), M428-M432.

Bateman, A.L. (1999). Understanding the process of grieving and loss: A critical social thinking perspective. *Journal of the American Psychiatric Nurses Association, 5*(5), 139-147.

Beck, A., Rush, A.J., Shaw, B.F., & Emery, G. (1979). *Cognitive theory of depression.* New York; Guilford Press.

Becker, J.V., & Johnson, B.R. (2008). Gender identity disorders and paraphilias. In R.E. Hales, S.C. Yudofsky, & G.O. Gabbard (Eds.), *The American Psychiatric Publishing textbook of clinical psychiatry* (5th ed.). Washington, DC: American Psychiatric Publishing.

Becker, J.V., & Stinson, J.D. (2008). Human sexuality and sexual dysfunctions. In R.E. Hales, S.C. Yudofsky, & G.O. Gabbard (Eds.), *The American Psychiatric Publishing textbook of clinical psychiatry* (5th ed.). Washington, DC: American Psychiatric Publishing.

Bellfield, B. & Catalano, J.T. (2009). Developments in current nursing practice. In J.T. Catalano (Ed.), *Nursing now! Today's issues, tomorrow's trends* (5th ed.). Philadelphia: F.A. Davis.

Black, D.W. & Andreasen, N.C. (2011). *Introductory textbook of psychiatry* (5th ed.). Washington, DC: American Psychiatric Publishing.

Blumenthal, M. (Ed.). (1998). *The complete German Commission E monographs: Therapeutic guide to herbal medicines.* Austin, TX: American Botanical Garden.

Bourgeois, J.A., Seaman, J.S., & Servis, M.E. (2008). Delirium, dementia, and amnestic and other cognitive disorders. In R.E. Hales, S.C. Yudofsky, & G.O. Gabbard (Eds.), *The American Psychiatric Publishing textbook of psychiatry* (5th ed.). Washington DC: American Psychiatric Publishing.

Bowlby, J. (1961). Processes of mourning. *International Journal of Psychoanalysis, 42,* 317-322.

Burgess, A. (2009). Rape violence. *Nursing Spectrum/NurseWeek CE: Course 60025.* Retrieved August 19, 2010 from http://ce.nurse.com/60025/Rape-Violence/.

Catalano, J.T. (2009). *Nursing now! Today's issues, tomorrow's trends* (5th ed.). Philadelphia: FA Davis.

Cheong, J., Herkov, M., & Goodman, W. (2009). Frequently asked questions about depression. *PsychCentral.* Retrieved November 15, 2009, from http://psychcentral.com/library/depression_faq.htm

Chess, S., Thomas, A., & Birch., H. (1970). The origins of personality. *Scientific American 223,* 102.

Child Welfare Information Gateway (CWIG). (2008). *What is child abuse and neglect?* Retrieved August 11, 2009, from http://www.childwelfare.gov/pubs/factsheets/whatiscan.cfm

Coeytaux, R.R., Kaufman, J.S., Kaptchuk, T.J., Chen, W., Miller, W.M., Callahan, L.F., and Mann, J.D. (2005). A randomized, controlled trial of acupuncture for chronic daily headache. *Headache, 45*(9), 1113-1123.

College and Association of Registered Nurses of Alberta (CARNA). (2005). *Professional boundaries for registered nurses: Guidelines for the nurse-client relationship.* Edmonton, AB: CARNA.

Coniglione, T. (1998). Our doctors must begin looking at the total person. *InBalance.* Oklahoma City, OK: The Balanced Healing Medical Center.

Corr, C.A., Nabe, C.M., & Corr, D.M. (2008). *Death and dying.* Florence, KY: Cengage Learning.

Council of Acupuncture and Oriental Medicine Associations (CAOMA). (2009). *Conditions treated by acupuncture and oriental medicine.* Retrieved November 14, 2009, from http://www.acucouncil.org/conditions_treated.htm

Cummings, J.L., & Mega, M.S. (2003). *Neuropsychiatry and behavioral neuroscience.* New York: Oxford University Press.

Curtis, C.M., Fegley, A.B., & Tuzo, C.N. (2009). *Psychiatric mental health nursing success.* Philadelphia: FA Davis.

Deglin, J.H., & Vallerand, A.H. (2009). *Davis's drug guide for nurses* (11th ed.). Philadelphia: FA Davis.

Dion, Y., Annable, L., Sandor, P., & Chouinard, G. (2002). Risperidone in the treatment of Tourette syndrome: A double-blind, placebo-controlled trial. *Journal of Clinical Psychopharmacology, 22*(1), 31-39.

Doenges, M.E., Moorhouse, M.F., & Murr, A.C. (2010). *Nurse's pocket guide: Diagnoses, prioritized interventions, and rationales* (12th ed.). Philadelphia: FA Davis.

Doenges, M.E., Moorhouse, M.F., & Murr, A.C. (2010). *Nursing diagnosis manual: Planning, individualizing, and documenting client care* (3rd ed.). Philadelphia: FA Davis.

Dopheide, J.A. (2001). ADHD Part 1: Current status, diagnosis, etiology/pathophysiology. American Pharmaceutical Association 148th Annual Meeting, San Francisco, CA, March 16-20, 2001.

Eisendrath, S.J., & Lichtmacher, J.E. (2009). Psychiatric disorders. In S.J. McPhee, & M.A. Papadakis (Eds.), *Current medical diagnosis and treatment* (48th ed.). New York: McGraw-Hill.

Engel, G.L. (1964). Grief and grieving. *American Journal of Nursing, 64,* 93–97.

Erikson, E.H. (1963). *Childhood and society.* New York: WW Norton.

Finkelman, A.W. (1997). *Psychiatric home care.* Gaithersburg, MD: Aspen Publications.

Foley, D.L., Eaves, L.J., Wormley, B., Silberg, J.L., Maes, H.H., Kuhn, J., & Riley, B. (2004). Childhood adversity, monoamine oxidase A genotype, and risk for conduct disorder. *Archives of General Psychiatry, 61*(7), 738-744.

Folstein, M.F., Folstein, S.E., & McHugh, P.R. (1975). "Mini-Mental State": A practical method for grading the cognitive state of patients for the clinician. *Journal of Psychiatric Research, 12*(3), 189-198.

Foroud, T., Gray, J., Ivashina, J., & Conneally, P.M. (1999). Differences in duration of Huntington's disease based on age at onset. *Journal of Neurology, Neurosurgery and Psychiatry, 66*(1), 52-56.

Freud, S. (1894/1962). The neuro-psychoses of defense. In Strachey, J. (Ed.), *Standard edition of the complete psychological works of Sigmund Freud, Vol 3.* London: Hogarth Press.

Friedmann, E., & Thomas, S.A. (1995). Pet ownership, social support, and one-year survival after acute myocardial infarction in the cardiac arrhythmia suppression trial. *American Journal of Cardiology, 76*(17), 1213-1217.

Gibbons, R.D., Hur, K., Brown, C.H., & Mann, J.J. (2009). Relationship between antiepileptic drugs and suicide attempts in patients with bipolar disorder. *Archives of General Psychiatry, 66*(12), 1354-1360.

Godenne, G. (2001). The role of pets in nursing homes...and psychotherapy. *The Maryland Psychiatrist, 27*(3), 5-6.

Gordon, M. (1994). *Nursing diagnosis: Process and application* (3rd ed.). St. Louis: Mosby–Year Book.

Haddad, P.M. (2001). Antidepressant discontinuation syndromes: Clinical relevance, prevention, and management. *Drug Safety, 24*(3), 183-197.

Halmi, K.A. (2008). Eating disorders: Anorexia nervosa, bulimia nervosa, and obesity. In R.E. Hales, S.C. Yudofsky, & G.O. Gabbard (Eds.), *The American Psychiatric Publishing textbook of clinical psychiatry* (5th ed.). Washington, DC: American Psychiatric Publishing.

Halstead, H. L. (2005). Spirituality in older adults. In M. Stanley, K.A. Blair, & P. G. Beare (Eds.), *Gerontological nursing: A health promotion/protection approach* (3rd ed.). Philadelphia: FA Davis.

Hare, C.B. (2006). Clinical overview of HIV disease. *InSite HIV Knowledge Base.* Retrieved November 9, 2009, from http://hivinsite.ucsf.edu

Harvard Medical School. (2005). The homeless mentally ill. *Harvard Mental Health Letter, 21*(11), 4-7.

Harvard Medical School. (2001). *Alcohol use and abuse.* Boston, MA: Harvard Health Publications.

Harvard Medical School. (2001). Bipolar disorder—Part I. *The Harvard Mental Health Letter, 17*(10), 1-4.

Hays, J.S., & Larson, K.H. (1963). *Interacting with patients*. New York: Holt, Rinehart, & Winston.

Hill, J. (2003). Early identification of individuals at risk for antisocial personality disorder. *British Journal of Psychiatry, 182*(suppl 44), s11-s14.

Hollander, E., Berlin, H.A., & Stein, D.J. (2008). Impulse-control disorders not elsewhere classified. In R.E. Hales, S.C. Yudofsky, & G.O. Gabbard (Eds.), *The American Psychiatric Publishing textbook of clinical psychiatry* (5th ed.). Washington, DC: American Psychiatric Publishing.

Ho, B.C., Black, D.W., & Andreasen, N.C. (2003). Schizophrenia and other psychotic disorders. In R.E. Hales & S.C. Yudofsky (Eds.), *The American Psychiatric Publishing textbook of clinical psychiatry* (4th ed.). Washington, DC: American Psychiatric Publishing.

Holt, G.A., & Kouzi, S. (2002). Herbs through the ages. In M.A. Bright (Ed.), *Holistic health and healing*. Philadelphia: FA Davis.

Hufft, A., & Peternelj-Taylor, C. (2003). Forensic nursing: A specialty for the twenty-first century. In J.T. Catalano (Ed.), *Nursing now! Today's issues, tomorrow's trends* (3rd ed.). Philadelphia: FA Davis.

International Association of Forensic Nurses (IAFN). (2009). *What is forensic nursing?* Retrieved November 13, 2009, from http://www.iafn.org/

International Association of Forensic Nurses (IAFN) and American Nurses' Association (ANA). (2009). *Forensic nursing: Scope and standards of practice*. Silver Spring, MD: ANA.

James, D.J., & Glaze, L.E. (2006). *Mental health problems of prison and jail inmates*. Bureau of Justice Statistics Special Report, September 2006.

Jensen, J.E., & Miller, B. (2004). *Home health psychiatric care: A guide to understanding home health psychiatric care as covered under Medicare Part A*. Seattle, WA: The Washington Institute for Mental Illness Research and Training.

Joint Commission, The. (2010). *The comprehensive accreditation manual for hospitals: The official handbook* (January, 2010). Oakbrook Terrace, IL: Joint Commission Resources.

Jonsson, S.A., Luts, A., Guldberg-Kjaer, N., & Brun, A. (1997). Hippocampal pyramidal cell disarray correlates negatively to cell number: Implications for the pathogenesis of schizophrenia. *European Archives of Psychiatry and Clinical Neuroscience, 247*(3), 120-127.

Joska, J.A., & Stein, D.J. (2008). Mood disorders. In R.E. Hales, S.C. Yudofsky, & G.O. Gabbard (Eds.), *The American Psychiatric Publishing textbook of clinical psychiatry* (5th ed.). Washington, DC: American Psychiatric Publishing.

Julien, R.M. (2008). *A primer of drug action: A comprehensive guide to the actions, uses, and side effects of psychoactive drugs* (11th ed.). New York: Worth Publishers.

Kaufman, D.M., & Zun, L. (1995). A quantifiable, brief mental status examination for emergency patients. *Journal of Emergency Medicine, 13*(4), 449-456.

King, B.M. (2009). *Human sexuality today* (6th ed.). Upper Saddle River, NJ: Pearson Education.

Kokman, E., Smith, G.E., Petersen, R.C., Tangalos, E., & Ivnik, R.C. (1991). The short test of mental status: Correlations with standardized psychometric testing. *Archives of Neurology, 48*(7), 725-728.

Kübler-Ross, E. (1969). *On death and dying*. New York: Macmillan.

Ladd, G.W. (1999). Peer relationships and social competence during early and middle childhood. *Annual Review of Psychology, 50,* 333-359.

Lagerquist, S.L. (2006). *Davis's NCLEX-RN Success* (2nd ed.). Philadelphia: FA Davis.

Ledray, L.E. (2001). Evidence collection and care of the sexual assault survivor: The SANE-SART response. *Violence against women.* Retrieved November 13, 2009, from http://www.mincava.umn.edu/documents/commissioned/2forensicevidence/2forensicevidence.html

Leiblum, S.R. (1999). Sexual problems and dysfunction: Epidemiology, classification, and risk factors. *The Journal of Gender-Specific Medicine, 2*(5), 41-45.

Linnet, K.M., Wisborg, K., Obel, C., Secher, N.J., Thomsen, P.H., Agerbo, E., &, Henriksen, T.B. (2005). Smoking during pregnancy and the risk for hyperkinetic disorder in offspring. *Pediatrics, 116*(2), 462-467.

Lubit, R.H., & Finley-Belgrad, E.A. (2008). Borderline personality disorder. *eMedicine Psychiatry.* Retrieved July 17, 2009, from http://emedicine.medscape.com/article/913575

Lutz, C.A., & Przytulski, K.R. (2010). *Nutrition and diet therapy evidence-based applications* (5th ed.). Philadelphia: FA Davis.

Lynch, V.A. (2006). *Forensic nursing.* St. Louis: Mosby.

Lynch, V.A., Roach, C.W., & Sadler, D.W. (2006). Education and credentialing for forensic nurses. In V.A. Lynch (Ed.). *Forensic nursing.* St. Louis: Mosby.

Mack, A.H., Franklin, J.E., & Frances, R.J. (2003). Substance use disorders. In R.E. Hales & S.C. Yudofsky (Eds.), *The American Psychiatric Publishing textbook of clinical psychiatry* (4th ed.). Washington, DC: American Psychiatric Publishing.

Mahler, M., Pine, F., & Bergman, A. (1975). *The psychological birth of the human infant.* New York: Basic Books.

Marangell, L.B., Silver, J.M., Goff, D.C., & Yudofsky, S.C. (2003). Psychopharmacology and electroconvulsive therapy. In R.E. Hales & S.C. Yudofsky (Eds.), *The American Psychiatric Publishing textbook of clinical psychiatry.* Washington, DC: American Psychiatric Publishing.

Merck Manual of Health and Aging. (2005). New York: Random House Publishing Group.

Minzenberg, M.J., Yoon, J.H., & Stein, D.J. (2008). Schizophrenia. In R.E. Hales, S.C. Yudofsky, & G.O. Gabbard (Eds.), *The American Psychiatric Publishing textbook of clinical psychiatry* (5th ed.). Washington, DC: American Psychiatric Publishing.

Murray, R.B., Zentner, J.P., & Yakimo, R. (2009). *Health promotion strategies through the life span* (8th ed.). Upper Saddle River, NJ: Prentice-Hall.

NANDA International (NANDA-I). (2009). *About NANDA International.* Retrieved January 27, 2009, from http://www.nanda.org/AboutUs.aspx

NANDA International (NANDA-I). (2009). *Nursing diagnoses: Definitions and classification, 2009-2011.* Hoboken, NJ: Wiley-Blackwell.

National Center for Complementary and Alternative Medicine (NCCAM). (2009). *Facts-at-a-glance and mission.* Retrieved January 13, 2010, from http://nccam.nih.gov/about/ataglance/

National Center for Complementary and Alternative Medicine (NCCAM). (2007). *Acupuncture: An introduction.* Retrieved January 13, 2010, from http://nccam.nih.gov/health/acupuncture/D404_BKG.pdf

National Coalition for the Homeless (NCH). (2007). *Who is homeless?* Retrieved September 3, 2009, from http://www.nationalhomeless .org/factsheets/who.html

National Coalition for the Homeless (NCH). (2008a). *How many people experience homelessness?* Retrieved September 3, 2009, from http:// www.nationalhomeless.org/factsheets/how_many.html

National Coalition for the Homeless (NCH). (2008b). *Why are people homeless?* Retrieved September 3, 2009, from http://www .nationalhomeless.org/factsheets/why.html

National Coalition for the Homeless (NCH). (2008c). *HIV/AIDS and homelessness.* Retrieved September 3, 2009, from http://www .nationalhomeless.org/factsheets/hiv.html

National Coalition for the Homeless (NCH). (2008d). *Homeless families with children.* Retrieved September 3, 2009, from http://www .nationalhomeless.org/factsheets/families.html

National Council of State Boards of Nursing (NCSBN). (2010). *Test plan for the National Council Licensure Examination for Registered Nurses.* Retrieved January 14, 2010, from http://www.ncsbn.org

National Institutes of Health (NIH). (2008). *The use of complementary and alternative medicine in the United States.* Bethesda, MD: NIH.

National Institute of Mental Health (NIMH). (2009). Borderline personality disorder: Raising questions, finding answers. Retrieved July 20, 2009, from http://www.nimh.nih.gov/health/publications/ borderline-personality-disorder-fact-sheet/index.shtml

National Institute of Mental Health (NIMH). (2009). *Autism spectrum disorders.* NIH Publication No. 08-5511. Retrieved January 14, 2010, from http://www.nimh.nih.gov/health/publications/autism/index.shtml

New Mexico AIDS Education and Training Center. (2009). *CD4 (T-cell) tests.* Retrieved November 9, 2009, from http://www.aidsinfonet.org

Oldham, J.M., Gabbard, G.O., Goin, M.K., Gunderson, J., Soloff, P., Spiegel, D., Stone, M., & Phillips, K.A. (2006). Practice guideline for the treatment of patients with borderline personality disorder. In *The American Psychiatric Association practice guidelines for the treatment of psychiatric disorders, Compendium 2006.* Washington, DC: American Psychiatric Publishing.

PDR for herbal medicines (4th ed.). (2007). Montvale, NJ: Thomson Healthcare Inc.

Peplau, H.E. (1962). Interpersonal techniques: The crux of psychiatric nursing. *American Journal of Nursing 62*(6), 50-54.

Peplau, H.E. (1991). *Interpersonal relations in nursing.* New York: Springer.

Pfeiffer, E. (1975). A short portable mental status questionnaire for the assessment of organic brain deficit in elderly patients. *Journal of the American Geriatric Society, 23*(10), 433-441.

Phillips, N.A. (2000). Female sexual dysfunction: Evaluation and treatment. *American Family Physician, 62*(1), 127-136, 141-142.

Piaget, J., & Inhelder, B. (1969). *The psychology of the child.* New York: Basic Books.

Popper, C.W., Gammon, G.D., West, S.A., & Bailey, C.E. (2003). Disorders usually first diagnosed in infancy, childhood, or adolescence. In R.E. Hales & S.C. Yudofsky, (Eds.), *The American Psychiatric Publishing textbook of clinical psychiatry* (4th ed.). Washington, DC: The American Psychiatric Publishing.

Pranthikanti, S. (2007). Ayurvedic treatments. In J.H. Lake & D. Spiegel (Eds.), *Complementary and alternative treatments in mental health care.* Washington, DC: American Psychiatric Publishing.

Prator, B.C. (2006). Serotonin syndrome. *Journal of Neuroscience Nursing, 38*(2), 102-105.

Presser, A.M. (2000). *Pharmacist's guide to medicinal herbs.* Petaluma, CA: Smart Publications.

Priesnitz, W. (2005). Are you dying to lose weight? *Natural Life Magazine, Vol. 84*(2). Retrieved January 13, 2010, from http://www.life.ca/nl/84/weight.html

Rabins, P., Bland, W., Bright-Long, L., Cohen, E., Katz, I., Rovner, B., Schneider, L., & Blacker, D. (2006). Practice guideline for the treatment of patients with Alzheimer's disease and other dementias of late life. In *American Psychiatric Association practice guidelines for the treatment of psychiatric disorders, compendium 2006.* Washington, DC: American Psychiatric Association.

Ramsland, K. (2009). *The childhood psychopath: Bad seed or bad parents?* Retrieved July 20, 2009, from http://www.trutv.com/library/crime/criminal_mind/psychology/psychopath/4.html

Registered Nurses' Association of British Columbia (RNABC). (2003). *Nurse-client relationships.* Vancouver, BC: RNABC.

Sadock, B.J., & Sadock, V.A. (2007). *Synopsis of psychiatry: Behavioral sciences/clinical psychiatry* (10th ed.). Philadelphia: Lippincott Williams & Wilkins.

Sagrestano, L.M., Rogers, A., & Service, A. (2008). HIV/AIDS. In B.A. Boyer & M.I. Paharia (Eds.), *Comprehensive handbook of clinical health psychology.* Hoboken, NJ: John Wiley & Sons.

Schatzberg, A.F., Cole, J.O., & Debattista, C. (2010). *Manual of clinical psychopharmacology* (7th ed.). Washington, DC: American Psychiatric Publishing.

Schoenen, J., Jacquy, J., & Lenaerts, M. (1998). Effectiveness of high-dose riboflavin in migraine prophylaxis: A randomized controlled trial. *Neurology, 50*(2), 466-470.

Schroeder, B. (2009). Getting started in home care. *Nursing Spectrum CE Courses.* Retrieved November 11, 2009, from http://ce.nurse.com/60085/Getting-Started-in-Home-Care/

Schuster, P.M. (2002). *Concept mapping: A critical-thinking approach to care planning.* Philadelphia: FA Davis.

Seligman, M. (1974). Depression and learned helplessness. In R. Friedman, and M. Katz, (eds.), *The psychology of depression: Contemporary theory and research.* Washington, DC: V.H. Winston & Sons.

Selye, H. (1956). *The stress of life.* New York: McGraw-Hill.

Siegel, J.M., Angulo, F.J., Detels, R., Wesch, J., & Mullen, A. (1999). AIDS diagnosis and depression in the Multicenter AIDS Cohort Study: The ameliorating impact of pet ownership. *AIDS Care, 11*(2), 157-170.

Skinner, K. (1979, August). The therapeutic milieu: Making it work. *Journal of Psychiatric Nursing and Mental Health Services, 17*(8), 38-44.

Skodol, A.E., & Gunderson, J.G. (2008). Personality disorders. In R.E. Hales, S.C. Yudofsky, & G.O. Gabbard (Eds.), *The American Psychiatric Publishing textbook of clinical psychiatry* (5th ed.). Washington, DC: American Psychiatric Publishing.

Soares, N., & Grossman, L. (2007, November 28). Somatoform disorder: Conversion. *Emedicine Journal, 2*(9). Retrieved March 19, 2009, from http://www.emedicine.com/PED/topic2780.htm

Steinberg, L. (2002). Yoga. In M.A. Bright (Ed.), *Holistic health and healing.* Philadelphia: F.A. Davis.

Sullivan, H.S. (1953). *The interpersonal theory of psychiatry.* New York: WW Norton.

Sullivan, H.S. (1956). *Clinical studies in psychiatry.* New York: WW Norton.

Sullivan, H.S. (1962). *Schizophrenia as a human process.* New York: WW Norton.

Tardiff, K.J. (2003). Violence. In R.E. Hales & S.C. Yudofsky (Eds.), *The American Psychiatric Publishing textbook of clinical psychiatry* (4th ed.). Washington, DC: The American Psychiatric Publishing.

Thomas, A., Chess, S., & Birch., H. (1970). The origin of personality. *Scientific American 223*(2), 102-109.

Townsend, M.C. (2011). *Essentials of psychiatric/mental health nursing* (5th ed.). Philadelphia: FA Davis.

Townsend, M.C. (2009). *Psychiatric mental health nursing: Concepts of care in evidence-based practice* (6th ed.). Philadelphia: FA Davis.

Trivieri, L., & Anderson, J.W. (2002). *Alternative medicine: The definitive guide.* Berkeley, CA: Celestial Arts.

U.S. Conference of Mayors (USCM). (2006). An American tragedy: Hunger, homelessness in the land of plenty. Retrieved September 3, 2009, from http://mayors.org/usmayornewspaper/documents/12_20_06/pg4_hunger_homeless_summary.asp

U.S. Conference of Mayors (USCM). (2008). *A status report on hunger and homelessness in America's cities: 2008.* Washington, DC: USCM.

U.S. Department of Agriculture (USDA) and U.S. Department of Health and Human Services (USDHHS). (2005). *Dietary guidelines for Americans 2005* (6th ed.). Washington, DC: USDA & USDHHS.

Voeller, K.K.S. (2004). Attention-deficit hyperactivity disorder (ADHD). *Journal of Child Neurology, 19*(10), 798-814.

Whitaker, J. (2000). Pet owners are a healthy breed. *Health & Healing 10*(10), 1-8.

Worden, J.W. (2009). *Grief counseling and grief therapy: A handbook for the mental health practitioner* (4th ed.). New York: Springer.

Yalom, I. (2005). *The theory and practice of group psychotherapy* (5th ed.). New York: Basic Books.

Yurkovich, E., & Smyer, T. (2000). Health maintenance behaviors of individuals with severe mental illness in a state prison. *Journal of Psychosocial Nursing and Mental Health Services, 38*(6), 20-31.

Yutzy, S.H. (2003). Somatoform disorders. In R.E. Hales & S.C. Yudofsky (Eds.), *The American Psychiatric Publishing textbook of clinical psychiatry* (4th ed.). Washington, DC: American Psychiatric Publishing.

Zinner, S.H. (2004). Tourette syndrome—much more than tics. *Contemporary Pediatrics, 21*(8), 38-49.

Subject Index

Note: Page numbers followed by "f" indicate figures; those followed by "t" indicate tabular material.

Drug Index

Note: Page numbers followed by followed by "t" indicate tabular material. Trade names appear in **bold**.

Nursing Diagnoses Index